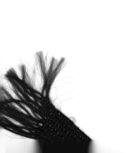

An Atlas of Planar and SPECT Bone Scans

Second Edition

An Atlas of Planar and SPECT Bone Scans

Second Edition

Edited by

Lawrence E Holder
MD

Professor of Radiology
University of Maryland School of Medicine
Director, Division of Nuclear Medicine
University of Maryland Medical Systems
22 South Greene Street
Baltimore, MD 21201-1595
USA

Ignac Fogelman
MD FRCP

Professor of Nuclear Medicine
Department of Nuclear Medicine
Guy's Hospital
St Thomas Street
London
UK

B David Collier
MD

Associate Professor of Radiology and
Orthopaedic Surgery
Director of Nuclear Medicine
Department of Radiology and Nuclear
Medicine
Froedtert Memorial Lutheran Hospital -
East
9200 W Wisconsin Avenue
Milwaukee, WI
USA

MARTIN DUNITZ

© **Martin Dunitz Ltd 2000**

First published in the United Kingdom in 2000
Martin Dunitz Ltd
The Livery House
7-9 Pratt Street
London NW1 0AE

A CIP catalogue record for this book is available from the British
Library.

ISBN 1-85317-469-6

Distributed in the United States by:
Blackwell Science Inc.
Commerce Place, 350 Main Street
Malden, MA 02148, USA
Tel: 1–800–215–1000

Distributed in Canada by:
Login Brothers Book Company
324 Salteaux Crescent
Winnipeg, Manitoba, R3J 3T2
Canada
Tel: 204–224–4068

Distributed in Brazil by:
Ernesto Reichmann Distribuidora de Livros, Ltda
Rua Coronel Marques 335, Tatuape 03440–000
Sao Paulo
Brazil

Composition by Scribe Design, Gillingham, Kent, UK
Printed and bound in Hong Kong

Contents

Dedication

This book is dedicated to Ms Nellie Kelty,
an inspirational colleague for an entire
professional career

Preface to the Second Edition

Since the publication of the First Edition in 1989, four significant changes in the practice of radionuclide bone imaging in nuclear medicine have occurred. The first has been the universal availability of Single Photon Emission Computed Tomography (SPECT) imaging and the application of SPECT to a wide variety of clinical problems in almost all anatomic areas. The second has been the quantum leap in reasonably priced computing power available for data processing and display. The third has been the widespread use of Computed Tomography (CT) and Magnetic Resonance Imaging (MRI) to problems of the musculoskeletal system, and the continued technological development of those modalities. The fourth has been the recognition that optimum patient management requires physiologic knowledge of bone metabolism as well as anatomic lesion detail.

The contents of the Second Edition reflect these changing realities and patterns of practice. The number of SPECT images has increased dramatically, and the anatomic detail available from these images has been emphasized. Normal three phase anatomy has been extensively illustrated. Correlation with available anatomic images from CT, MR and contrast angiography as a means to learn SPECT anatomy and the vascular anatomy of the radionuclide angiogram and blood pool images of the three phase technique have been stressed. Better anatomic localization of abnormal tracer accumulation not only aids in diagnosis, but is extremely important in patient management. The correlation of the physiologic data available from the three phases of the bone scan and SPECT images, with the anatomic findings on plain radiographs, CT and MR images, are helpful in most cases. In some areas of practice, such as trauma and tumor imaging, the use of correlative images are essential.

The basic plan of presentation of the images is disease centered with emphasis on clinical presentation. However, within most chapters images are arranged anatomically. The main index is organized to guide the reader to all the images in a particular anatomic area when the presenting complaint is vague or uncertain. Detailed, cross-referenced indices have been included to make this atlas even easier to use in specialized situations such as pediatrics, sports medicine, and imaging techniques.

Acknowledgments

It is impossible to acknowledge all of our colleagues and co-workers who in some way contributed to the production of this Atlas or to the education of the authors in the area of radionuclide bone imaging. We are extremely grateful to them all.

Ms Sally Kim in Baltimore coordinated the editorial efforts required. Without her organizational skills and meticulous attention to detail this work would not have been completed. The basis of this Atlas is the images it contains. These have been for the most part produced by the outstanding technologist staffs at the University of Maryland Medical Systems in Baltimore, the Medical College of Wisconsin in Milwaukee, and Guy's Hospital in London. Their dedication to quality is recognized and appreciated. Dave Crandall of the Audiovisual Section at the University of Maryland Department of Radiology photographed many of the images. Ms Harriet Hill typed much of the manuscript. Many colleagues, too numerous to mention individually, provided patient information, thoughtful discussion, and education in pathology, pathophysiology and correlative imaging. We thank them all.

The combination of prints, film, slides, and digital images were splendidly handled by Ms Tanya Wheatley and the rest of the staff at Martin Dunitz and Mr John Gardiner at Scribe Design. We appreciate their patience and efforts during our learning experience, as we entered the digital imaging publication era.

Bone imaging basics

1

Introduction

The bone scan is the most universally performed nuclear medicine imaging procedure. It is most often used as a high sensitivity examination when patients complain of pain of potentially osseous origin and in the staging of breast, prostate, and other cancers. In most clinical situations the bone scan outperforms conventional X-ray for the detection of skeletal pathology. At other times the bone scan provides information about bone metabolism that complements the anatomical detail available from conventional X-ray, computed tomography (CT), or magnetic resonance imaging (MRI).

Current clinical bone scanning has developed since the clinical introduction of technetium-99m (^{99m}Tc)-labeled tracers in 1980, and has progressed alongside improvements in imaging techniques. Each new generation of gamma cameras has provided the nuclear medicine practitioner with improved bone scan images. The use of single photon emission computed tomography (SPECT) enhances the planar bone scan by providing cross-sectional anatomical detail and image contrast. The radionuclide angiogram (RNA) and the blood pool or tissue phase images (BP) of the three-phase technique provide additional physiologic information useful for both diagnosis and management decisions.

This atlas considers in detail adult bone scanning with technetium-99m-labeled diphosphonates, and also includes the most commonly encountered problems in the pediatric and adolescent patient. The mechanisms of tracer uptake (pp. 1,2), techniques for performing the many variations of planar imaging including the RNA, the BP and whole body (WB) studies, and for SPECT imaging (pp. 3,4), and a variety of clinical considerations important for obtaining the most diagnostic images (pp. 5–11) complete this first chapter. Chapter 2 includes a carefully structured presentation of normal bone scans, normal variants, artifacts, and pitfalls. Frequently encountered, more or less characteristic global scan 'patterns' which should suggest either a specific entity or category of abnormality are illustrated in

Chapter 3. In addition a section on 'focal' pattern recognition, which allows the identification of specific individual bones, is included. The broad categories of clinical problems are covered in specific chapters: trauma (Chapter 4), primary (Chapter 5) and metastatic (Chapter 6) tumor, arthritis (Chapter 7), infection (Chapter 8), metabolic disease (Chapter 9), and a group of miscellaneous lesions (Chapter 10). The grouping of lesions by anatomic area within each chapter and the extensive indexing by anatomic areas will be useful in evaluating areas of abnormal osseous uptake when the underlying etiology is unknown.

Mechanisms of tracer uptake

Bone scanning is almost exclusively performed using ^{99m}Tc-labeled diphosphonate (Figure 1.1) which shows exquisite sensitivity for skeletal abnormality. The technique has the limitation that scan appearances may be nonspecific; however, in many clinical situations recognizable patterns of scan abnormality are seen which often suggest a specific diagnosis.

The mechanism of tracer uptake on to bone is not fully understood but it is believed that diphosphonate is absorbed on to the surface of bone, with particular affinity for sites of new bone formation in which smaller crystals have relatively more surface area available for tracer interaction (Figures 1.2 and 1.3). It is thought that diphosphonate uptake on bone primarily reflects osteoblastic activity but is also dependent on skeletal vascularity. Thus bone scan images provide a functional display of skeletal activity. As functional change in bone occurs earlier than gross structural change, the bone scan will often detect abnormalities before they are seen on an X-ray. Similarly the functional or metabolic significance of early bone marrow edema changes visualized on MR images can be elucidated. Any diphosphonate which is not taken up by bone is excreted via the urinary tract, and in a normal study the kidneys are clearly visualized on the

Figure 1.1

Chemical structure of diphosphonate compounds used for bone scanning. At the present time MDP is the most widely used agent. HEDP, hydroxyethylidene diphosphonate; MDP, methylene diphosphonate; HMDP, hydroxy-methylene diphosphonate; DPD, dicarboxypropane diphosphonate.

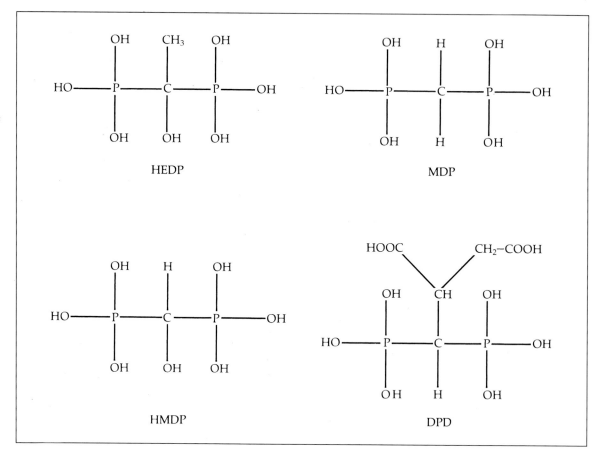

Figure 1.2

Mechanism of diphosphonate uptake on bone.

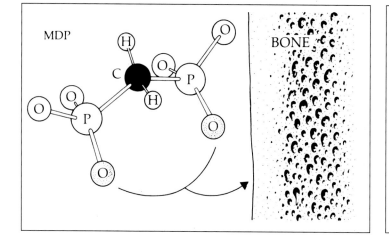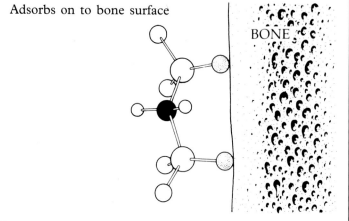

bone scan; indeed there are many examples of renal pathology which have been detected for the first time on the bone scan.

It is also recognized that, on occasion, there may be uptake of ^{99m}Tc-labeled on diphospho- nate at non-skeletal sites. There have been many situations reported where this can occur, but it is believed that in all cases the common factor is the presence of local microcalcification or hydroxyapatite crystal formation.

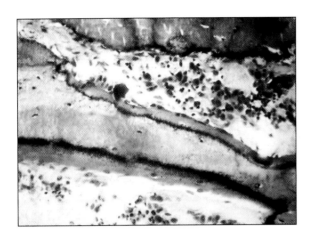
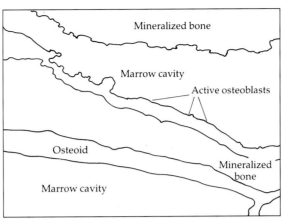

Figure 1.3

Microautoradiograph of rabbit bone showing adsorption of ³H-HEDP on bone surfaces. The heavy concentration of silver grains is at the interface between osteoid and bone, i.e., at the site where mineralization occurs.

Bone scan techniques

Protocols

A variety of bone scanning options is available. Which one or ones are used as part of the initial examination and which ones may be used as a supplement to answer specific questions will be the bone imaging physician's choice. Many nuclear medicine departments will have several 'standard protocols', each used for specific clinical situations. Protocols also vary with the specific imaging equipment available. Tables 1.1 and 1.2 outline some of these protocols in use at the University of Maryland Medical Center.

Table 1.1 Imaging options for radionuclide bone imaging

Option	Purpose	Recommendation
RNA	Evaluate vascular flow	Any focal area of new or suspicious pain, recent surgery, abnormal radiographic lesion
BPs	Assess regional perfusion, relative vascularity	Any focal area of new or suspicious pain, recent surgery, abnormal radiographic lesion
WB BPs	Assess perfusion to entire body	Multiple area of pain, trauma, widespread disease
WB delays	Evaluate distribution of bone metabolism	Every bone scan, especially patients for metastatic work-up
Delayed spots	Further define area of interest or abnormal uptake	Unclear, or poorly defined area, need 90° (orthogonal) images
SPECT	Increase lesion contrast, localization	Abnormal focus unresolved, normal scan especially head, neck, spine, and pelvis
Delayed 5–24 h	Increased target to background ratio, for increased soft tissue clearance, eliminate obscured pelvic bones	DSs for poor soft tissue clearance, full bladder

Abbreviations: RNA, radionuclide angiogram; SPECT, single photon emission computed tomography; DS, delayed spot image..

Table 1.2 Imaging protocol with XLFoV camera

Image	Matrix	ACQ parameters	Collimator
RNA	64 × 64	1.0 sec/frame; 90 frames	General purpose or high resolution★
BPs	256 × 256	1000 K CTS/head (max 5 min); torso	General purpose or high resolution★
	256 × 256	400 K CTS/head (max 5 min); Extremities	
WB BP	2048 × 512	16 cm/min	General purpose or high resolution
WB delay	2048 × 512	10 cm/min	High, ultra-high resolution
SPECT	128 × 128	128 steps; 30 sec/step	High, ultra-high resolution
Bone spots	256 × 256	1000 K CTS/head (max 10 min); torso 400 K CTS/head (max 10 min); extremities	High, ultra-high resolution

Abbreviations: CTS, counts; K, 1000.
★If logistically difficult to change collimators.
(Reproduced with permission from Kelty N et al, Technical considerations for optimal orthopedic imaging. *Semin Nucl Med* 1997; **27**: 328–33.)

At the University of Maryland RNA and BP images are obtained whenever there is a focal area of pain or other symptom, foci of prior surgery or trauma, or a known anatomic lesion for which a functional assessment has been requested. Multiple foci of concern might lead to a WB BP examination. SPECT imaging is used both to provide cross-sectional anatomic detail and to improve image contrast. Using SPECT it is possible to separate underlying and overlying distributions of activity into sequential tomographic planes.

Quality control

Detailed discussions of image resolution, contrast and noise in planar and SPECT imaging, the imaging physics related to SPECT acquisition and processing, or the technical aspects of image display are beyond the scope of this clinical atlas. It must suffice to emphasize that meticulous care and effort in image acquisition, including patient positioning and the elimination of patient movement and the continuous quality control of imaging equipment, are necessities to obtain 'diagnostic' images (Tables 1.3–1.5).

Figure 1.4

Posterior view bone scans of the thoracolumbar spine, obtained with the collimator (a) in close apposition to the patient's back, (b) 13 cm from the back, and (c) 25 cm from the back. As the collimator is moved away from the patient, spatial resolution decreases and image clarity deteriorates.

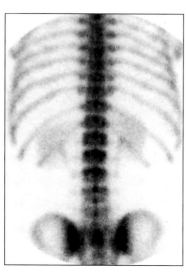
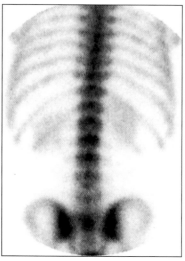
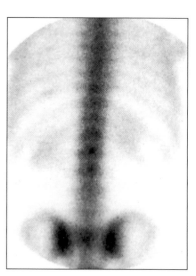

a   b   c

Table 1.3 Technical imaging parameters

Item	*Effect*	*Recommendation*
Collimator	Count rate and resolution	Flow and BPs (all purpose); WB, spots, and SPECT (high resolution)
Matrix size in pixels	Resolution	Flow: 64 × 64 Blood pools: 256 × 256 WB: 2048 × 512 Spots: 256 × 256 SPECT: 128 × 128
Counts	Image statistics	BPs and delays: extremities 400 K CTS, torso 1000 K CTS per head
Time/Speed	Image statistics	RNA: 1.0 sec frames; can be reframed to reduce noise, and allow for anatomic recognition of structures. WB: 10 cm/min scan speed SPECT: 128 steps, 30 sec/step
Table attenuation	Statistics	Know imaging tables' limitations, when possible placing the detector directly against the patient
Distance	Resolution	Keep detectors as close as possible
Acquisition zoom	Change of image size, usually to magnify	Acquire counts only from area of interest, hardware process, changes pixel size; can increase resolution if initial pixel size is too big compared with system resolution
Magnification or processing zoom	Magnifies acquired images	Electronic magnification after acquisition for definition of smaller areas or multiple lesions, resolution; visual perception enhanced by larger size

Abbreviations: K, 1000.
(Reproduced with permission from Kelty N et al, Technical considerations for optimal orthopedic imaging. *Semin Nucl Med* 1997; **27**: 328–33.)

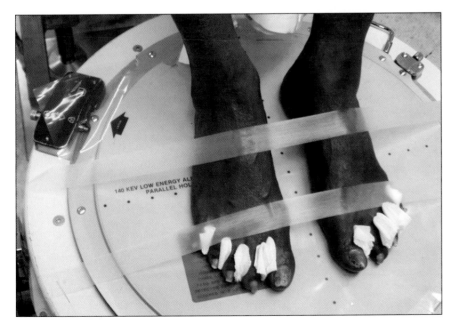

Figure 1.5

Position for plantar view. Thin plastic sheet protects collimator face from contamination. Cotton pledgets separate toes and tape decreases patient movement.

Table 1.4 Global causes of image degradation

Pitfall	*Result*
Over 5 cm collimator-to-patient separation	Loss resolution
Wrong energy windows	Loss resolution
Low count study	'Grainy' scan
^{99m}Tc-MDP impurities	Increased background activity and soft tissue uptake
Renal failure	Increased background activity
Slight patient motion	Loss resolution
Obesity	Increased background and scattered activity

Table 1.5 Quality control schedule

Item	*Frequency*	*Comment*
Flood field	Daily	Detects nonuniformities, PMT shifts, contamination
Bar phantom	Weekly	Evaluate spatial resolution and linearity
Energy peak position and resolution	Quarterly	Verify energy calibration
Isotope peaking	Each study	Correct energy and window settings
Center of rotation	Monthly	Assures SPECT imaging accuracy
Collimators	Daily Quarterly	Visual inspection for defects and scratches Flood field on all collimators
Monitors	Daily	Intensity and contrast drifting, scaling problems
Imaging devices	Daily	Intensity and contrast drifting, CRT problems
Peripheral devices	Daily	Safety pads, imaging tables, cassettes, EKG

Abbreviations: CRT, cathode ray tube; EKG, electrocardiogram; PMT, photomultiplier tube.
(Reproduced with permission from Kelty N et al, Technical considerations for optimal orthopedic imaging. *Semin Nucl Med* 1997; **27**: 328–33.)

Clinical considerations

Worksheet

This clinical atlas emphasizes the 'interrogation' of the obtained images. Diagnoses are based on recognition of the distribution and characteristics of tracer uptake. As used in routine clinical practice this approach requires close cooperation between the technology staff and the nuclear physician or radiologist. Knowing the specific clinical question being asked by the referring physician, the patient's signs and symptoms, pertinent prior interventions or lesions, and review of correlative images guide the staff in obtaining the most revealing images. The old cliché 'if you cannot see it, you cannot diagnose it' is very true for bone imaging, and can be further expanded to state that the lesion must be precisely localized before it can be diagnosed. To these ends, Tables 1.6–1.9 include some items that have been useful to the authors.

Table 1.6 Focused bone imaging history

Questions	Rationale
History of any prior trauma or surgery, biopsy, hardware, cardiac zipper sign, or CABG	Physiologic uptake or photon-deficient areas
History of any acute bone trauma, surgery, or fractures	Pathologic uptake
Medications: antibiotics, steroids, i.m. injections	For understanding osteomyelitis, AVN, soft tissue uptake, i.e. cause and effect
Chemotherapy (date of last treatment)	Flare response, renotoxic
Radiation therapy (date of last treatment and to what area or areas)	Flare response, portal effect
Correlative image history	Superimpose physiologic information from RNBI on anatomic lesion
Recent radioisotope procedure	Abnormal accumulations/sites

Abbreviations: AVN, avascular necrosis; CABG, coronary artery bypass graft; i.m., intramuscular; RNBI, radionuclide bone imaging.
(Reproduced with permission from Kelty N et al, Technical considerations for optimal orthopedic imaging. *Semin Nucl Med* 1997; **27**: 328–33.)

Table 1.7 Positioning for radionuclide bone imaging

Technique on view	Purpose/comment
Orthogonal view	90° image of the lesion increases specificity of location
Oblique/Lateral	Allows separation between lesion and normal bone, helpful with shine-through lesions
SPECT imaging	Gives increased contrast imaging for lesion detection and localization
Postvoid	Eliminates bladder activity which can obscure pelvic bones
Squat shot	Pelvic bone imaging, separates bladder
Upright imaging	Allows organ and soft tissue to drop slightly to help differentiate nonosseous uptake from bone uptake, i.e. kidney and rib overlap, pleural effusion
Creative imaging	Arms over head, separate scapula and ribs Internal/External rotation of arms to give rotation to the humeral head Slight internal rotation of lower legs to separate tibia and fibula overlap on anterior lower leg views. Use posterior view to see fibula best Hyperextend the neck to allow closer positioning to shoulders, clavicles, and sternoclavicular joints without creating rotation sometimes caused by patients turning the head Extensive use of pillows, wedge sponges, rolled blankets, and such to elevate, attain symmetry, or for patient support and comfort Lead shields to cover injection sites of infiltrated doses to minimize scatter, to block a full bladder in a patient unable to void, or to shield hot lesions adjacent to AOI needing high resolution, so that image statistics for the AOI are not masked by the counts or scatter from the hotter lesion Multiheaded camera systems have allowed further creativity for focused imaging
Gauze/Cotton between the digits	Clearly separates toes/fingers when imaging extremities; use wide tape to keep hands or feet immobile for the imaging

Abbreviation: AOI, area of interest.
(Reproduced with permission from Kelty N et al, Technical considerations for optimal orthopedic imaging. *Semin Nucl Med* 1997; **27**: 328–33.)

Table 1.8 Patient positioning for SPECT imaging

Bony structure	Special positioning	Comments
Knees	5–7.5 cm pad between knees; secure knees with straps to prevent motion. Secure feet in neutral position to prevent rotation	For obese patients both knees may not fit in field of view
Hips and pelvis	Empty bladder before examination. Position hips symmetrically and secure knees and/or feet to prevent motion	Bladder filling during examination creates artifacts
Lumbar spine	Keep arms out of field of view. A pillow under the knees may relieve back pain	Patients with back pain often move during the examination
TMJ	Secure neck in comfortable hyperextension. Instruct patient not to talk	Check lateral view to be sure the chin is in the field of view

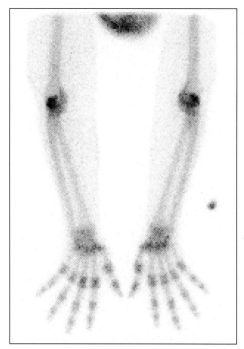

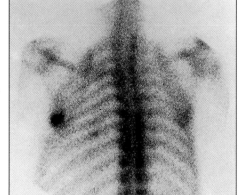

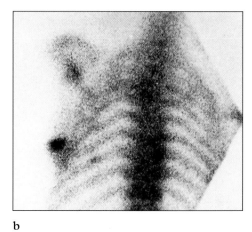

a   b

Figure 1.6

One position for imaging of the elbows, forearms, and hands, when the patient is prone on the WB table. Outstretched extremity over the head prone on collimator face.

Figure 1.7

Lesion of scapula or rib? Bone scan views: (a) posterior thorax and (b) with arm elevated. A lesion is seen in the left chest on (a) but it is not clear whether it is associated with a rib or the scapula. With the arm elevated, it is apparent that the lesion is in the scapula.

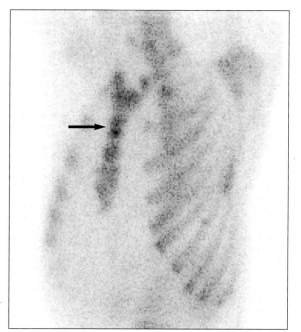
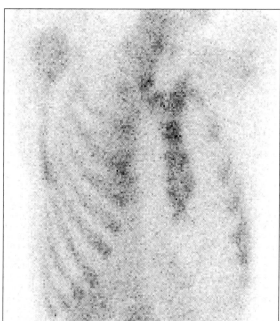

a   b

Figure 1.8

DS. Oblique views (a) LAO and (b) RAO to demonstrate details of the sternum. Focal increase, often linear, at the manubrial body junction (arrow) is a normal variant.

Teaching point

Even in patients with physical constraints that limit movement, creative positioning will in most cases allow imaging in at least one plane and often in the orthogonal plane needed to localize an abnormal focus of tracer uptake. The imager can combine the positional data from paired images, for example, an RAO and LAO, or LPO and RPO to replace a lateral view, as the orthogonal view for an anterior or posterior image.

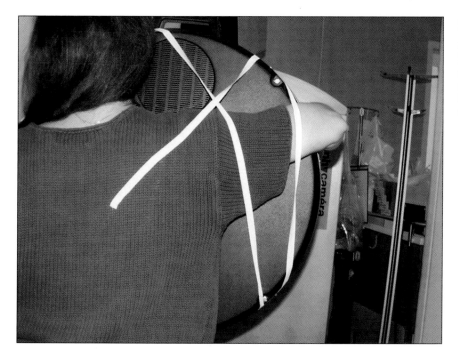

Figure 1.9

Creative positioning. Patients are often more comfortable standing upright. Tape for immobilization should be used.

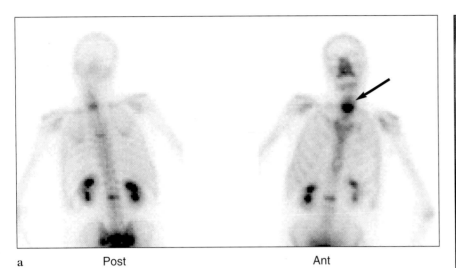

a   Post   Ant

Figure 1.10

Uptake in thyroid cartilage. (a) WB anterior. Location of neck uptake can be suspected by comparing the relative intensities on anterior (arrow) and posterior views. (b) Lateral radiograph demonstrates the calcified cartilage (arrow), which also illustrates value of correlative images.

Teaching point

Symmetrical positioning is important both for anatomic symmetry, especially in young patients with physeal activity, and also for comparing relative intensity of uptake on anterior and posterior views.

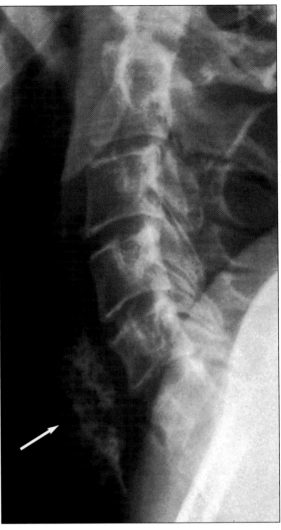

b

Figure 1.11

Lead shielding, to obtain high-quality spot views of hands when patient confined to supine position.

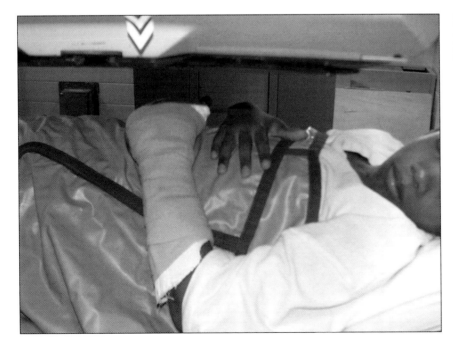

Table 1.9 Correlative imaging guidelines

Rule	*Purpose*	*If/Then condition*
Pre-examination: patient's imaging history is reviewed, pertinent films are obtained and reviewed; or at a minimum the reports are reviewed	Comparison to the other imaging examinations can aid in the specificity of the diagnosis. They may also aid in positioning for the RNA, BPs, and/or DS imaging	If clinical indication is to detect acute osteomyelitis, the bone scan is abnormal suggesting an acute process, and a prior radiograph does not explain the uptake, then our standard of care is to obtain a radiograph within 24 hrs of the scan
Post-examination: when there is abnormal bone uptake a correlative radiograph, CT scan, or MR image can be beneficial	May aid in anatomic localization of the abnormal bone uptake, and add specificity. It is also necessary to respond to the specific clinical question about the physiologic or metabolic activity of an anatomic lesion	If clinical indication is for a noninfectious acute process, and the bone scan is abnormal suggesting an acute abnormality, and if a prior radiograph does not aid in answering the question, then a radiograph within 1 week of the scan is required
		If clinical problem is subacute or chronic, and the bone scan is abnormal, but does not suggest an acute process, and old radiographs explain the bone scan abnormality, then new films are not typically necessary; or if bone scan is abnormal and suggests an acute process not explained by prior radiographs, then new films can be obtained

Normal anatomy, variations, artifacts and pitfalls

2

In order to recognize an abnormal bone scan, the physician must be familiar with the appearance of the normal bone scan and commonly seen variants. In addition the most common artifacts encountered during image acquisition and interpretation, as well as a variety of pitfalls often secondary to normal physiologic handling of tracer, must be considered. Although normal anatomy and variations are emphasized throughout the text, this chapter provides a framework upon which to apply normal anatomy to scan analysis and differential diagnosis.

Normal planar imaging

Planar imaging includes the three-phase RNB scan with an RNA, BP or tissue phase images, and DS or WB scans. WB BP, early fixation phase, and 24-hour post-injection delayed images are additional planar imaging options.

Three phase imaging

Head

Figure 2.1

Normal head and neck, anterior. (a) RNA. Five seconds per view. Right axillary and subclavian vein seen on all four images suggests elongated bolus or slow flow. Faint visualization of neck arteries (primarily carotid arteries on anterior view) (arrowhead), middle cerebral arteries (thin arrow), and anterior cerebral arteries (short arrow). Second and third frames demonstrate capillary and venous phase activity with sagittal sinus (thick arrow). (b) BP image obtained immediately following RNA without moving the patient or changing camera position. Activity represents a combination of tracer in the intravascular spaces and in extravascular, extracellular spaces. Sagittal sinus (long arrow). Central mid-line activity projected over the nose (arrow) represents a combination of oropharyngeal and nasal mucosal tissues. (c) DS, head and neck. To compare with (a) and (b). (d) X-ray, contrast arteriogram, anterior, arterial phase. (I₃) Internal carotid artery, cavernous portion within the venous sinus; (I₄) internal carotid artery, cerebral portion within the cranial subarachnoid space; (M) middle cerebral artery; (A) anterior cerebral artery.

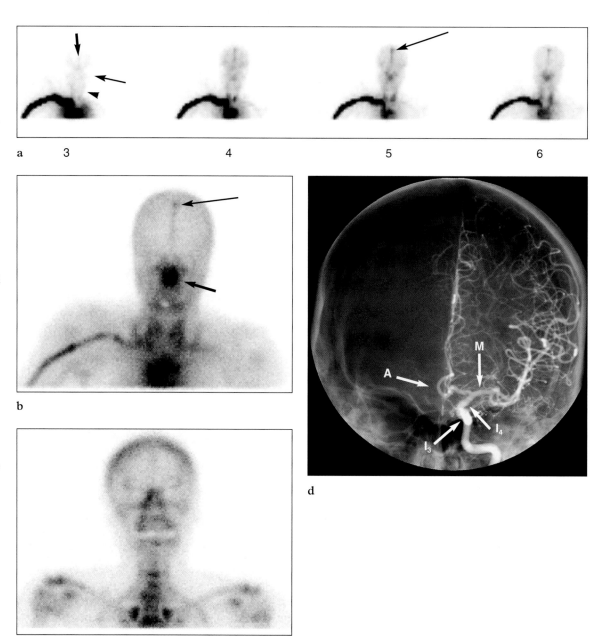

a   3   4   5   6

b

c

d

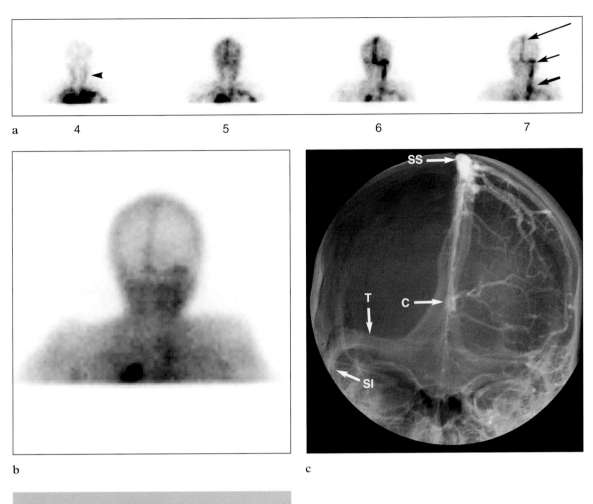

a   4   5   6   7

b

c

Figure 2.2

Normal head and neck, posterior. (a) RNA. Neck vessels on posterior view (arrowhead) also represent a combination of carotid and vertebral arteries with a greater contribution from the much larger carotid vessels. The sagittal sinus (long arrow) is better seen on posterior view. There is often asymmetry in sinus drainage with the right sigmoid sinus (thin arrow) often much larger than the left. In the associated jugular vein (thick arrow) asymmetry is common. **(b)** BP. Depending on head position, a result of neck flexion or camera angle, the sigmoid sinus and neck vessels are more or less visualized. **(c)** X-ray, contrast angiograms, anterior projection, venous phase image. (SS) Superior sagittal sinus; (C) confluence of sinuses; (T) transverse sinus; (SI) sigmoid sinus, which will flow into internal jugular vein (not shown).

Teaching point

Five-second RNA images are often a good compromise between temporal resolution and spatial resolution requirements. With digital acquisition techniques, one second per frame images can be obtained and viewed with less temporal resolution if needed.

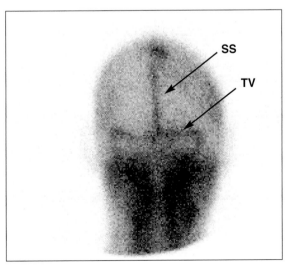

Figure 2.3

BP, posterior. In another patient, different angulation demonstrates both the sagittal sinus (SS) and the transverse sinuses (TV).

Upper trunk

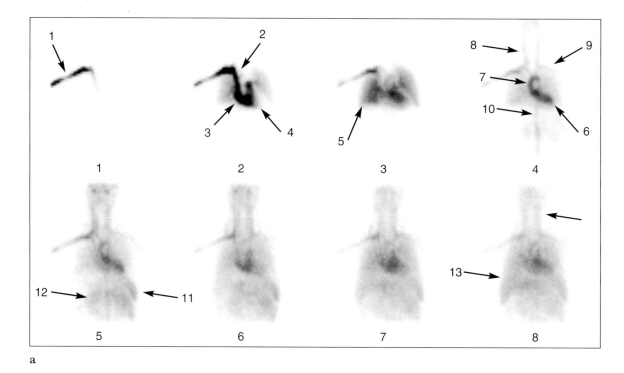

a

Figure 2.4

Normal upper trunk (chest and neck), anterior. (a) RNA, five-second sequential images. (1) Axillary/subclavian vein, (2) superior vena cava, (3) right atrium, (4) right ventricle, (5) lungs, (6) left ventricle, (7) aortic arch, (8) right carotid artery, (9) left subclavian artery, (10) abdominal aorta, (11) spleen, (12) kidney, (13) liver. **(b)** BP. (4) Right ventricle, (6) left ventricle, (11) spleen, (12) kidney, (13) liver, (14) oropharyngeal region. **(c)** X-ray, contrast venogram, anterior chest. (1) Axillary/subclavian vein, (2) superior vena cava, (3) right atrium, (4) right ventricle region, and (5) catheter passing through left brachiocephalic vein. **(d)** X-ray, contrast arteriogram, right main pulmonary artery injection. The main pulmonary artery and branches are well seen. **(e)** X-ray, contrast arteriogram, aortic arch injection. (1) Right brachiocephalic artery, (2) right common carotid artery, (3) subclavian artery, (4) right vertebral artery, (5) left common carotid artery, and (6) left brachiocephalic artery. (All angiograms in chapter two courtesy of Dr Geoffrey Hastings, Baltimore, Maryland.)

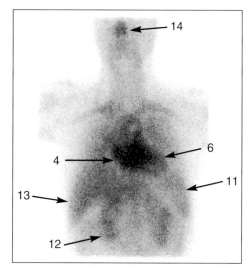

b

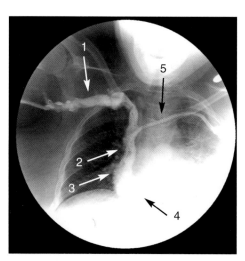

c

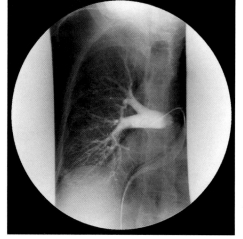

d

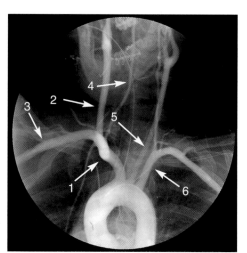

e

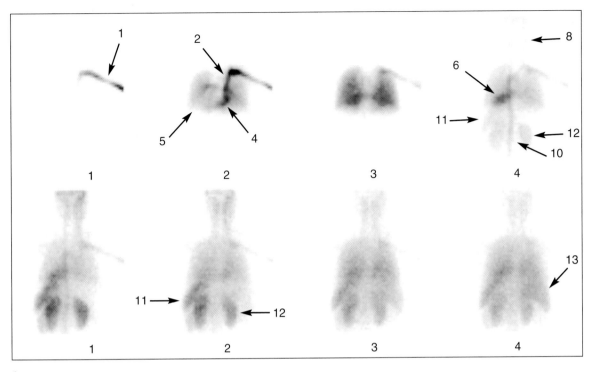

a

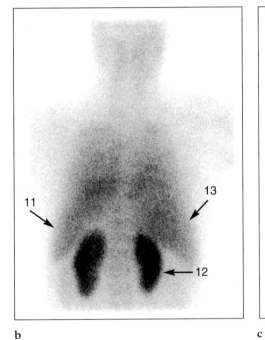

b

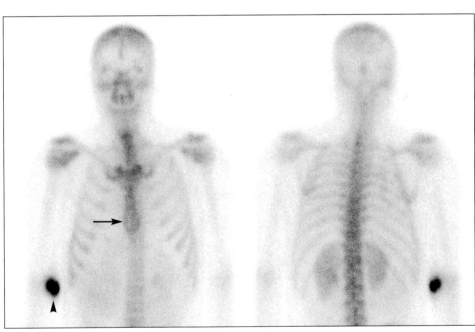

c   Ant   Post

Figure 2.5

Normal upper trunk (neck, chest, shoulders, thoracic spine, upper abdomen), posterior. (a) RNA. (1) Right subclavian vein, (2) superior vena cava, (4) right ventricle, (5) lungs, (6) left ventricle, (8) carotid arteries, (10) abdominal aorta, (11) spleen, (12) kidneys, (13) liver. (b) BP image (11) spleen, (12) kidneys, (13) liver. (c) DS, portion of a WB scan. Anterior (left image) and posterior (right image). This image is presented to correlate the position of the RNA and BP activity in Figures 2.2 and 2.5 (a and b), with the underlying osseous anatomy. Incidentally noted is some central thinning of the sternum with decreased activity, a normal variation that should not be mistaken for a pathologic photon deficiency.

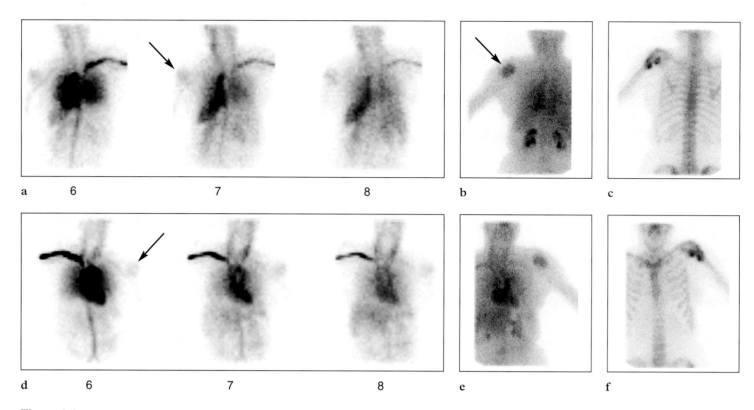

a   6   7   8   b   c

d   6   7   8   e   f

Figure 2.6

Leiomyosarcoma, left proximal humerus. Abnormal three-phase study of shoulder region to compare with normal images in Figures 2.1–2.5. All other structures are normal. (**a**) RNA, posterior. Mild relatively focal increased tracer about the left shoulder (arrow). (**b**) BP, left shoulder, posterior. Moderately intense, focal, increased activity (relative vascularity) (arrow). (**c**) DS, left shoulder. Two intense focal areas of increased tracer. (**d**) RNA, anterior. Mild focal increased relative vascularity slightly less prominent on anterior view (arrow). (**e**) BP, left shoulder, anterior. (**f**) DS, left shoulder, anterior.

Lower trunk

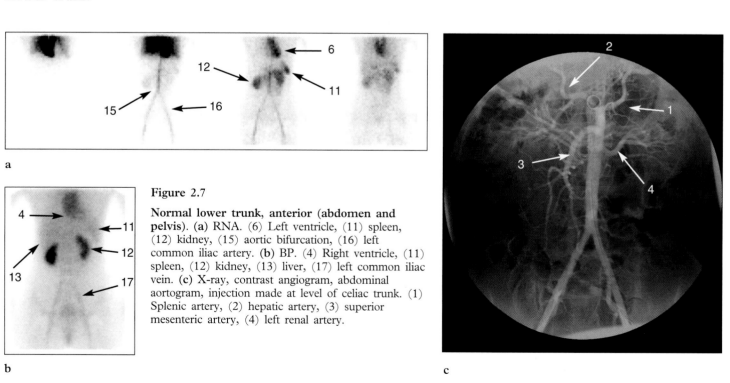

a

b

Figure 2.7

Normal lower trunk, anterior (abdomen and pelvis). (**a**) RNA. (6) Left ventricle, (11) spleen, (12) kidney, (15) aortic bifurcation, (16) left common iliac artery. (**b**) BP. (4) Right ventricle, (11) spleen, (12) kidney, (13) liver, (17) left common iliac vein. (**c**) X-ray, contrast angiogram, abdominal aortogram, injection made at level of celiac trunk. (1) Splenic artery, (2) hepatic artery, (3) superior mesenteric artery, (4) left renal artery.

c

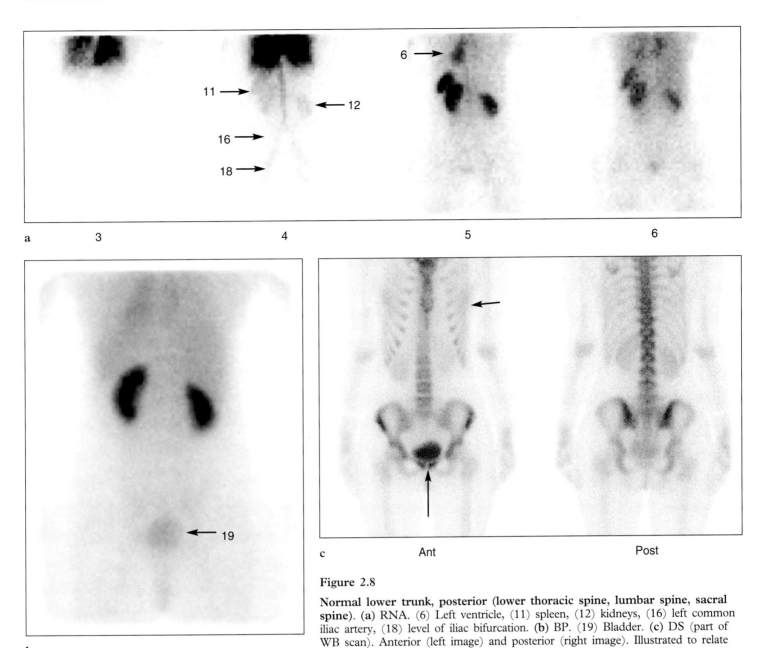

a   3   4   5   6

b

c   Ant   Post

Figure 2.8

Normal lower trunk, posterior (lower thoracic spine, lumbar spine, sacral spine). (a) RNA. (6) Left ventricle, (11) spleen, (12) kidneys, (16) left common iliac artery, (18) level of iliac bifurcation. **(b)** BP. (19) Bladder. **(c)** DS (part of WB scan). Anterior (left image) and posterior (right image). Illustrated to relate the underlying osseous structures to the activity on the RNA and BP images. Incidental nonspecific mild bilateral breast uptake (arrow). Normal photon deficiency (long arrow) represents the cartilage at the symphysis.

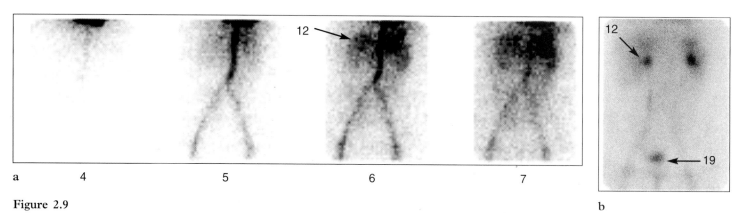

a   4   5   6   7

b

Figure 2.9

Normal lower trunk, anterior. (a) RNA. Resolution can vary significantly depending on the amount of adipose tissue present. In this case renal detail (12) is decreased. **(b)** BP. In patients with very rapid renal excretion or if the BP image acquisition is even slightly delayed, renal pelvic activity (12) can be more prominent than parenchymal activity, and bladder (19) can also be seen.

Figure 2.10

Normal posterior lower trunk (lumbosacral spine), posterior. (a) RNA. Renal outline (11) is better seen on posterior view than anterior. With a tight bolus injection the renal artery perfusion can often be seen (11b). **(b)** BP. Slight prominence to the renal pelvis (11) is normal. On the posterior view, faint visualization of the ureters can often be seen (arrowheads), bladder (19). **(c)** X-ray, contrast angiogram. Flush aortogram injection made just above the level of the renal arteries. Round catheter tip marker (20) is at the level of the T12 intervertebral disk space with origin of the right renal artery (5) at the L1–2 interspace. (1) Splenic artery, (4) left renal artery.

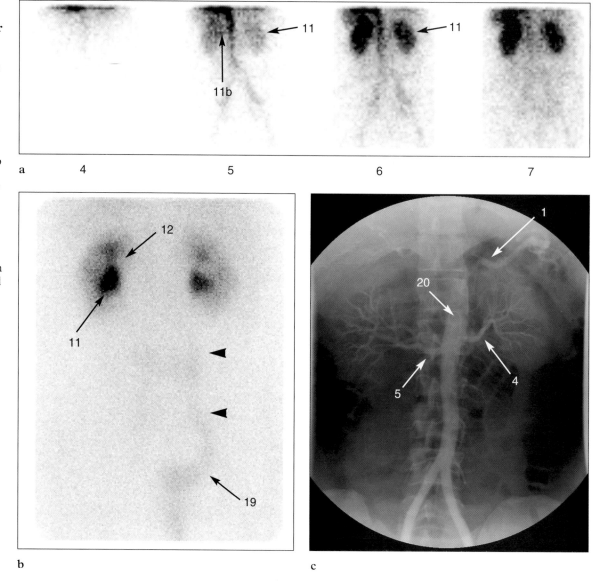

a   4   5   6   7

b   **c**

Pelvis and hips

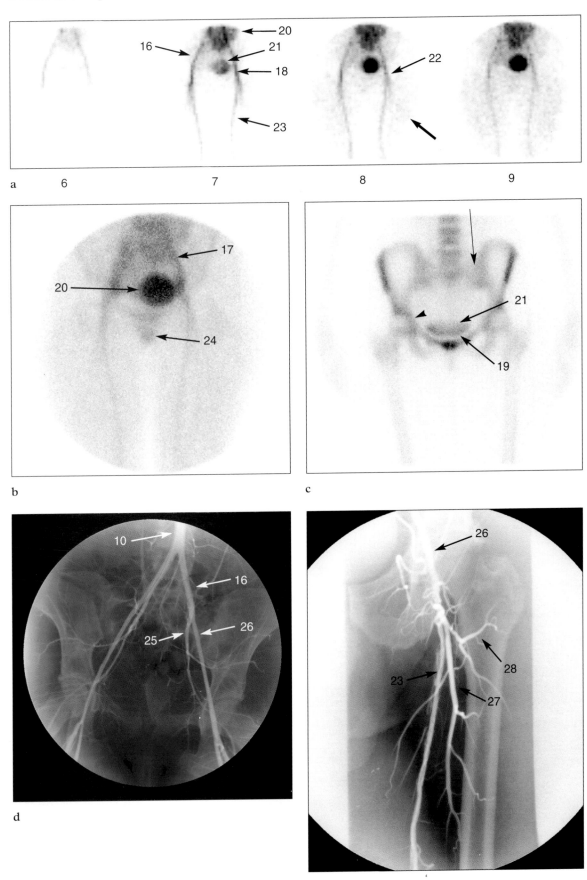

Figure 2.11

Normal pelvis and hips, anterior. 21-year-old female, actively menstruating. **(a)** RNA. Normally, there is no increased perfusion to the hip region (thick arrow). (16) Right common iliac artery, (18) region of common femoral artery, (20) nonspecific intestinal perfusion, (21) uterus, (22) region of common femoral bifurcation, (23) superficial femoral artery. **(b)** BP. (17) Common iliac vein region, (20) uterus, (24) external genitalia. **(c)** DS, pelvis and hips. (19) Bladder, (21) region of uterus. Note the relative tracer uptake in the acetabular regions (arrowhead) and SI joint regions (thin arrow) in this 21-year-old patient. **(d)** X-ray, contrast arteriogram, pelvis. (10) Lower abdominal aorta, (16) left common iliac artery, (25) internal iliac artery, (26) external iliac artery. **(e)** X-ray, contrast arteriogram, left hip region. (26) Left external iliac artery, (23) superficial femoral artery, (27) deep femoral artery, (28) lateral circumflex femoral artery.

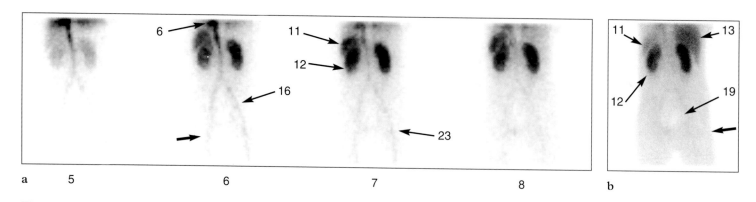

a 5   6   7   8   b

Figure 2.12

Normal pelvis and hips, posterior. (a) RNA, pelvis and hips, posterior. XLFOV camera. RNA. Five seconds per image. Normally there is no increased perfusion to the hip region (thick arrow). (6) Tip of left ventricle seen at top of image, (11) spleen, (12) kidney, (16) right common iliac artery, (23) right superficial femoral artery. (b) BP, pelvis, posterior. XLFOV camera. Image obtained immediately following the last RNA frame. Region of the hip (thick arrow). (11) Spleen, (12) kidney, (13) liver, (19) bladder, which on these early images appears as a photon-deficient region.

Femurs

Figure 2.13

Normal femurs. (a) RNA, femurs, anterior. (27) Superficial femoral artery, (23) deep femoral artery. (b) BP, femurs, anterior. (29) Saphenous vein, (30) popliteal vein, (31) popliteal artery. Note relative photon deficiency associated with popliteal fossa region, which is normal. (c) BP, femurs, posterior. Venous structures less well defined on posterior view. Popliteal fossa not included in field of view. (d) X-ray, contrast angiogram, arterial phase image, mid-femur level. (23) Deep femoral artery, (27) superficial femoral artery.

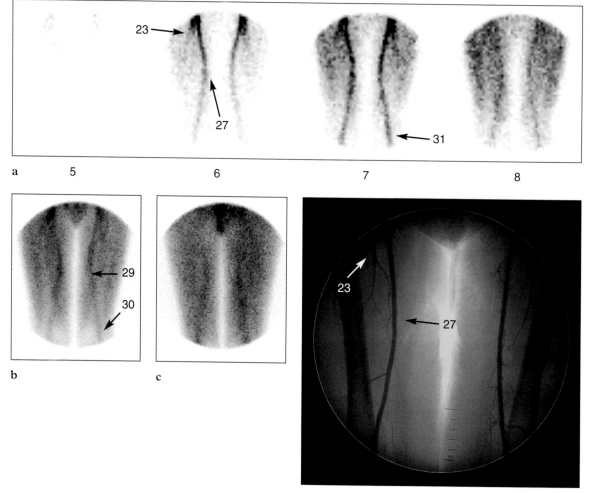

a 5   6   7   8

b   c

d

Knees and legs

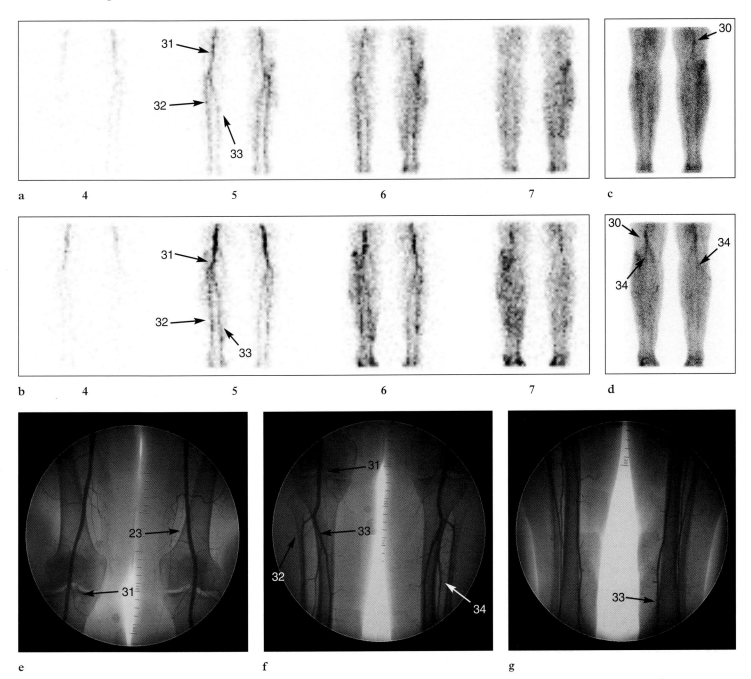

Figure 2.14

Normal knees and legs. (a) RNA, knee and leg, anterior. (31) Popliteal artery, (32) anterior tibial artery, (33) posterior tibial artery. **(b)** RNA, knee and leg, posterior. (31) Popliteal artery, (32) anterior tibial artery, (33) posterior tibial artery. Better definition of popliteal and posterior tibial artery on posterior RNA. **(c)** BP, knee and leg, anterior. (30) Popliteal vein. **(d)** BP, knee and leg, posterior. (30) Popliteal vein, (34) lesser saphenous vein. **(e)** X-ray, contrast arteriogram, arterial phase about the knees, digital subtraction technique. (23) Femoral artery, (31) popliteal artery. **(f)** X-ray, contrast arteriogram, knee and upper leg, arterial image, digital subtraction technique. (31) Popliteal artery, (32) anterior tibial artery, (33) posterior tibial artery, (34) peroneal artery. **(g)** X-ray, contrast arteriogram, lower leg, arterial phase, digital subtraction technique. (33) Posterior tibial artery.

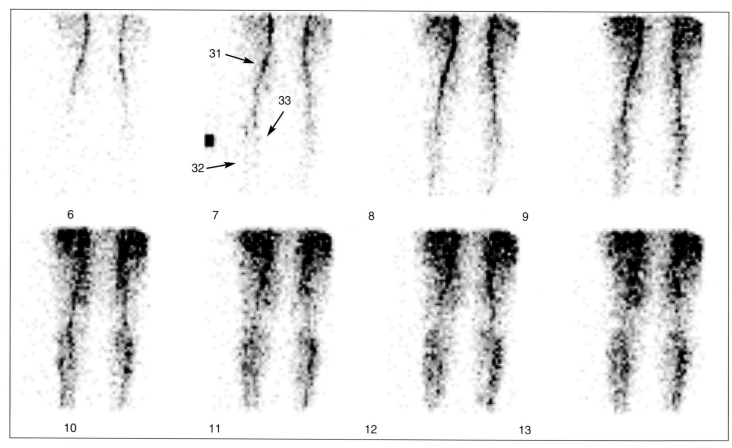

6   7   8   9

10   11   12   13

a

Figure 2.15

Normal knees, anterior.
(a) RNA. (31) Popliteal
artery, (32) anterior tibial
artery, (33) posterior
tibial artery. Later
venous and capillary
phase images as well as
BP image (b) accentuate
the normal photon
deficiency often
associated with the
popliteal fossa. (b) BP,
knees, anterior. Photon
deficiency associated with
popliteal region (arrow).

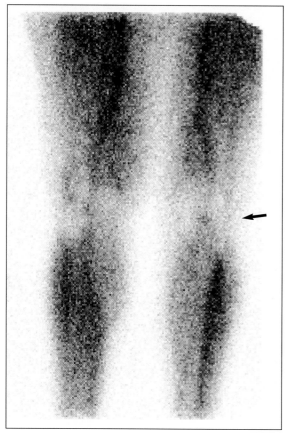

b

Ankle and foot

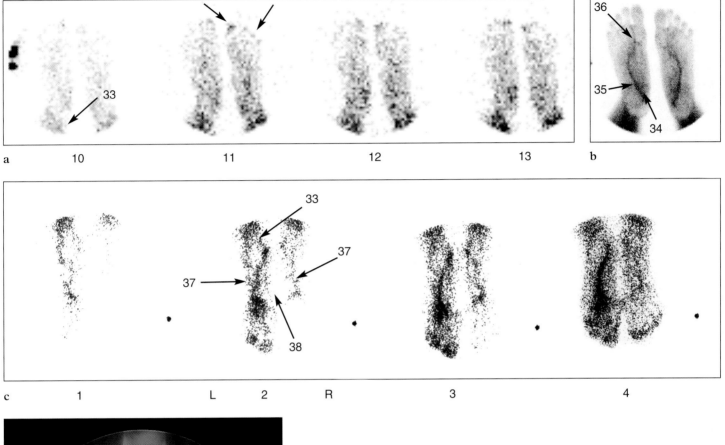

a   10   11   12   13   b

c   1   L   2   R   3   4

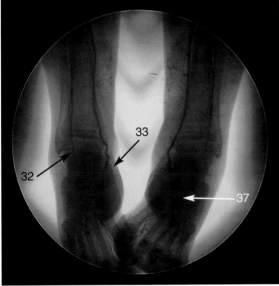

d

Figure 2.16

Normal ankle and foot, plantar views. (a) RNA. Not an atypical RNA of the foot. (33) Region of posterior tibial artery at the ankle where it branches into medial and lateral plantar arteries. The regions supplied by the plantar and dorsal digital arteries are identified, although the individual vessels are not usually seen. **(b)** BP, plantar. Obtained without moving the patient, immediately after images in **(a)**. The higher counts provide much better spatial resolution. (34) Posterior tibial vein, (35) lateral plantar vein, (36) dorsalis pedis vein. **(c)** RNA, plantar. A different patient from **(a)** and **(b)**. Shown to demonstrate variations in the arterial flow and visualization of the distal portions of the foot. Vascular soft tissue lesion underlying the MTP region of the left foot with increased flow through the vessels supplying that area. (33) Posterior tibial artery, (37) large lateral plantar artery, (38) smaller medial plantar artery is the other branch of the posterior tibial artery. **(d)** X-ray, contrast, arteriogram, lower leg, anterior, digital subtraction technique. (32) Distal aspect of anterior tibial artery with its medial continuation as the dorsalis pedis artery, (33) posterior tibial artery at the level of its branching into larger lateral plantar and smaller medial plantar artery, (37) lateral plantar artery.

Teaching point

Normal RNA and BP images of the foot have significant variability. Not only is this an area of lower blood flow, but its distance from the site of injection results in significant loss of bolus effect.

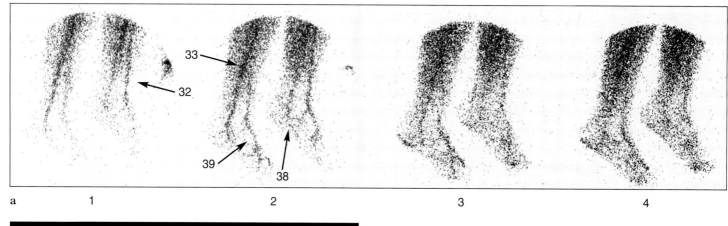

a   1   2   3   4

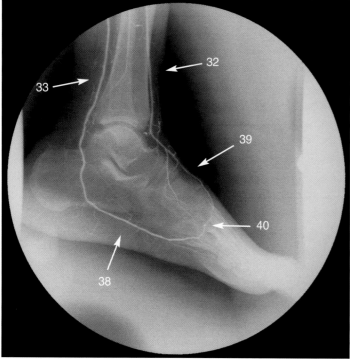

b

Figure 2.17

Normal ankle and foot, lateral. (a) RNA, left medial, right lateral. (32) Anterior tibial artery, (33) posterior tibial artery, (38) lateral plantar artery, (39) dorsalis pedis artery. **(b)** X-ray, contrast arteriogram, lateral view. (32) Anterior tibial artery, (33) posterior tibial artery, (38) lateral plantar artery, (39) dorsalis pedis artery, (40) plantar arch.

Figure 2.18

Normal wrist and hands. (a) RNA, hand and wrist, palmar. (41) Radial artery, (42) ulnar artery, (43) volar arch, probably superficial, (44) volar arch, probably deep, (45) common digital artery area. **(b)** BP, hand and wrist, palmar view. (46) Cephalic vein (radial vien), (47) basilic vein (anterior ulnar vien), (48) superficial dorsal veins, (49) increased uptake represents normal relative increased vascularity of the tissues of the thenar eminence. **(c)** DS, hand and wrist, palmar view. (49) Thenar eminence region. Relative vascularity present on the BP images has decreased. (50) Pisiform, (51) head of metacarpal, (52) base of proximal phalanx. Radioactive marker (arrowhead) indicates right hand. **(d)** RNA, palmar. Analog images, five seconds per view, from another patient. (41) Radial artery, (42) ulnar artery, (43) volar arch, probably superficial, which is more often the continuation of the ulnar artery, (45) common digital artery area. **(e)** X-ray, contrast angiogram, arterial phase, hand and wrist, from a different patient. The radial artery does not fill. (42) Ulnar artery, (43) volar arch, probably superficial, (45) palmar digital arteries, (46) metacarpal arteries.

Wrist and hand

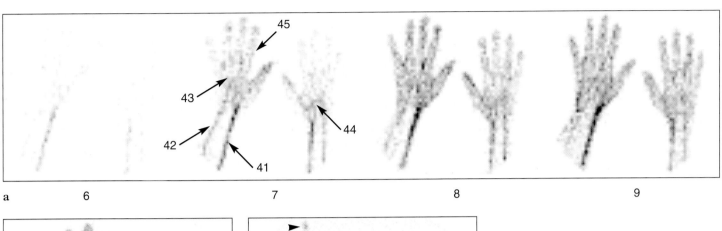

a   6   7   8   9

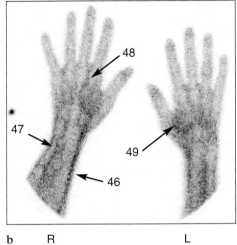

b   R   L

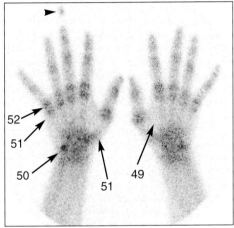

c   R   L

Teaching point

Normal RNA images of the hand also have wide variability because of the low-flow state, but there is less degradation of the bolus than in RNA images of the foot. It has also been our experience that digital RNA images have less detail than comparable analog angiographic images.

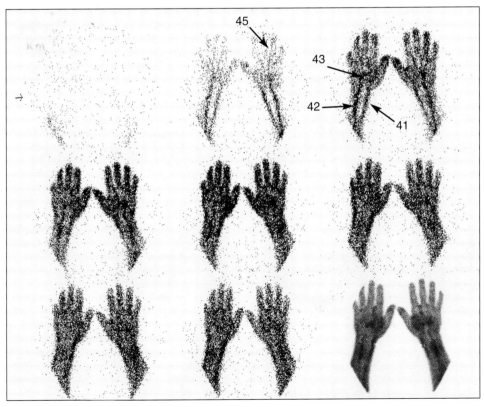

d

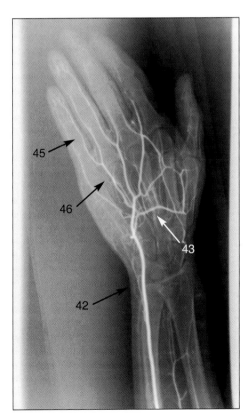

e

Blood pool

Whole body

Figure 2.19

Normal BP, WB: 35-year-old male. Anterior (left image) and posterior (right image). Activity is already seen in normal renal calices, renal pelvis, and bladder. Cephalic vein (arrows), median cubital vein (arrowhead), sagittal sinus (long arrow), transverse sinuses (thin arrow).

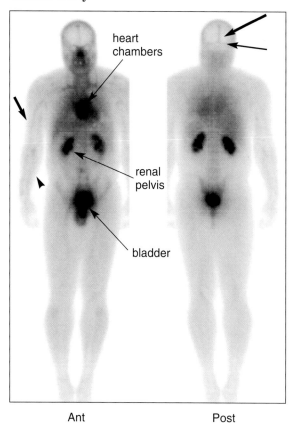

heart chambers

renal pelvis

bladder

Ant   Post

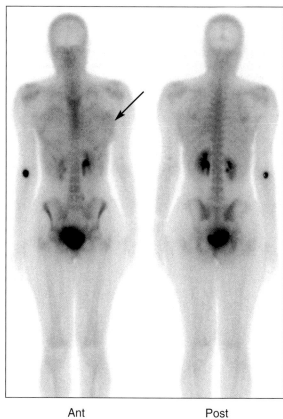

Ant   Post

Figure 2.20

Normal, BP, WB. 23-year-old female. Anterior (left image) and posterior (right image). Injection site (arrow). Slight head movement (thin arrow) appreciated best on anterior view obscures some detail.

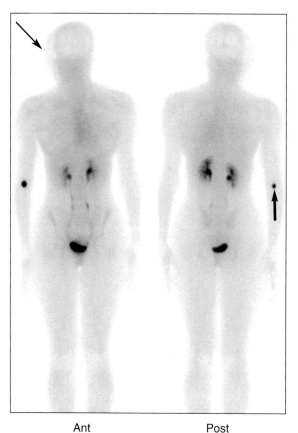

Ant   Post

Figure 2.21

Early fixation phase. WB, 20 minutes post-injection, same patient as in Figure 2.20. Anterior (left image) and posterior (right image). Incidental increased tracer uptake in breast tissue (thin arrow). Note early fixation of tracer predominantly in axial skeleton.

Teaching point

Well-defined osseous uptake on images obtained more than 5–10 minutes post-injection most likely represents early fixation phase activity rather than increased relative vascularity, which would be seen in the typical BP or tissue phase image obtained immediately following injection of tracer. This occurs because the half-time of tracer movement from the vascular to extravascular, extracellular spaces is 1–2 minutes and half-time of tracer movement from extravascular, extracellular spaces to the hydration shell of the bone crystal is approximately 30 minutes.

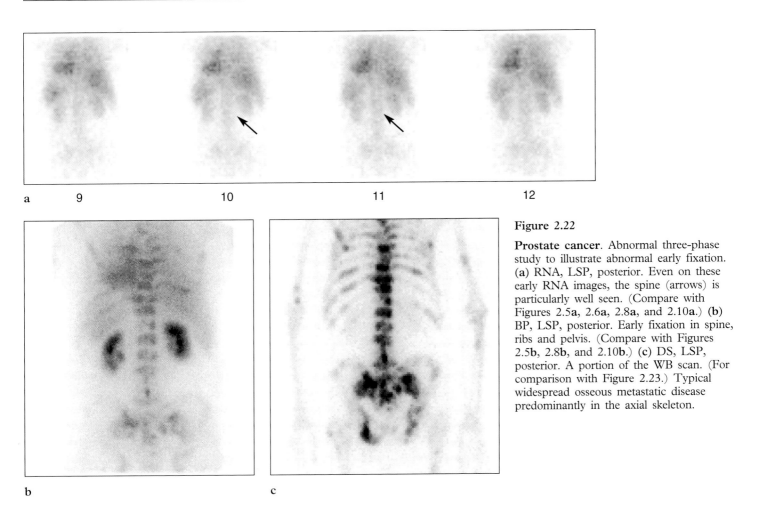

a   9   10   11   12

b   c

Figure 2.22

Prostate cancer. Abnormal three-phase study to illustrate abnormal early fixation. (a) RNA, LSP, posterior. Even on these early RNA images, the spine (arrows) is particularly well seen. (Compare with Figures 2.5a, 2.6a, 2.8a, and 2.10a.) (b) BP, LSP, posterior. Early fixation in spine, ribs and pelvis. (Compare with Figures 2.5b, 2.8b, and 2.10b.) (c) DS, LSP, posterior. A portion of the WB scan. (For comparison with Figure 2.23.) Typical widespread osseous metastatic disease predominantly in the axial skeleton.

Delayed images

Whole body or 3 hour

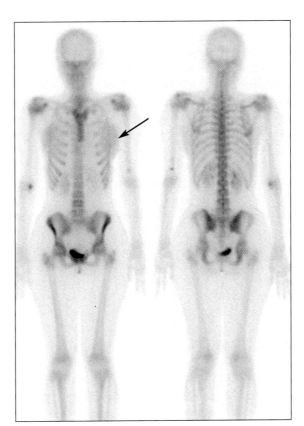

Figure 2.23

Normal WB, 3 hours following injection: 23-year-old female, same patient as Figure 2.21. Incidental normal tracer uptake in breast tissue (thin arrow).

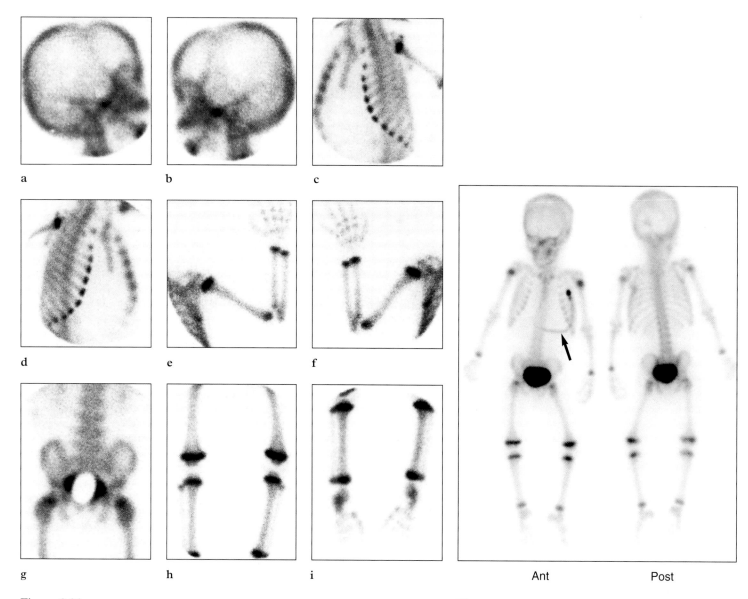

Ant   Post

Figure 2.24

Normal WB bone scan using multiple spot technique: 6-month-old female. (**a**) Skull, RL and (**b**) skull, LL. Note photon deficiency of the anterior fontanel and mild uptake associated with sutures. (**c**) Chest, LAO. (**d**) Chest, RAO. (**e**) Right arm, posterior. (**f**) Left arm, posterior. (**g**) Lumbar spine and pelvis, anterior. (**h**) Knees and legs, anterior. (**i**) Lower leg and feet, anterior. Note physeal activity throughout the skeleton.

Figure 2.25

Normal WB scan: 6-month-old female. Incidental-retained tracer in the Hickman catheter (arrow) on anterior view.

Teaching point

More growth in the upper extremity occurs from the epiphyses at the proximal humerus and distal radius, whereas, in the lower extremity, growth occurs most at the distal femur and proximal tibia. The normal physiologic uptake in the physes reflects this differential growth rate.

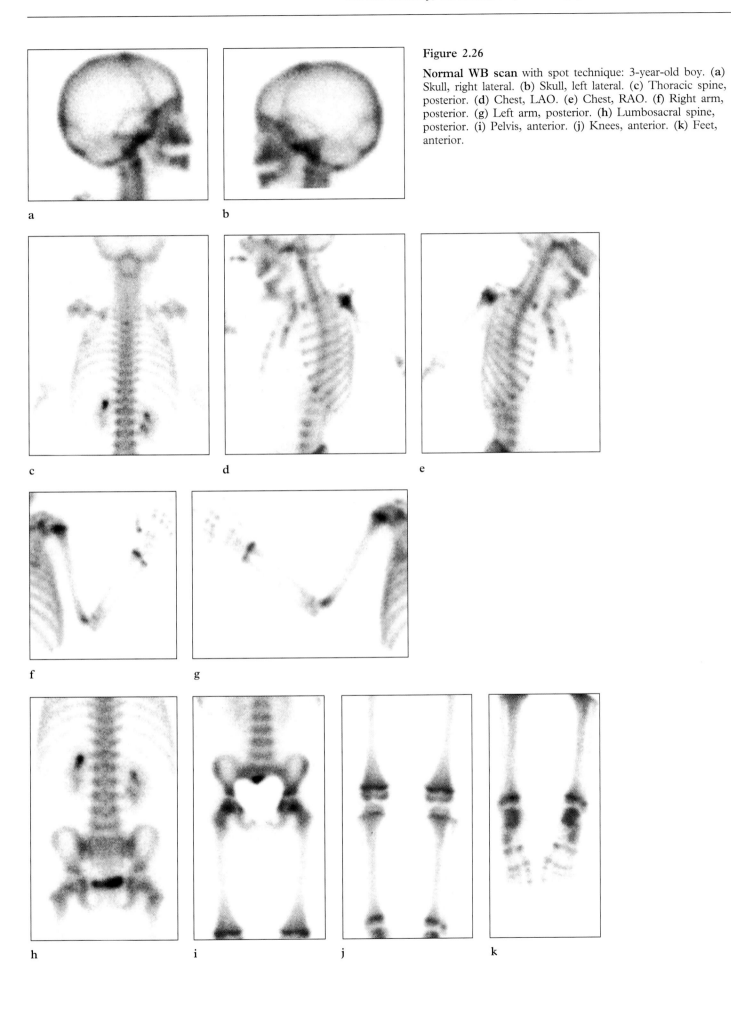

Figure 2.26

Normal WB scan with spot technique: 3-year-old boy. (**a**) Skull, right lateral. (**b**) Skull, left lateral. (**c**) Thoracic spine, posterior. (**d**) Chest, LAO. (**e**) Chest, RAO. (**f**) Right arm, posterior. (**g**) Left arm, posterior. (**h**) Lumbosacral spine, posterior. (**i**) Pelvis, anterior. (**j**) Knees, anterior. (**k**) Feet, anterior.

Figure 2.27

WB bone scan: 6-year-old male.

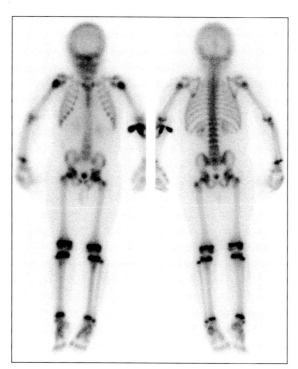

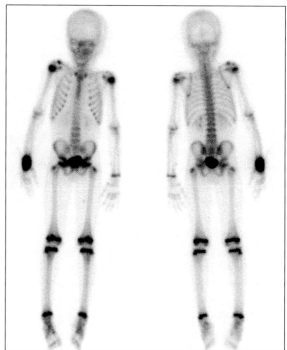

Figure 2.28

Normal WB bone scan: 8-year-old male.

Figure 2.29

Normal WB bone scan: 12-year-old male. Note the progressive changes in the relative epiphyseal activity when compared with younger patients. In addition, those epiphyses, which are still open, are better defined.

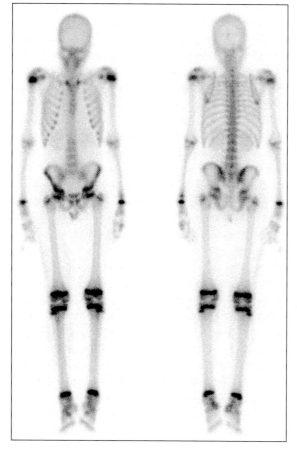

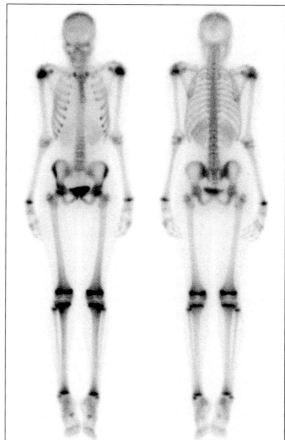

Figure 2.30

Normal WB bone scan: 13½-year-old female.

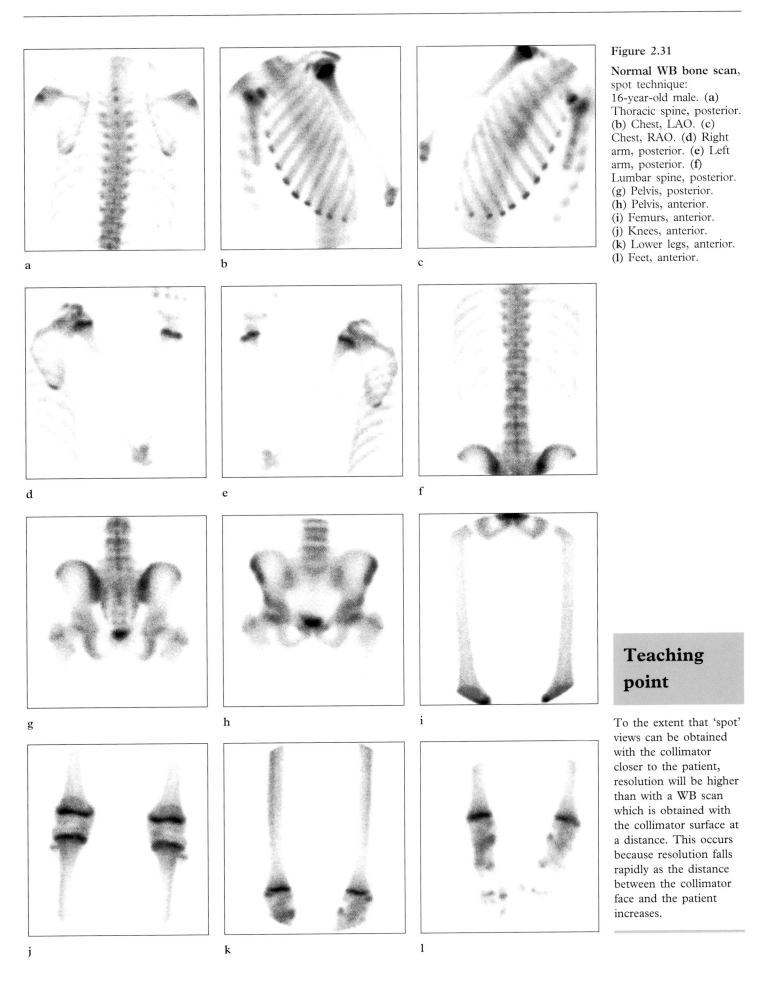

Figure 2.31

Normal WB bone scan, spot technique: 16-year-old male. **(a)** Thoracic spine, posterior. **(b)** Chest, LAO. **(c)** Chest, RAO. **(d)** Right arm, posterior. **(e)** Left arm, posterior. **(f)** Lumbar spine, posterior. **(g)** Pelvis, posterior. **(h)** Pelvis, anterior. **(i)** Femurs, anterior. **(j)** Knees, anterior. **(k)** Lower legs, anterior. **(l)** Feet, anterior.

Teaching point

To the extent that 'spot' views can be obtained with the collimator closer to the patient, resolution will be higher than with a WB scan which is obtained with the collimator surface at a distance. This occurs because resolution falls rapidly as the distance between the collimator face and the patient increases.

Figure 2.32

Normal WB bone scan: 22-year-old female. Note the absence of physeal activity when compared to WB scans on teenagers in Figures 2.29–2.31.

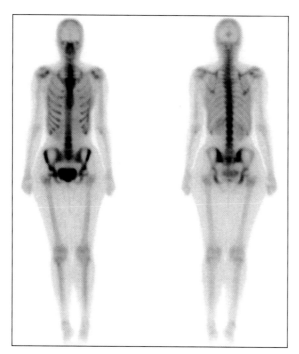

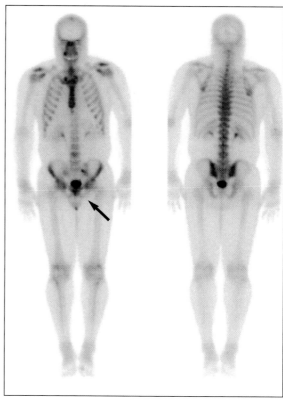

Figure 2.33

Normal WB bone scan: 26-year-old male.

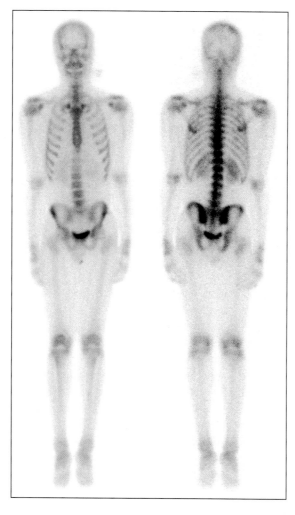

Figure 2.34

Normal WB bone scan: 35-year-old male. Some mild external genitalia and urine contamination activity (arrow).

Teaching point

When examining young adults, in whom there is no history of malignancy, arthritis, or trauma, slight increased tracer uptake can be seen at asymptomatic juxta-articular sites in the hands, feet, and knees. In the authors' experience, no patient with this combination of clinical and scintigraphic findings has had significant skeletal pathology. After careful evaluation of history and clinical data, X-ray correlation in these circumstances is usually unwarranted.

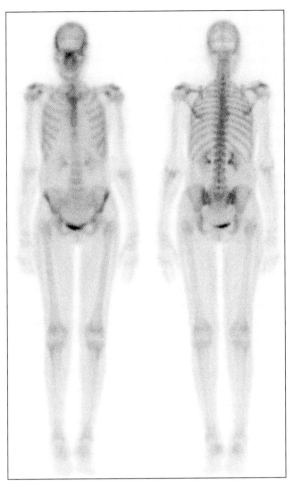

Figure 2.35

Normal WB bone scan: 53-year-old female. Incidental slight relative retention of tracer in soft tissues is normal variation.

Figure 2.36

Normal WB bone scan: 59-year-old male. Costal cartilage calcification (thin arrow) is not uncommon as patients get older. There is a photon deficiency overlying the proximal left femur, which represents a coin in the patient's pocket (long arrow).

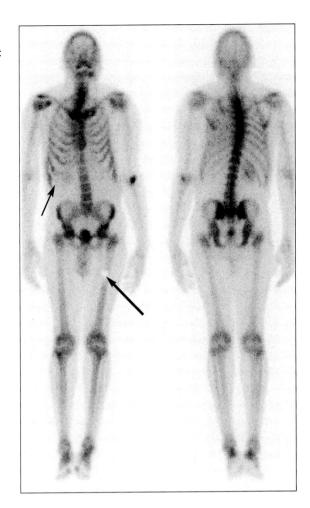

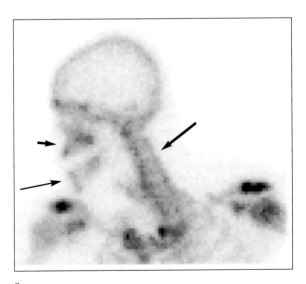

a

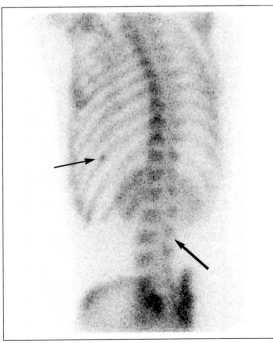

b

Figure 2.37 a and b

Multiple orthogonal spot views. Invaluable aid for anatomic localization of abnormal tracer uptake. **(a)** DS. Skull, lateral and CSP oblique. The anterior to posterior extent of the maxilla (short arrow) and mandible (thin arrow). Oblique cervical spine (long arrow). **(b)** DS, TSP and LSP, LPO. Incidental healing rib fracture (thin arrow). Facet regions (long arrow).

continued

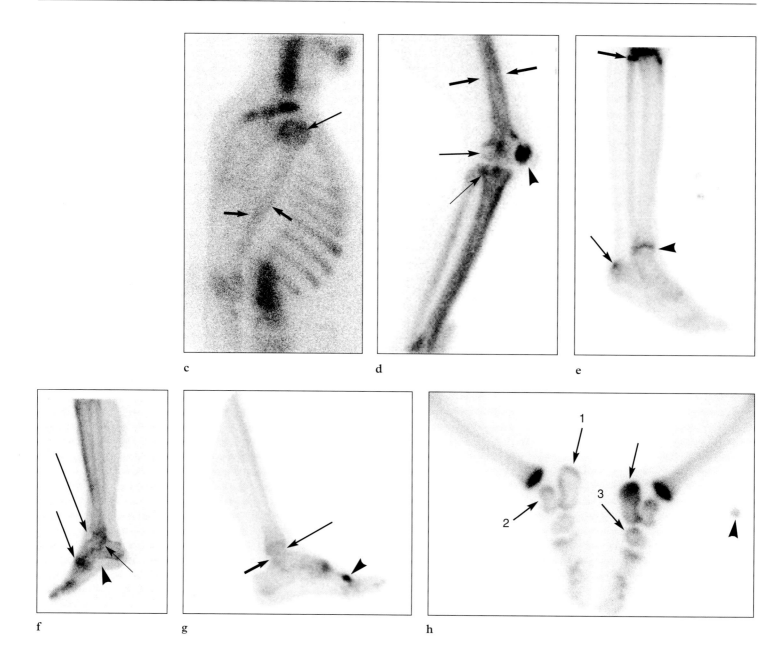

c d e

f g h

Figure 2.37 c–h

(c) DS, shoulder and humerus, seen on lateral chest. Although the shoulder joint is usually better defined on SPECT imaging, the glenohumeral joint (thin arrow) and the anterior and posterior cortices (thick arrows) are well seen. (d) DS. Lower femur and knee, lateral. The anterior and posterior femoral cortex (thick arrows), the patella (arrowhead), the posterior inferior condylar surface of the femur (arrow), and the tibiofibular joint (thin arrow) are well seen. The anterior and posterior tibia cortex can be defined. Usually separate anterior and posterior fibular cortices cannot be defined. (e) DS, lower leg and ankle, lateral. In this adolescent the proximal fibular epiphysis (arrow) is seen, as is the distal tibial epiphysis (arrowhead). The definition of the anterior and posterior tibial cortices as well as the fibula is appreciated. Minimal increased tracer at the insertion of the Achilles tendon is present in this patient who

was resolving a mild Achilles tendonitis. (f) DS, lower leg and ankle, lateral. In this adult, there is mild uptake in the tibiotalar joint region (arrow), in the posterior subtalar joint region (thin arrow), and in the navicular cuneiform region (long arrow). In asymptomatic adults, the significance of this minor uptake is uncertain. The plantar arch (arrowhead) is used to define the calcaneal cuboid joint region. (g) DS, lower leg and ankle, medial view. The tibiotalar joint region can be seen (arrows). Healing first metatarsal stress fracture (arrowhead). (h) Three year old, DS, ankle and foot, lateral. The right-sided marker is noted (arrowhead). The posterior right calcaneous is abnormal (thin arrow). Image shown to demonstrate the high-resolution detail which can be obtained of the individual bones of the hind and mid-foot in this age group. (1) Calcaneous, (2) talus, (3) cuboid.

Normal SPECT

SPECT imaging increases lesion contrast and isolates activity in the plane of interest. For large or anatomically complex structures more accurate localization of lesions is often possible. In addition smaller, less intense areas of abnormal tracer uptake, which are silent on planar imaging, can be detected with SPECT. Since inherent spatial resolution is better with planar imaging, for relatively small and superficial structures SPECT should not be substituted for high-resolution planar imaging. In the authors' institutions, SPECT supplements planar imaging. Correlative imaging with transaxial CT and transaxial, sagittal, and coronal MR images aids in understanding the normal SPECT appearance and also in the anatomic localization of foci of abnormal uptake. The evaluation of 3-D volumetric reprojection images displayed in cine or movie mode is an integral part of study analysis, often providing an important clue to lesion detection or localization.

Head

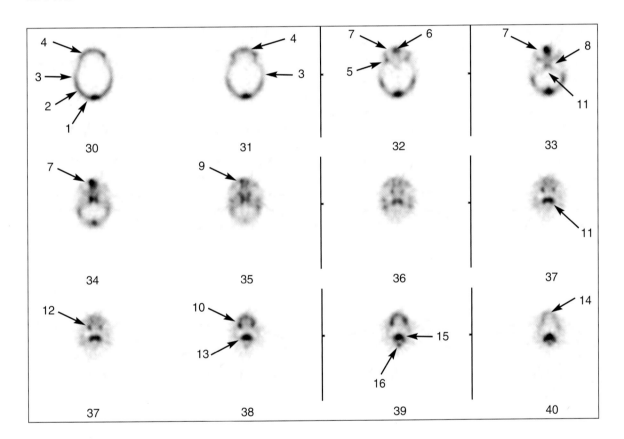

Teaching point

During data acquisition for SPECT imaging of the head, most often the camera must be positioned at some distance from the head, so that resolution is decreased below theoretical limits.

Figure 2.38

Normal head SPECT. Transaxial sections acquired 128 × 128 × 128, Hann filter, displayed 2 pixel thick slices from cranial to caudal. (1) Occipital bone, (2) parietal bone, (3) temporal bone, squamosal portion, (4) frontal bone, (5) greater wing sphenoid, orbital process, (6) nasal bone and frontal process of maxilla cannot be individually identified, (7) orbit, appears as photon deficiency bordered laterally by greater wing of sphenoid, (8) middle cranial fossa, (9) maxillary sinus bordered laterally by zygoma, (10) maxilla, (11) clivus, (12) mandible, ramus, (13) C1 vertebra, (14) mandible, (15) vertebral body C2, (16) spinous process C2.

Figure 2.39

Normal transaxial CT images, from cranial to caudal. Representative images. Appreciate that transaxial CT images are routinely obtained parallel to the supraorbitomeatal plane. Transaxial nuclear medicine images (Figure 2.38) are obtained parallel to the infraorbitomeatal plane. (1) Occipital bone, (2) parietal bone, (3) temporal bone, squamosal portion, (4) frontal bone, (6) nasal bone and front of maxilla, (7) orbit, (8) middle cranial fossa, (10) maxilla, (11) clivus, (12) mandible, ramus, (13) C1 vertebra, (15) vertebral body C2, (16) spinous process C2, (17) dens of C2, (18) frontal sinus.

Teaching point

The relatively different transaxial planes of section of routine nuclear medicine images, which are more horizontal than the oblique CT images, must be kept in mind when performing correlative image analysis.

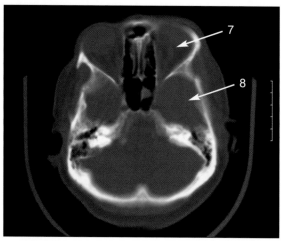

a

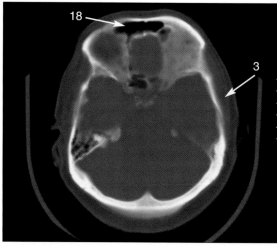

b

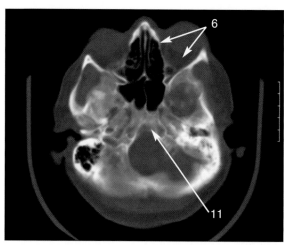

c

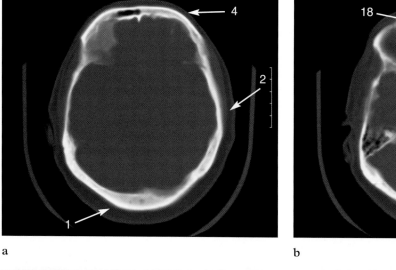

d

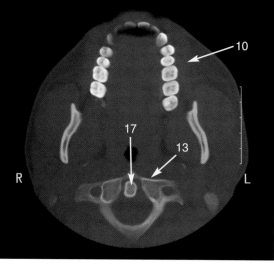

e

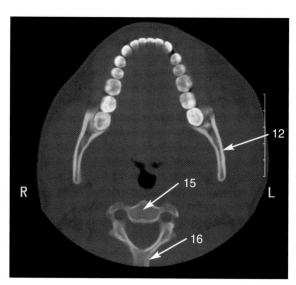

f

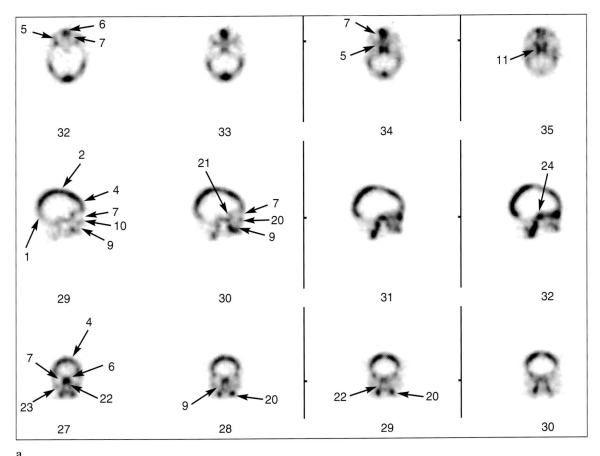

a

b

Figure 2.40

Normal skull SPECT, triangulation display. 128 × 128 × 128 acquisition, Hann filter, displayed 2 pixels thick. Transaxial images (top row) displayed from cephalad to caudad, for orientation purposes. Sagittal images (middle row) displayed from right to left, and coronal images (bottom row), displayed from anterior to posterior. (1) Occipital bone, (2) parietal bone, (4) frontal bone, (5) sphenoid, greater wing, orbital process, (6) nasal bone and frontal process of maxilla, cannot be separated, (7) orbit, appears as photon deficiency, (8) middle cranial fossa, appears as photon deficiency, (9) maxillary sinus, appears as photon deficiency, (10) maxilla, (11) clivus, (12) mandible, ramus, (14) mandible, (19) nasopharyngeal activity, (20) maxillary teeth, activity associated with, (21) sellar region, (22) sphenoid, lesser wing, (23) maxilla, frontal process, (24) TMJ.

Teaching point

Triangulation display in which pixels, representing an anatomic area, can be simultaneously located in all three planes is a valuable diagnostic aid.

Figure 2.41

Normal head coronal images. (a–c)
Direct CT, and (**d**) MR, T1 weighted.
Displayed from anterior to posterior.
Correlative images for Figure 2.40. (4)
Frontal bone, (7) orbit, (9) maxillary sinus,
(10) maxilla, (12) mandible, ramus, (23)
maxilla, frontal process, (25) pituitary gland,
as gray soft-tissue density, (26) sphenoid
sinus. The cortex of the floor of the sella
(roof of the sphenoid sinus) and air in
sphenoid sinus are both black on this image
and therefore cannot be separately
identified. (**e**) Sagittal images. MR, T1
weighted. Displayed from mid-line to lateral.
(7) Orbit, (9) maxillary sinus, (11) clivus
(gray represents marrow), (17) dens of C2,
(18) frontal sinus. On these images the
cortex of the skull appears black with the
marrow appearing gray. White signal
represents fat in the scalp. Air appears
black.

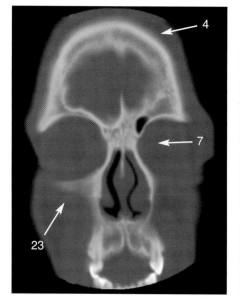

a

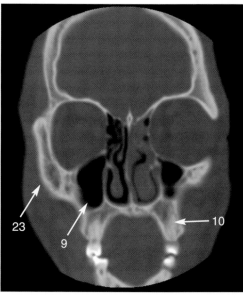

b

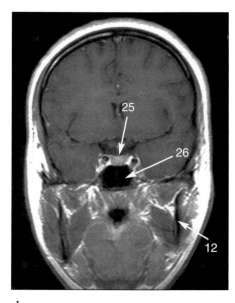

c

d

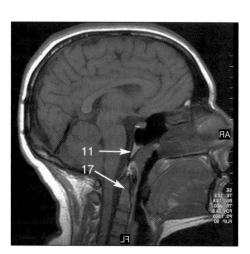

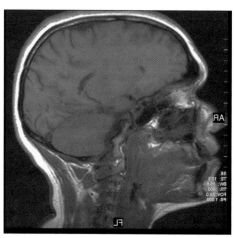

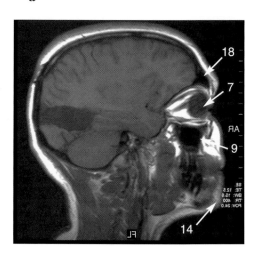

e

Shoulder

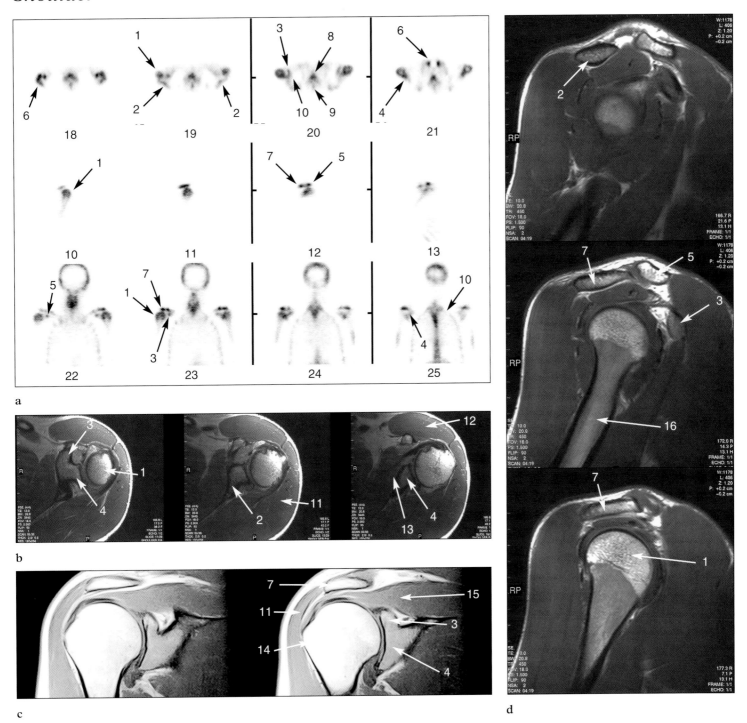

Figure 2.42

Normal shoulder. (a) SPECT, triangulation display. Transaxial images (top row) displayed from superior to inferior, sagittal images (middle row), displayed from right lateral to medial, and coronal images (bottom row) displayed from anterior to posterior. 128 × 128 × 128 acquisition, iterative reconstruction, displayed 3 pixels thick. (1) Humeral head, (2) scapula, spine, (3) scapula, coracoid process, (4) scapula, glenoid, (5) clavicle, lateral end, (6) clavicle, medial end (note that the more anteriorly located medial end of the clavicle is not seen on the coronal images which are more posterior), (7) acromion process, (8) T3, vertebral body, (9) T2, vertebra, spinous process, (10) lung apex, appears as a photon-deficient region. (b) Transaxial images. MR, T1 weighted. Displayed from cephalad to caudad. (1) Humeral head, marrow appears gray. The cortex is black. (2) Scapular spine, (3) coracoid process, (4) glenoid, (11) deltoid muscle, (12) pectoralis muscle, (13) subscapular muscle. (c) Coronal images. MR, T1. (3) Coracoid process, (4) glenoid, (7) acromion process, (11) deltoid muscle, (14) greater tuberosity, marrow is gray, overlying cortex is black, (15) supraspinatus muscle. (d) Sagittal images. MR, T1 weighted. Displayed medial to lateral. (1) Humeral head, (2) scapular spine, (3) coracoid process, (5) clavicle, lateral end, (7) acromion process, (16) humeral shaft marrow. Surrounding cortex appears black.

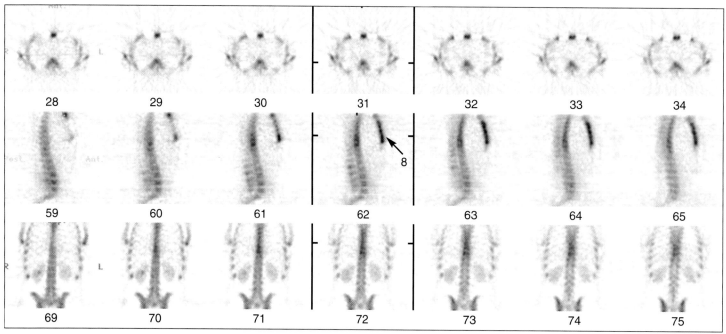

d

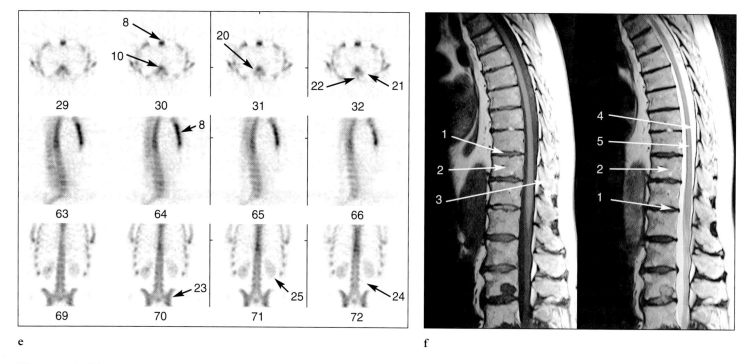

e   f

Figure 2.45 d–h

(**d**) SPECT, triangulation display, transaxial images (top arrow) centered at approximately T8, displayed cephalad to caudad. Sagittal images (middle row) displayed from right to left and coronal (bottom row) displayed from anterior to posterior. 128 × 128 × 128 acquisition with Hann filter. Displayed 1 pixel thick slice. (**e**) SPECT, triangulation display. Magnified view. Transaxial images through approximately T7 vertebra. Coronal images (bottom row) begin at the posterior portion of the vertebral body and extend more posteriorly. (8) Sternum, (10) T7 vertebral body, (20) pedicle region, (21) lateral mass region, (22) spinous process, (23) medial ilium, (24) C3 transverse process, (25) kidney. (**f**) Sagittal image. MR, T1 (left image) and T2 (right image) mid-line. (1) Intervertebral disk space, (2) vertebral body, (3) spinous process, (4) spinal fluid, (5) spinal cord. (**g**) X-ray, localizer film to select CT image planes. Without localizer lines (left image) and with localizer lines (right image). (**h**) Transaxial, CT, sequential images through T8 vertebra, from cephalad to caudad. This was a thoracic CT scan displayed and photographed with bone windows. The lung is black surrounding the soft tissues of the heart and mediastinal structures. (3) Spinous process, (4) scapula, (8) sternum, (12) rib, (26) transverse process, articulating with the rib anterior to it. The rib also articulates with the vertebral body at the costovertebral junction. (27) Lamina, (28) facet joint made up of the more posteriorly located inferior articular facet of the upper vertebrae and the more anteriorly located superior articular facet of the lower vertebrae.

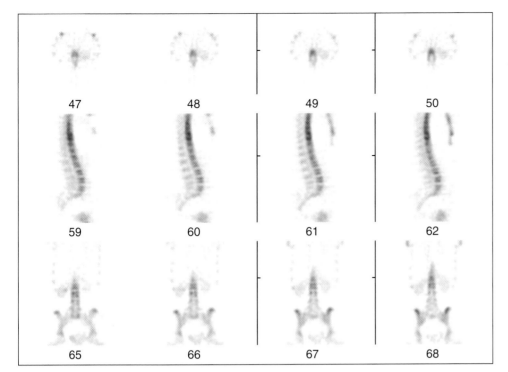

a

b

Figure 2.48

Normal lumbar spine. Slight 32-year-old female. (a) SPECT, triangulation display with transaxial images (top row) through L1 vertebra, sagittal images (middle row) centered at mid-line, and coronal images (bottom row) more posteriorly centered in the vertebral canal. (b) Transaxial images from same patient as (a). Centered through L5 vertebra. (28) Lamina, (29) ilium, wing. Note the variation in this patient's transaxial images compared with the patient in Figure 2.47.

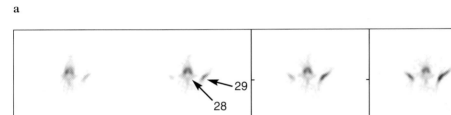

a   b   c

Figure 2.49

Normal lumbosacral spine: 6-mm thick slices with very heavy (smoothed) filter. This example illustrates the wide variation in filter possibilities and display available. (a) SPECT, lumbosacral spine, coronal, and (b) sagittal. Normal anatomy, including SI joints on coronal and the spinous processes seen on the mid-line sagittal image. (c) SPECT, transaxial image through L3 vertebral body. Note the relationship of the body to the spinal canal and posterior structures.

Teaching point

The iterative reconstruction technique deals better with noise, such as bladder-filling artifact, which creates significant problems with the filtered back-projection algorithm. As increased computing power becomes widely available, this technique may be used more commonly in routine nuclear medicine practice.

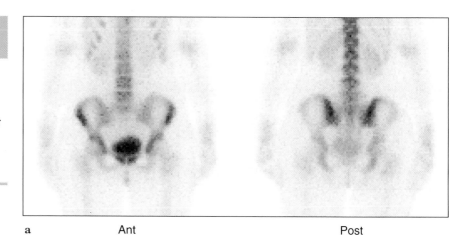

a   Ant   Post

Pelvis

Figure 2.50 a–c

Normal lower lumbar spine and pelvis. (a) DS. Portion of WB scan for orientation and reference. Anterior (left image) and posterior (right image). **(b–d)** SPECT study. 128 × 128 × 128 acquisition. Iterative reconstruction, OSEM with three iterations and six subsets. **(b)** Sagittal images from right to mid-line. For anatomic reference. (8) Sternum, (11) L5 vertebral body, (32) bladder, (33) symphysis, (34) L4–L5 intervertebral disk space, appears as photon deficiency. **(c)** SPECT, sequential transaxial images from L5 caudal to hips. (11) L5 vertebra, (29) ilium, wing, (30) sacrum, (31) S1 vertebral body, (37) S4 vertebra, (38) ilium, (39) S4 vertebral body, (40) superior pubic ramus, (41) ischium, (42) femoral head.

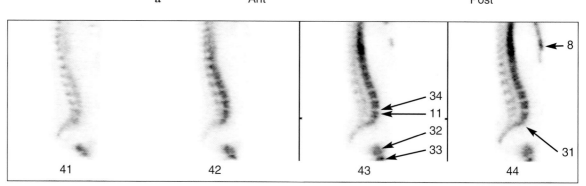

b

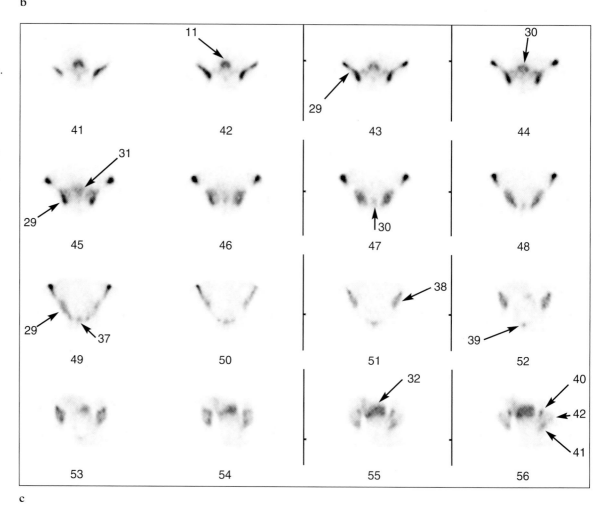

c

continued

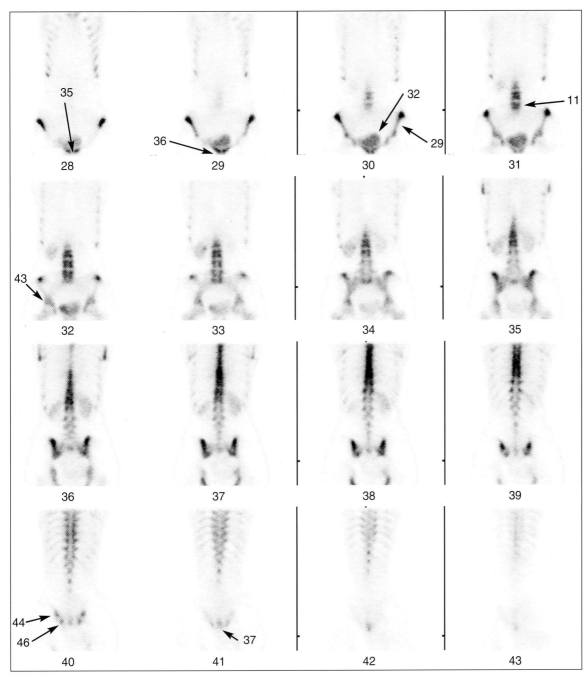

d

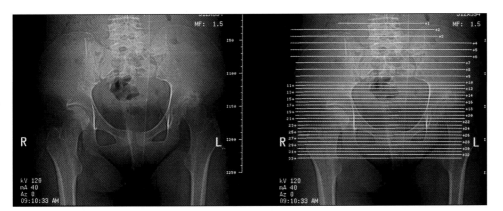

e

Figure 2.50 d and e

(**d**) SPECT sequential coronal images from front to back. (11) L5 vertebra, (29) ilium, wing, (32) bladder, (35) photon deficiency of cartilage symphysis, (36) pubis, (37) S4 vertebral body, (43) acetabulum, (44) ilium, posterior, (46) sacrum, alae. (**e**) X-ray, pelvis, localizer film to select CT image planes. Without localizer lines (left image) and with localizer lines (right image).

continued

Figure 2.50 f

(f) CT, pelvis, transaxial. Sequential 0.5 cm images. This was a pelvic CT examination, filmed and photographed using bone windows. Iliac crest to hips, from cephalad to caudad. (29) Iliac wing, (31) S1 vertebra, body, (52) S3 vertebra, body, (53) SI joint (SIJ), (54) sacral foramina, (55) coccyx.

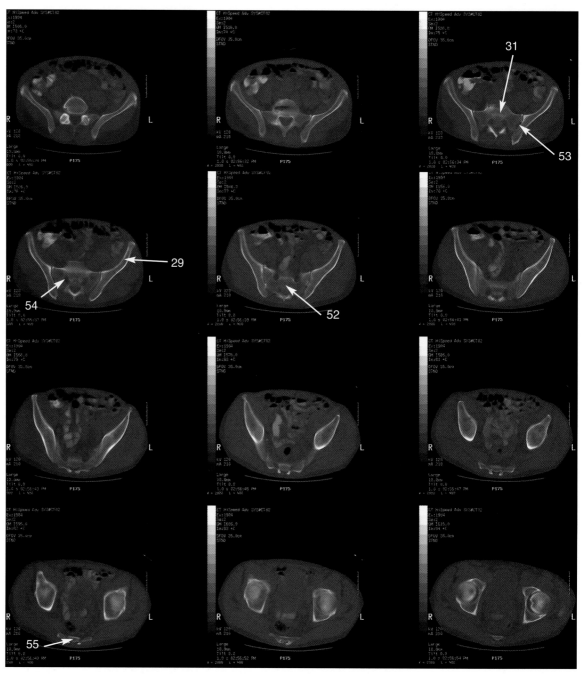

f

Hips

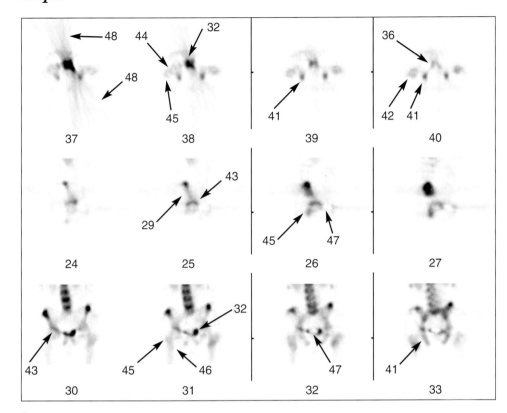

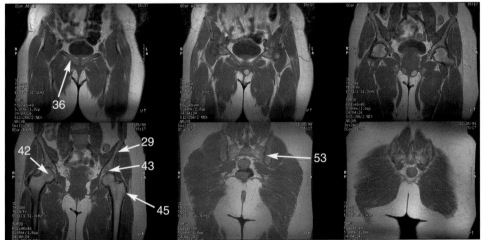

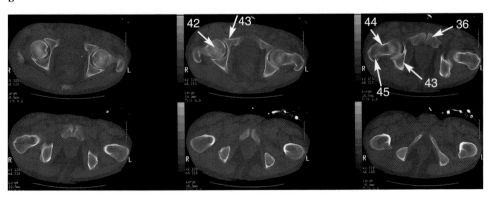

Figure 2.51

Normal adult hips. (a) SPECT. 128 × 128 × 128 acquisition, Hann filter, displayed 1 pixel thick. Transaxial images (top row) from superior to inferior. Sagittal (middle row) and coronal (bottom row). (29) Ilium, wing, (32) bladder, (36) symphysis, (41) ischium, (42) femur, (43) acetabulum, (44) femur, neck, (45) femur, greater trochanter, (46) femur, lesser trochanter, (47) Foley catheter in bladder, (48) streak artifact secondary to changing counts in the bladder during acquisition. (Compare bladder region on these filtered back projection images with the iterative reconstruction in Figure 2.50.) (b) Pelvis and hips. MR, T1, coronal, displayed from anterior to posterior. Label numbers after (c). (c) Hips. CT, transaxial. Sequential 0.5 cm contiguous slices displayed from upper acetabulum through proximal femur. (29) Ilium, (36) superior pubic ramus at symphysis, (42) femur, head, (43) acetabulum, (44) femur, neck, (45) femur, greater trochanter, (53) SI joint.

Figure 2.52

Normal hips, 8-year-old male. 128 × 128 × 128 acquisition, reconstructed with Butterworth 6.25 filter, displayed 2 pixels thick. SPECT, triangulation display. (32) Bladder, (40) pubis, (41) ischium, (49) physeal plate, proximal femur, (50) apophysis, greater trochanter, (51) ischial tuberosity.

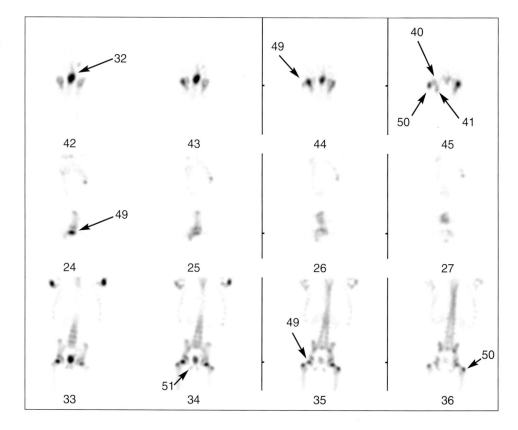

Knees

Figure 2.53 a–c

Normal adult knees. (a) Knees, 3-D volumetric reprojection images. Selected views from 0° to 70°. 128 × 128 × 128 acquisition, XLFOV camera, 4.1 mm per pixel. Butterworth 6.22 filter reconstruction. Smoothed appearance in this patient gives suboptimal definition of anterior, posterior, medial, and lateral tibial and femoral cortices and also the photon deficiency representing femoral tibial joint space. The oblique views separate the patellar femoral joint and also the fibular head from the tibia at the proximal tibiofibular joint. Identification numbers at end of legend. (b) Knees, SPECT, triangulation display. Transaxial images (top row) through patellar femoral joint, displayed cephalad to caudad, sagittal images (middle row) displayed from lateral to mid-line, and coronal images (bottom row) displayed from anterior to posterior. (c) Knee, SPECT, sequential transaxial images, 1 pixel thick slices displayed from cephalad to caudad.

continued

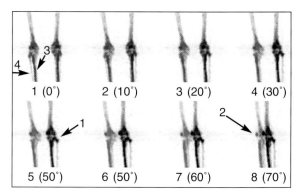

a

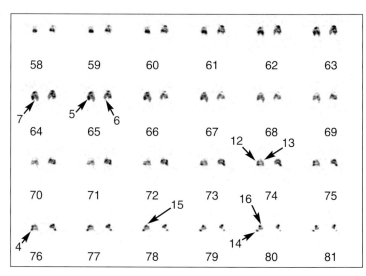

b

c

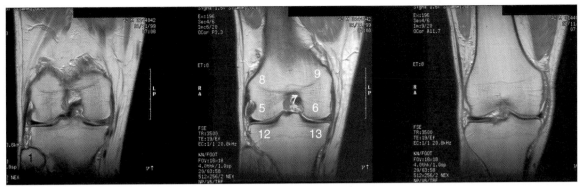

d

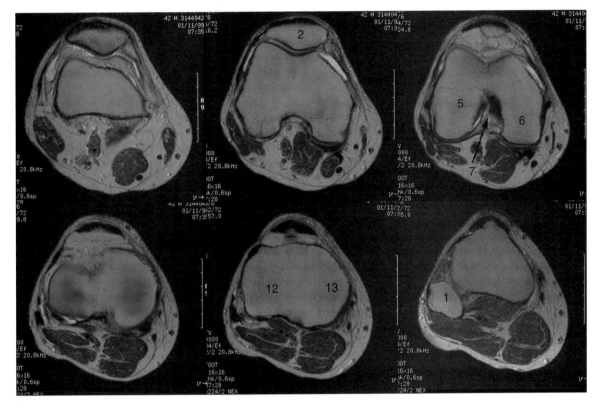

e

Figure 2.53 d–f

(d) Knee, MR, T1, coronal. Displayed from posterior (left image) to anterior (right-most image). (e) Knee, MR, T1, transaxial images. Displayed from cephalad to caudad. (f) Knee, MR, T1, sagittal. Displayed from medial (left image) to lateral (right-most image). These are taken with slight obliquity. The right-most sagittal image should be correlated with the left coronal image in (d), visualizing the plane of section passing superiorly to inferiorly through the femur, tibia, and then fibula. (1) Fibular head, articulating with tibia at proximal tibiofibular joint, (2) patella, (3) ANT tibial cortex, (4) fibula shaft, (5) lateral femoral condyle, (6) medial femoral condyle, (7) intercondylar notch, (8) lateral epicondyle, (9) medial epicondyle, (10) anterior tibial cortex, (11) posterior tibial cortex, (12) lateral proximal tibia (subarticular), (13) medial proximal tibia (subarticular), (14) proximal fibula, distal to proximal tibiofibular joint, (15) proximal tibial shaft with central photon deficiency representing marrow cavity, (16) tibial tubercle region.

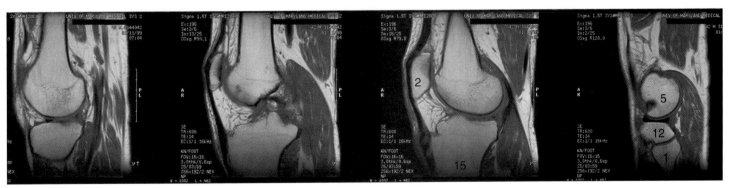

f

Figure 2.54

Normal knees in 8-year-old male. (**a** and **b**).
SPECT, 128 × 128 × 128 acquisition, reconstructed
with Hann filter and displayed 1 pixel thick.
Sequential transaxial images (top row) from superior
to inferior, sagittal (middle row) from lateral to mid-
line, and coronal (bottom row) from front to back.
The presence of intense physeal uptake can create
problems in reconstruction. For identification
numbers, see end of legend. (**c**) Knee, MR, T1
representative sagittal in another patient, a few years
older than the patient in (**a**) and (**b**). The regions of
the physes are still apparent in the distal femur (17)
and proximal tibia (18). (2) Patella, (5) lateral
femoral condyle (appears much less intense than the
physis just above it), (6) medial femoral condyle
(appears similar to lateral femoral condyle, with
relatively less uptake than the intense physeal
activity), (7) intercondylar notch, appears as photon
deficiency, (10) proximal tibial cortex, (17) physeal
plate, distal femur, (18) physeal plate, proximal tibia,
(19) fibular physes, (52) femoral shaft.

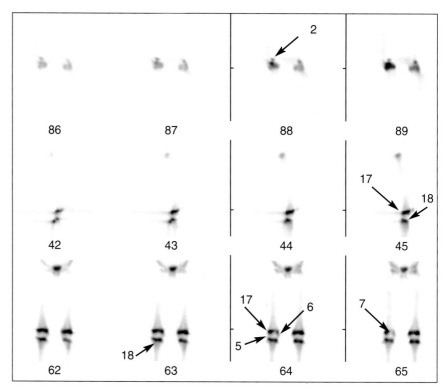

a

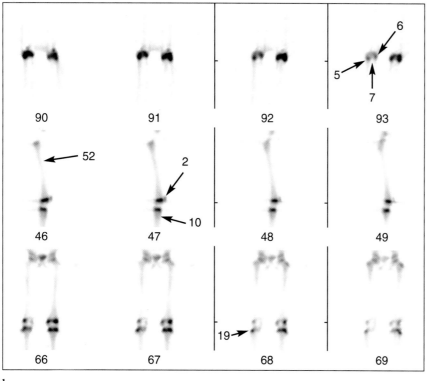

b

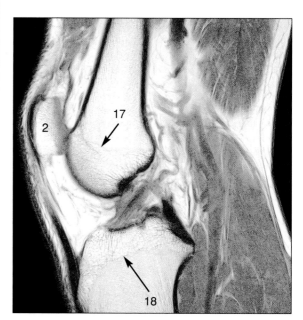

c

Legs

Figure 2.55

Normal legs, 46-year-old male. Incidental tracer in skin, of uncertain significance, allows anatomic localization. Planar images included for comparison. (**a**) DS legs anterior view and (**b**) DS, right leg, lateral view. For reference and orientation. Anterior tibial cortex (short arrow) and fibula (long arrow) are well seen on lateral image, but, in this patient with some nonspecific swelling, the posterior tibial cortex is not optimally visualized. Lateral tibial cortex (thick arrow) and medial tibial cortex (thin arrow) are seen on anterior image. The outline of the skin (arrowheads) is not usually seen. (**c**) Sequential transaxial images from upper to mid-leg. Skin uptake (arrowheads) outlines the extremity. The relative size of the tibia (long arrow) compared with the fibula (short arrow) is appreciated. The anterior increased tracer is accentuation of activity at the tibial tubercle. Occasionally, in larger patients, a photon deficiency representing the tibial marrow cavity can be appreciated. (**d**) Legs, MR, T1, transaxial. Selected images from proximal to distal. (1) Fibular head, at the proximal tibiofibular joint level. (12) Proximal tibia, (19) mid-fibula. Note the separation of the tibia and fibula in mid-leg. Note also the small marrow cavity (white signal) surrounded by cortex (black signal on T1 MR images). (20) Distal tibia at ankle, (21) lateral malleolus, which on these images is initially seen adjacent to distal tibia, and more distally is lateral to the talus (T), which is just coming into the plane of section, (22) medial malleolar extension of the tibia.

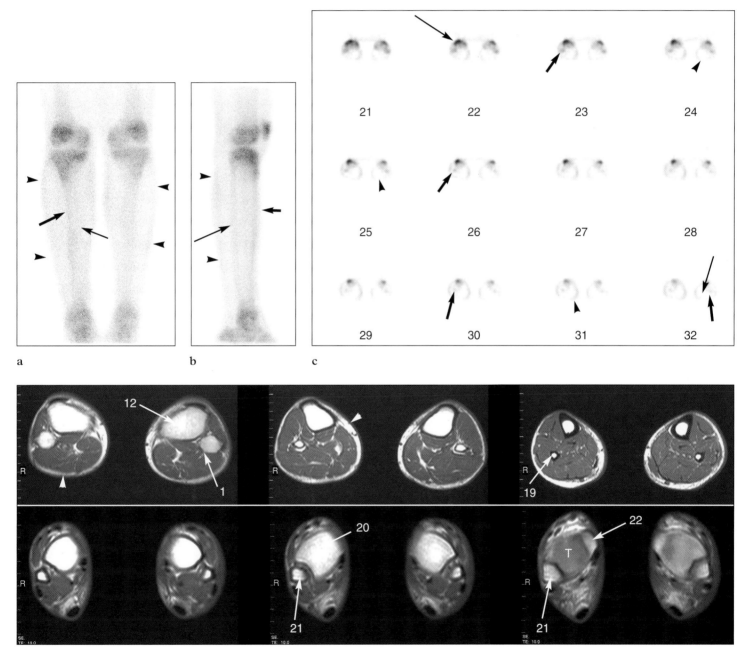

a   b   c

d

Ankle and foot

SPECT of the ankle and foot is always a challenge. The small size of the structures, the inability to place the camera close to the surface during rotation, and the efforts needed to immobilize the extremity are all reasons for decreased resolution. Data acquisition is usually done with the patient in a comfortable position to minimize movement. The initial reconstruction (Figure 2.56a) is then reoriented using oblique angle or free angle reorientation software which is generally available on most computer systems. The foot is reoriented on the sagittal image, first with the sole horizontal (Figure 2.56b) so that the transaxial sections are of the long axis of the foot and second with the tibiotalar joint horizontal (Figure 2.56c) so that the coronal image is along the short axis of the foot. Even with these reorientation efforts and the use of multiple different reconstruction algorithms, often localization of abnormal foci will have to be described as 'in the region of'.

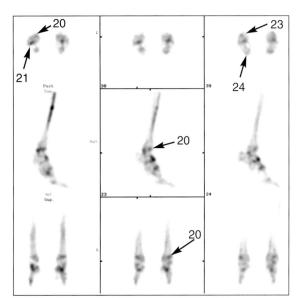

a

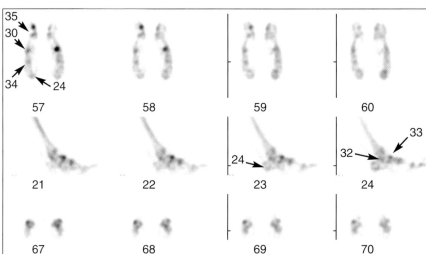

b

Figure 2.56 a–c

Normal ankle and foot. (a) SPECT, reconstructed as acquired. Butterworth 6.22 filter, triangulation display. Transaxial images (top row), displayed from cephalad to caudad, represent long axis through the upper portion of the ankle and hind-foot. Coronal images (bottom row), displayed posterior to anterior, are oblique. Identification numbers at end of legend. (b) SPECT, oblique angle reorientation of images in (a), with sole of foot horizontal. Transaxial images (top row) represent the long axis of the foot. (c) SPECT, oblique angle reorientation of images in (a), with tibiotalar joint horizontal. Coronal images (bottom row) represent short axis of the ankle and foot. Identification numbers are found at end of legend for Figure 2.57.

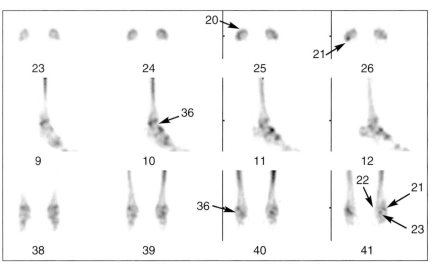

c

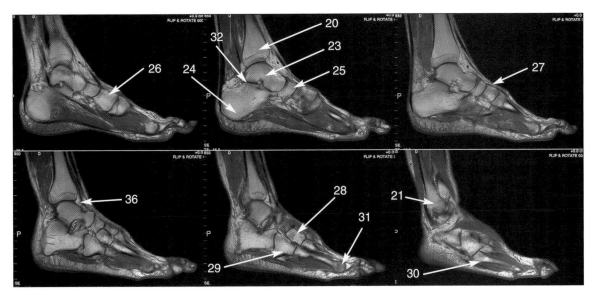

a

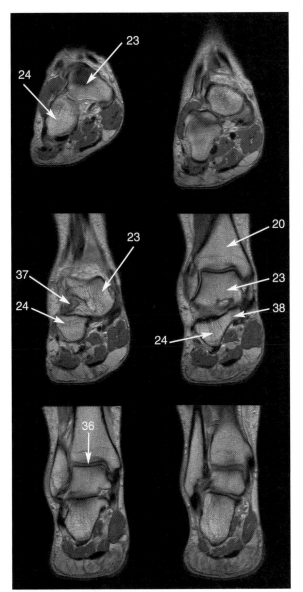

b

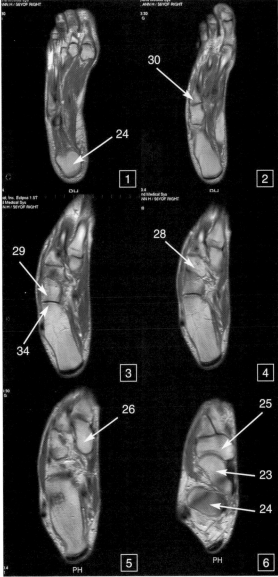

c

Figure 2.57 a–c

(a) MR, T1, sagittal. Displayed from medial to lateral. Marrow is gray and cortex is black. (b) MR, proton density-weighted image, coronal (short axis), displayed from anterior to posterior. (c) MR, T1, transaxial (long axis) displayed from plantar to dorsum. Image 1 is at the anterior subtalar joint, image 3 at the tarsal tunnel between the talus and calcaneous, image 4 at the sustentaculum tali, and images 5 and 6 at the posterior subtalar joint. (20) Distal tibia, (21) lateral malleolus, (22) medial malleolus, (23) talus, (24) calcaneous, (25) navicular, (26) medial cuneiform, (27) middle cuneiform, (28) lateral cuneiform, (29) cuboid, (30) fifth metatarsal, base, (31) fifth metatarsal, head, (32) posterior subtalar joint region, (33) talonavicular joint region, (34) calcaneal cuboid region, (35) MTP joint region, (36) tibiotalar joint region, (37) tarsal tunnel, (38) sustentaculum tali.

Variants of normal

Skull

Figure 2.58

Hyperostosis frontalis.
(a) DS, skull, lateral.
Mild-to-moderate
increased tracer involving
portions of the frontal
bone is typical of
hyperostosis. (b) X-ray,
skull, lateral. If clinically
relevant, the diagnosis
can be confirmed on a
plain X-ray.

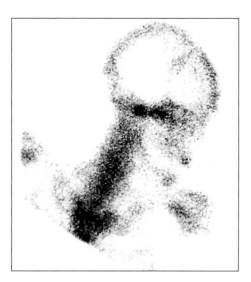

a

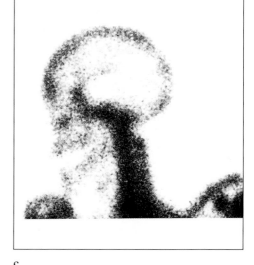

b

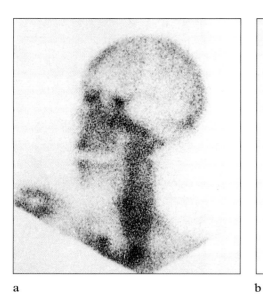

a

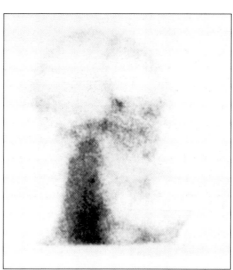

b

c

Figure 2.59

Skull sutures. (a–c) DS, skull, lateral views from three different patients. It is common to
see a focal area of increased tracer uptake which corresponds to the pterion, the site of
confluence of the frontal, parietal, temporal, and sphenoid bones. However, tracer uptake
may be seen extending along individual sutures.

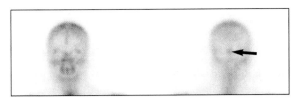

a

Figure 2.60

External occipital protuberance. (a) DS. Portions of a WB scan. Anterior (left image) and posterior (right image). Minimally intense round area of increased tracer seen on posterior view (arrow). **(b)** SPECT, triangulation display. Skull. The SPECT technique accentuates even these normal variations in tracer uptake (arrow).

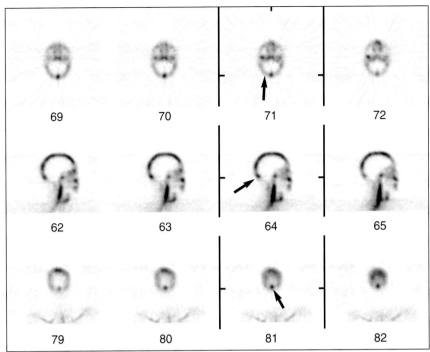

b

Neck

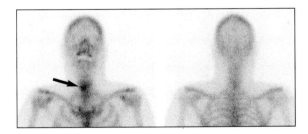

Figure 2.61

Thyroid cartilage uptake. DS, head and neck, from portion of WB bone scan. Anterior (left image) and posterior (right image). The uptake is clearly seen on the anterior view (arrow) but not seen on the posterior view.

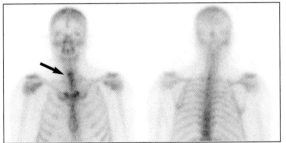

a

Figure 2.62

Thyroid cartilage uptake. (a) DS, portion of a WB bone scan. Anterior (left image) and posterior (right image). The uptake in the region of the thyroid cartilage on the anterior view (arrow) is less obvious than in Figure 2.61. **(b)** SPECT, head and neck, triangulation display. The thyroid cartilage uptake is well seen on all three planes. Transaxial (upper image), mid-line sagittal (middle image), and coronal through the mid-portion of the thyroid cartilage (lower image).

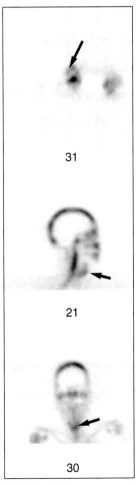

b

Chest

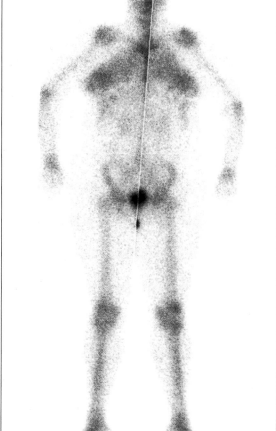

R   Ant   L

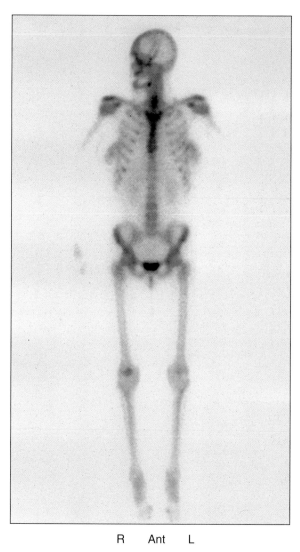

R   Ant   L

Figure 2.63

Breast uptake. WB, 3 hours post-injection. Anterior. Symmetrical intense breast uptake. Incidental finding in the patient being imaged for an athletic injury. (Images courtesy of Dr Neil Borelli, Westminster, Maryland.)

Figure 2.64

Breast uptake, DS. Portion of WB scan, anterior view. Moderate intense bilateral breast uptake.

Figure 2.65

Costal cartilage uptake. DS, portion of WB scan. Anterior (left image) and posterior (right image). Uptake in the costal cartilages (arrows) is most often seen in elderly patients as the cartilages calcify.

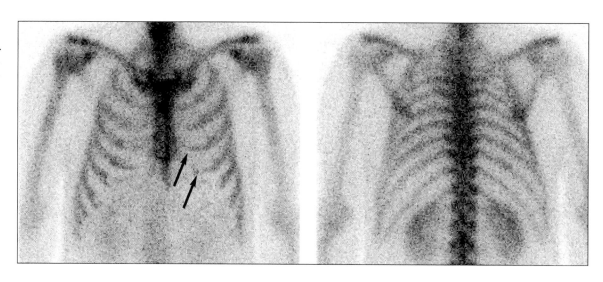

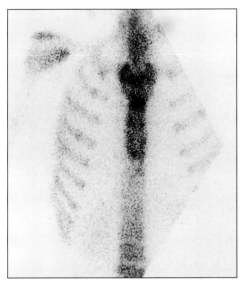

Figure 2.66

Normal angle of Louis uptake. Focal uptake in a linear orientation between the manubrium and body of the sternum is a common variant.

Teaching point

Uptake of tracer at the angle of Louis which is not minimal and linear requires careful clinical evaluation, since the sternum is a common site for metastatic disease, infection, and trauma.

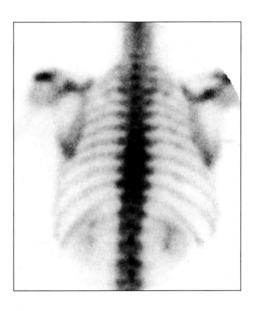

Figure 2.67

Stippled ribs. DS, thoracic spine, posterior. Prominent activity in the posterior ribs at the mid-clavicular level is thought to be due to increased tracer uptake at sites of muscle insertion.

Upper extremity

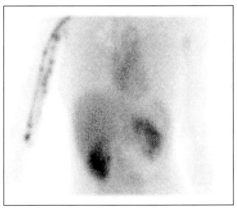

a

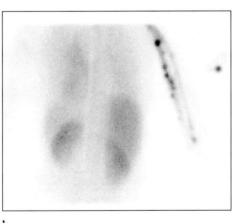

b

Figure 2.68

Venous retention. Injection made in vein in right antecubital fossa. **(a)** BP, arm, anterior and **(b)** BP, arm, posterior. Punctate areas of increased tracer throughout the veins.

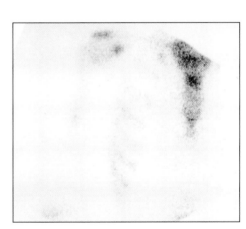

Figure 2.69

Deltoid insertion. DS, right arm, anterior. Minimal intense focal increased uptake in the upper third of the right humerus. This corresponds to the region of the deltoid muscle insertion and is a normal variant.

Teaching point

Although venous retention is most often a normal variant, when seen it should prompt clinical evaluation of the extremity for signs of infection or thrombosis.

Teaching point

When there is pronounced uptake in the upper third of the humerus, clinical evaluation is required, particularly if there is recent trauma or known primary malignancy.

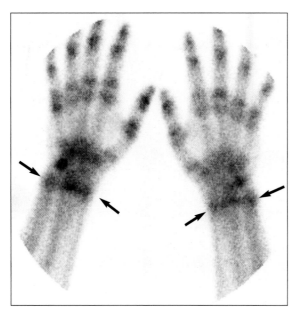

a

Figure 2.70

Residual physeal activity. Normal 32-year-old male.
(a) DS, hand and wrist, palmar view. Minimal
activity is seen in the physis for both distal radius and
ulna (arrows). (b) X-ray, wrist, PA. Growth plates
are fused.

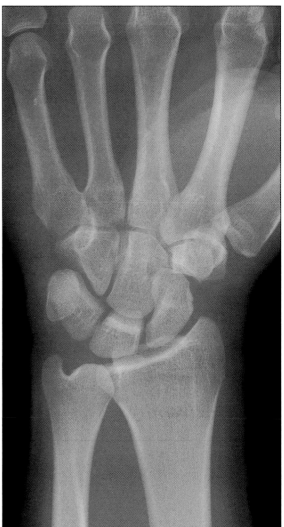

b

Spine

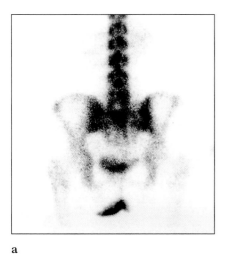

a

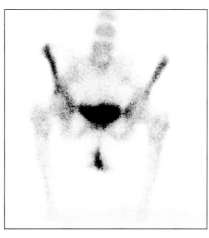

b

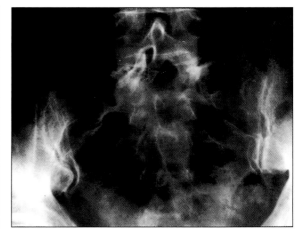

c

Figure 2.71

Spina bifida. (a) DS, lumbosacral spine, posterior and (b) DS, pelvis, anterior.
Small photon-deficient area associated with the L5–SI region. (c) X-ray,
lumbosacral junction, AP view. Spina bifida identified.

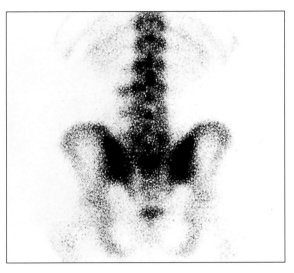

a

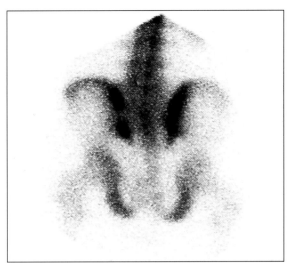

a

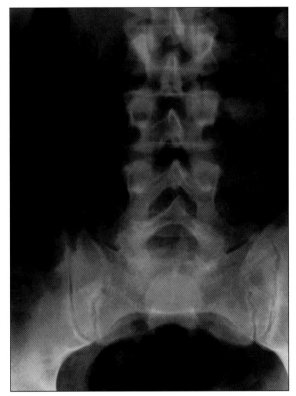

b

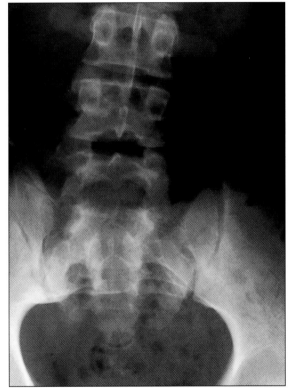

b

Figure 2.72

Large lumbar transverse process. (a) DS, lumbar spine, posterior. Mild-to-moderate asymmetric increased tracer involving the L3 and L4 lumbar transverse processes. **(b)** X-ray. Lumbar spine, AP. The developmental increase in the left L3 and L4 transverse processes is noted.

Figure 2.73

Sacralization of fifth lumbar vertebra. (a) DS, lumbo-sacral spine, posterior. Asymmetric uptake with mild increase on the left creating less sharpness in the upper part of the SI joint. **(b)** X-ray, lumbosacral region, PA view. 'Sacralization' of a large left-sided transverse process of L5 is noted.

Lower extremity

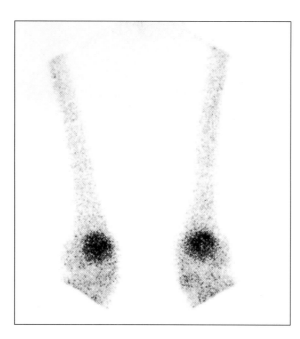

Figure 2.74

'Hot' patellar sign. DS, knees, anterior. Increased tracer homogeneously throughout both patellae. In asymptomatic patients this finding should be considered a normal variation. It should be confirmed on lateral views.

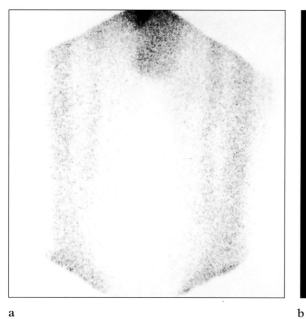

a

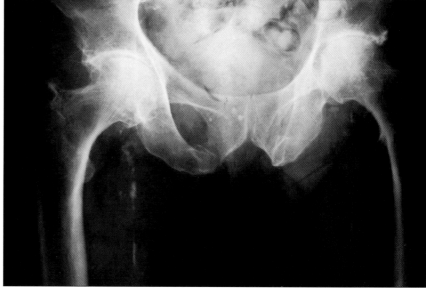

b

Figure 2.75

Vascular calcification uptake. (a) DS, femurs, anterior. Mild linear increased tracer medial to the femurs identified bilaterally. (b) X-ray, pelvis and upper femurs, AP. Vascular calcifications corresponding to the abnormal tracer uptake.

Figure numbers 2.76–2.78 are intentionally absent.

Artifacts

Artifacts in medical imaging can be defined as deviations from normal, which do not represent disease, normal physiologic, or normal anatomic variations in tracer uptake. One of the authors (DC) has used the term artifact interchangeably with the term deceptions, which included every deviation from a standard image appearance that could be mistaken for the pathology being investigated. In this atlas many such abnormal foci of tracer accumulation will be considered in separate sections: Normal variations (Chapter 2), Common diagnostic pitfalls (Chapter 2), Post-traumatic changes (Chapter 4), Urinary excretion variations (Chapter 10), and Non-osseous accumulations, secondary to a variety of etiologies.

In this section, we use the term artifact more narrowly to mean foci of nonphysiologically based increased uptake (such as associated with the mechanics of tracer injection) or photon deficiencies secondary to attenuation by synthetic objects or equipment failures (such as a faulty photomultiplier tube). Most such artifacts are easy to confirm through patient history, physical examination, or review of the performance of the study including camera set-up, injection of tracer, data acquisition, and processing. Only a few of many possible examples are included.

Planar

Chest

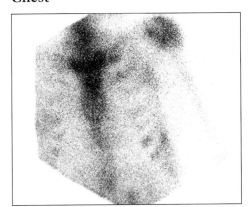

a

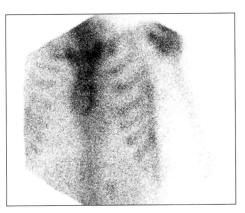

b

Figure 2.79

Breast prosthesis. (a) DS, chest, slight LAO. There is poorly defined relative photon deficiency overlying the region of the left third and fourth anterior ribs. **(b)** DS, chest, slight LAO, after prosthesis removed. The definition of the third and fourth ribs is now similar to the adjacent ribs.

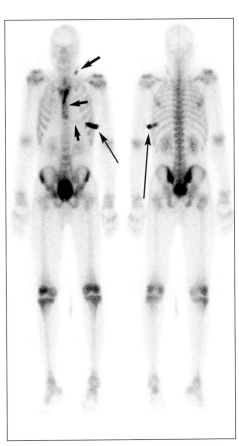

a

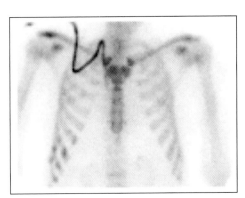

b

Figure 2.80

Retention. (a) Hickman catheter, tracer retention. Injection made through Hickman catheter. WB. Intense uptake at the injection port (thin arrow) inferolaterally as well as mild retention along the course of the entire catheter (short arrows). **(b)** Central venous catheter, retention. More commonly seen central venous line. DS, chest, anterior.

Teaching point

^{99m}Tc-MDP and many other commonly used radiopharmaceuticals will adhere to plastic catheters.

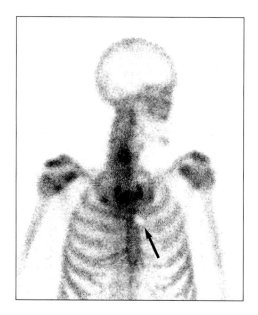

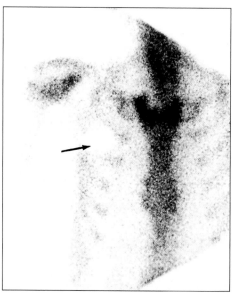

Figure 2.81

Metal medallion overlying sternum. DS, part of WB scan. Anterior. Small, well-defined photon deficiency (arrow) overlies the upper left portion of the sternum.

Figure 2.82

Pacemaker defect. Well-defined photon deficiency (arrow) overlies the right upper chest laterally. Compare this attenuation from a metal object with attenuation from a nonmetallic prosthesis in Figure 2.79.

Teaching points

An abnormality, either photon deficient or with increased tracer, that has sharp margins or a proportional geometric shape should raise the question of an artifact.

Obtaining a comprehensive clinical history will often elucidate the etiology of an artifact.

Abdomen

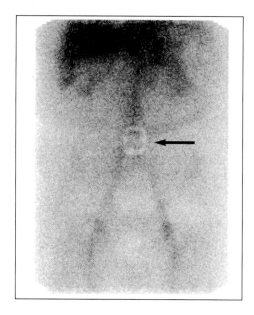

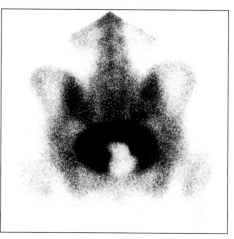

a   b

Figure 2.84

Barium in rectum. The patient was one-week post-barium meal (upper GI) examination. (a) DS, pelvis, anterior and (b) DS, pelvis, lateral. Large photon deficiency corresponds to the rectum.

Figure 2.83

Metallic belt buckle. BP, abdomen, anterior. Well-defined geometric square-shaped photon deficiency (arrow).

Bladder

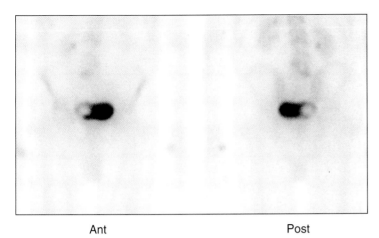

Ant   Post

Figure 2.85

Foley catheter in bladder. DS, portion of WB scan. Anterior (left image) and posterior (right image). The well-defined smooth circular photon deficiency represents the balloon of the catheter filled with saline.

Extremity

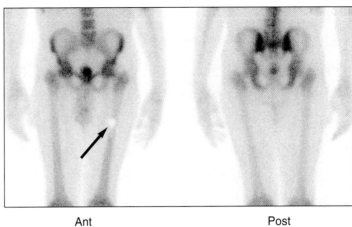

Ant   Post

Figure 2.86

Metal coin. DS, part of WB scan. Anterior (left image) and posterior (right image). Well-defined, smooth, circular photon deficiency (arrow) seen only on anterior view.

SPECT

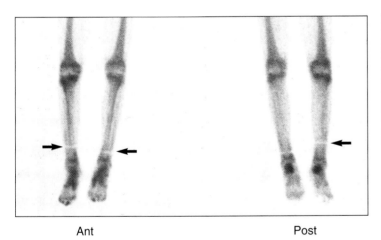

Ant   Post

Figure 2.87

Shackle sign. DS, lower extremity, part of WB bone scan. Anterior (left image) and posterior (right image). Well-defined, sharply marginated, horizontally oriented, linear areas of photon deficiency just above the ankles (arrows) seen on both anterior and posterior views. These represented the shackles in place on this prisoner who was being imaged.

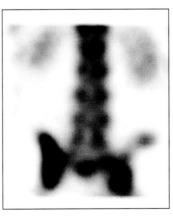

a   b

Figure 2.88

Positional asymmetry. Normal young adult volunteer with slight levoscoliosis. (**a**) SPECT, lumbar spine, selected coronal image. The asymmetry is most marked in the SI joint regions. (**b**) DS, lumbar spine and upper pelvis, posterior. The levoscoliotic curve is better appreciated.

Teaching point

Precise symmetric distribution of tracer uptake or of photon-deficient regions is often artifactual.

Teaching point

Anatomic asymmetry is contrasted with positional asymmetry, which can be corrected with oblique angle or free angle reorientation software available on most computer systems.

Figure 2.89

Low count acquisition. Projection images acquired at 2 seconds per image rather than 20 seconds per projection, as was the case for Figure 2.49. SPECT, selected coronal image. Note the 'grainy' appearance due to inadequate counting statistics.

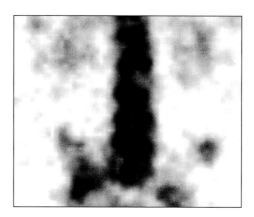

Teaching point

When a lower count study is obtained for any reason, the study can often be reprocessed using a smoother filter to obtain clinically useful information.

Figure 2.90

'In and out of field of view' artifact. SPECT data were intentionally acquired with the left knee positioned so that it was partially outside the field of view when the camera was in front and behind. SPECT, selected transaxial image. This is a type of incomplete angular sampling artifact.

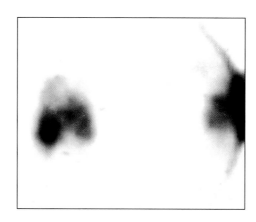

Teaching point

Routine acquisition quality control using either movie mode (cine) viewing of projection data or sinogram analysis should be done prior to every reconstruction.

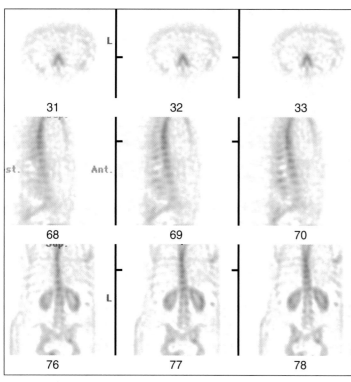

a

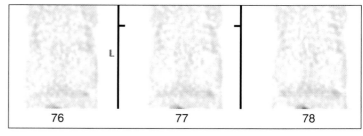

b

Figure 2.91

180° posterior acquisition. (a) SPECT, triangulation display. Transaxial images (upper row), sagittal images displayed right to left (middle row), and coronal images displayed front to back (lower row) demonstrate the detail of the posterior spinal structures and lack of detail in anterior rib and sternal structures. Compare with Figure 2.45(**d** and **e**). (b) SPECT, selected anterior coronal images. More anterior sections illustrate the lack of detailed information available from the anatomic structures furthest from the camera during acquisition. Compare with posterior coronal images in (**a**).

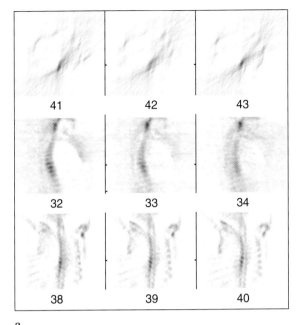

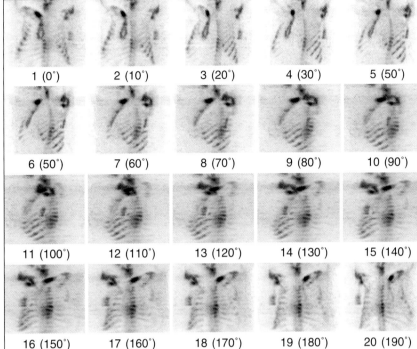

a

b

Figure 2.92

Incomplete angular sampling artifact. The patient could not lie still and acquisition was terminated after only 27 stops per head of the dual detector camera system, with 54 total stops available for reconstruction. Routine set-up was for 128 stops using a 128 × 128 acquisition matrix for 30 seconds per stop. Reconstruction with routine Hann filter, with images displayed 1 pixel thick. (a) SPECT, upper trunk, triangulation display. Transaxial sections (upper row) through the mid-thoracic spine, sagittal mid-line (middle row), and coronal images (bottom row). The coronal images demonstrate the patient's oblique position during acquisition. (b) 3-D volumetric reprojection images, selected views from 0° to 190°.

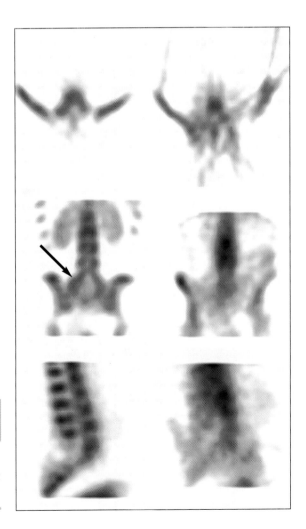

Figure 2.93

Motion artifact. SPECT, transaxial (top row), coronal (middle row), and sagittal (bottom row) obtained while the patient was moving (right column) and repeated after emphasizing to the patient the importance of remaining immobile during data acquisition (left column). Incidental normal bony fusion mass (arrow on coronal view) in this patient two years after L5–S1 fusion surgery.

Teaching point

Patient motion causes inconsistent projection data in SPECT acquisition. The inconsistency produces blur of image details (poor spatial resolution) and spreading of counts outside the true anatomic boundary in reconstructed images.

Figure 2.94

Bladder filling artifact. (a) DS, selected sequential projection images from SPECT acquisition. 128 × 128 × 128, XLFOV camera, 30 seconds per stop. Image 65 is the first image from head 1 and image 64 is the last image from head 2. Note the size of the bladder on the early image (thin arrow) and on the later image (thicker arrow). (b) Lumbar spine, SPECT, triangulation display. Transaxial images (top row), sagittal images (middle row), and coronal images (bottom row), are all through the plane of the bladder. Note streaky bladder-filling artifact (arrows) on transaxial and sagittal sections. (c) 3-D volume rendered reprojection images, selected views from anterior to steep oblique. Note the artifact reproduced on certain projections (arrows).

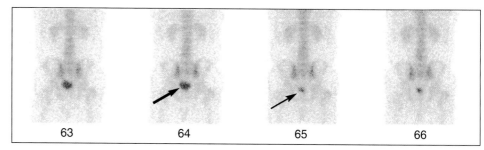

a

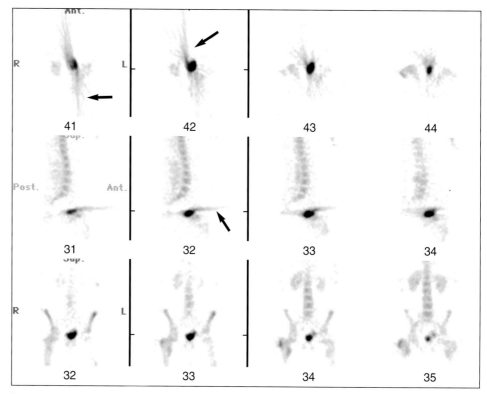

b

Teaching point

Bladder filling during acquisition leads to 'bladder-filling artifact' during reconstruction using filtered back projection technique. This is secondary to inconsistent projection data.

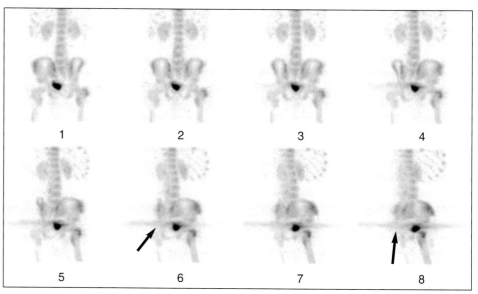

c

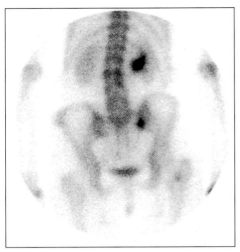

a

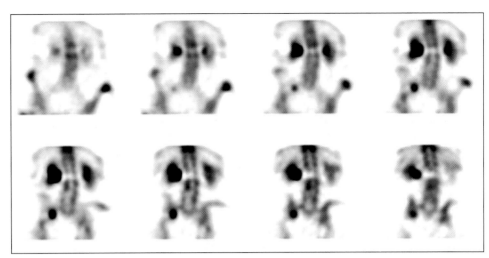

b

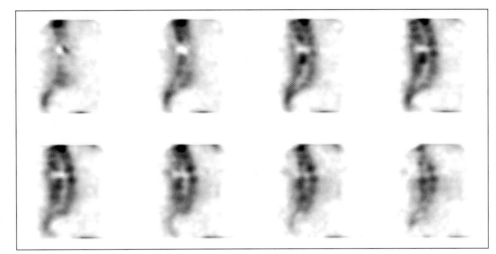

c

Figure 2.95

Photon-deficient reconstruction artifact secondary to intense activity in extrarenal pelvis. (a) DS, lumbosacral spine, posterior. (b) SPECT, lumbar spine, coronal. (c) SPECT, lumbosacral spine, sagittal. Photon-deficient L2 region is a reconstruction artifact.

Teaching point

The cold (photon-deficient) area appearing next to a very hot object (intense uptake) is caused by the sharp edge of the ramp filter used in SPECT image reconstruction with the filtered back-projection algorithm.

Pitfalls

This section is designed to emphasize that, during routine image analysis, variations of normal anatomy, nonpathologic physiologic alterations, and unusual presentations of common problems must always be kept in mind to minimize false-positive or false-negative interpretations. Only a few of many possible examples are included.

Figure 2.96

Infiltration, left external jugular injection site. DS, portion of WB scan. Anterior (left image) and posterior (right image). Analog image acquisition. Very intense uptake. Mild nonspecific uptake in left breast in patient three days post-biopsy with cancer diagnosis.

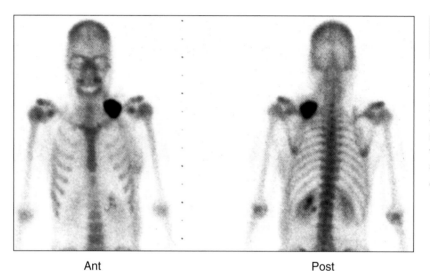

Ant   Post

Teaching point

The site of injection should be recorded for each study for potential later correlation with foci of activity secondary to partial extravascular infiltration of the administered dose.

Figure 2.97

Lymph node uptake. (a) WB. Anterior (left image) and posterior (right image). Partially excluded from the field of view by a lead shield, the injection site over the dorsum of the right hand is seen as an intense focus of uptake on the posterior image. The subtle, mild, round focus of increased tracer lateral to the ribs in the right axilla is best seen on anterior view. (b) DS, chest, arms up. The focus of activity moves with the axillary soft-tissue structures.

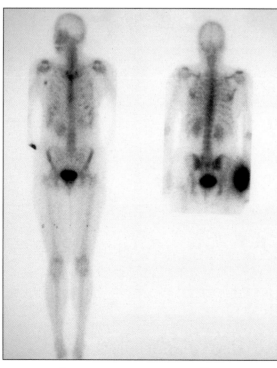

a   Ant   Post

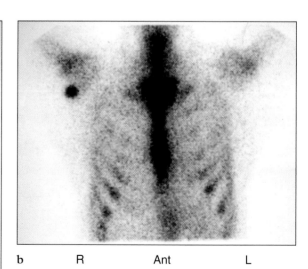

b   R   Ant   L

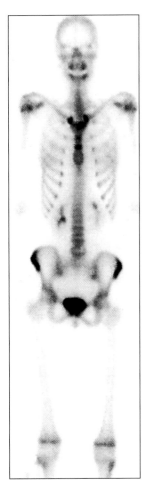

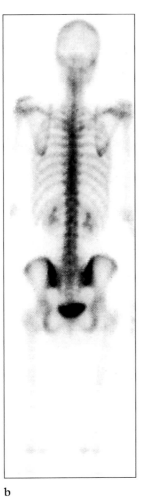

a

b

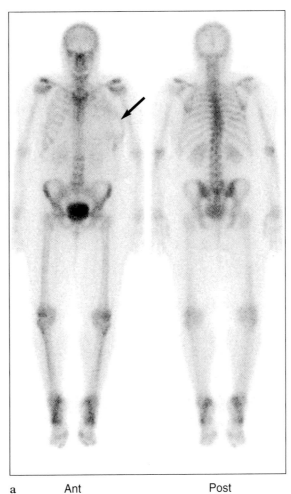

a Ant Post

Figure 2.99

Breast reconstruction. (a) WB. Asymmetric activity in the anterior chest region projecting lateral to the thorax (arrow) with decreased anterior rib activity. (b) DS, chest, anterior, obtained with arms extended. The more prominent soft-tissue (arrow) is better seen extending off the chest wall. The ribs are also better defined (thin arrow) but are still attenuated.

Figure 2.98

Shine-through. Normal, but asymmetric, intense, medial clavicular uptake in 16-year-old female. (a) WB, anterior and (b) WB, posterior. The posterior image is taken with very slight right posterior obliquity, so that the right medial clavicle is projected to the right of the spine, whereas the left medial clavicle is obscured by the spine.

Teaching point

When unable to distinguish 'shine-through' from a true rib lesion on a posterior view bone scan, a posterior oblique view can be obtained. A true lesion will remain in the same anatomic position within the rib, while 'shine-through' will either change in position or disappear.

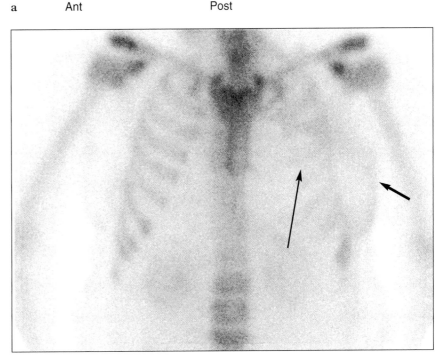

b

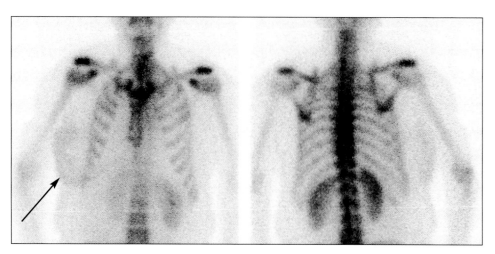

Figure 2.100

Breast cancer. DS, portion of WB bone scan. Anterior (left image) and posterior (right image). Significant asymmetric breast uptake on the right side (arrow) in a patient with a large cancer.

Teaching point

Although the range of normal physiologic breast uptake is wide and intensity of uptake variable, asymmetries in distribution and intensity need to be correlated with history and physical examination.

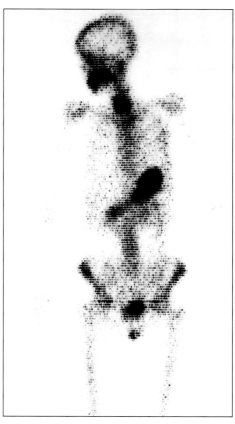

Figure 2.101

Free pertechnetate. WB, anterior. Tracer uptake in the mouth, salivary gland, thyroid, and stomach regions.

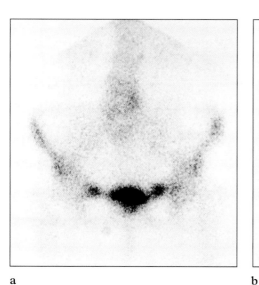

a

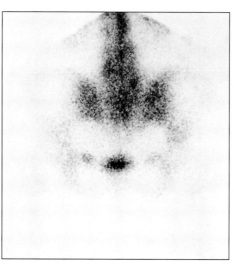

b

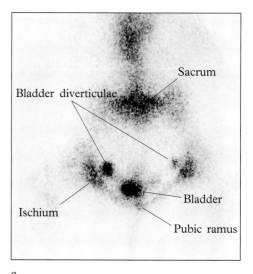

c

Figure 2.102

Bladder diverticula. (a) DS, pelvis, anterior. (b) DS, pelvis, posterior and (c) squat view with labels. On the anterior and posterior views of the pelvis, focal areas of increased tracer uptake are seen on each side of the bladder, overlying the superior pubic rami. The squat view clearly separates these areas from bone and confirms that they represent bladder diverticula.

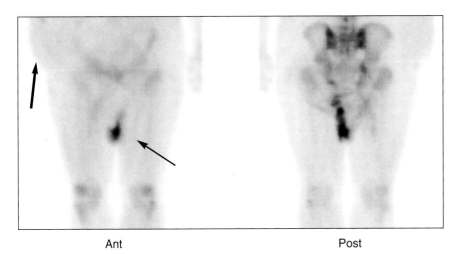

Ant   Post

Figure 2.103

Urine contamination. WB, portions of WB bone scan. Anterior (left image) and posterior (right image). The urine contamination on the anterior view (arrow) involves the lateral portion of the left scrotum extending inferomedially. This could be mistaken for the curvilinear activity of acute epididymitis. Incidentally noted is asymmetric appearance (thick arrow) of the patient's abdominal soft tissues. This was a large panniculus, which had rolled to the right side.

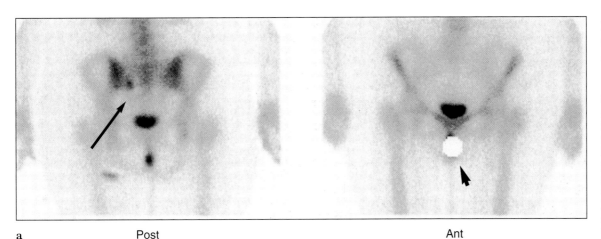

a   Post   Ant

b

Figure 2.104

Urine contamination. (a) DS, pelvis. Posterior (left image) and anterior (right image). There is a small focus of mild-to-moderate, round, increased tracer overlying the lower portion of the left SI joint on the posterior view (thin arrow). This is not seen on the anterior view. Incidental photon deficiency is associated with lead shield over urinary contamination in the genital area (arrowhead). (b) SPECT, selected transaxial views. The focus of abnormal tracer is seen posteriorly (arrow), clearly separated from bony structures.

Teaching point

The potential for urinary activity accounting for extra-osseous foci of tracer accumulation around the pelvis should always be considered. Removing clothing, cleaning the skin, and obtaining views in multiple projections are usually sufficient for confirmation.

Figure 2.105

Normal physeal activity. Anterior and lateral views obtained within minutes of each other. Collimator at a distance (left images) and very close (right images) to the surface of the knee. Resolution varies directly with collimator–object distance.

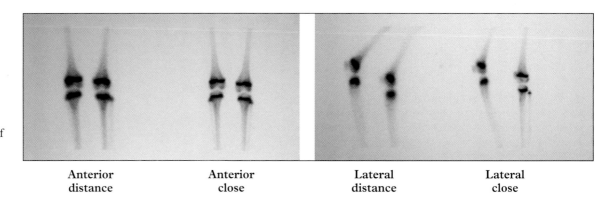

| Anterior distance | Anterior close | Lateral distance | Lateral close |

Teaching point

Technical factors and study performance designed to obtain the highest-quality images should be emphasized. See Figures 2.105 and 2.110.

Figure 2.106

Tourniquet effect. 22-year-old female with left arm and neck pain. Injection made in right antecubital fossa. **(a)** RNA, palmar view, five seconds per image. Mild relatively increased tracer to the right forearm and hand when compared with the left. **(b)** BP, hand and wrist, palmar. Obtained immediately after the RNA images without moving the patient or camera. Very minimal asymmetry with slight increase on the right when compared with the left. Marker (arrowhead) indicates right side. **(c)** DS, hand and wrist, palmar view. Mild nonspecific joint uptake in right third MCP joint and second and third PIP joints is nonspecific. Otherwise there is general symmetry in right-to-left uptake. Patient's pain is on the left secondary to bone bruise in distal carpal row, which on this view is in the region of the trapezoid capitate junction.

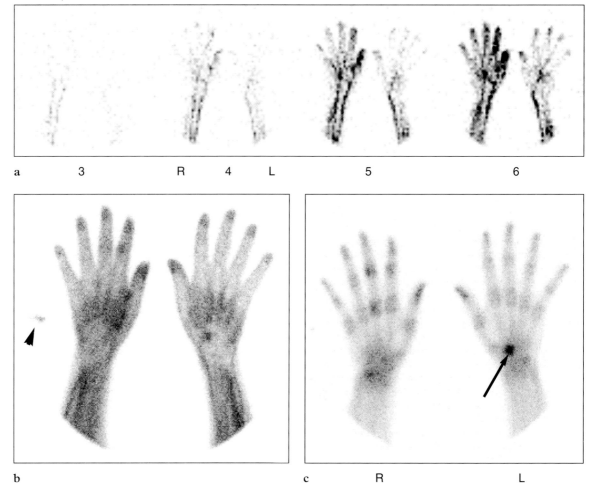

a   3   R   4   L   5   6

b

c   R   L

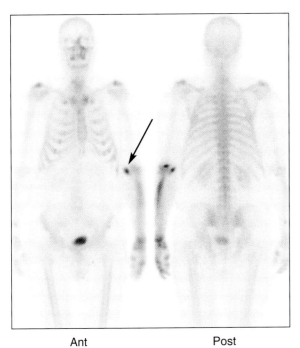

Ant   Post

Figure 2.107

Intra-arterial injection. WB, upper portion only
shown. Anterior (left image) and posterior (right
image). Inadvertent intra-arterial injection into the left
antecubital fossa with minimal extravascular
infiltration (thin arrow). Diffuse relative increased
tracer throughout all the bones supplied distal to the
injection site.

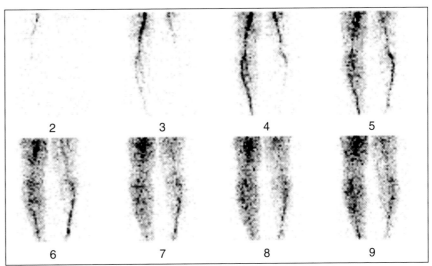

2   3   4   5

6   7   8   9

a

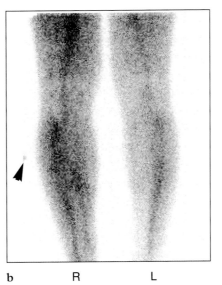

b   R   L

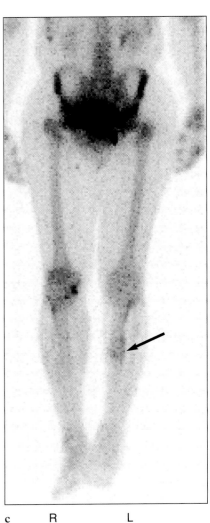

c   R   L

Figure 2.108

Anatomic asymmetry. Muscle
wasting in left lower leg following
traumatic lesion. **(a)** RNA, lower leg,
anterior view, five seconds per image.
Decreased muscle mass with slight
delayed perfusion to the left calf region.
(b) BP, legs, anterior view. The size
and volume of soft tissue in the left
calf compared with the right are noted.
Marker (arrowhead) indicates right
extremity. **(c)** WB, portion of WB
scan, anterior view. The volume of soft
tissue in the left extremity is smaller
than the right. The visualized bones,
however, are normally metabolic. The
area of healing of a fracture (arrow) is
noted.

Figure 2.109

Incorrect isotope peak. (a) WB. Acquired with standard protocol with camera peaked to ^{57}Co. (b) WB, obtained within minutes of the image in (a), with camera peaked to ^{99m}Tc.

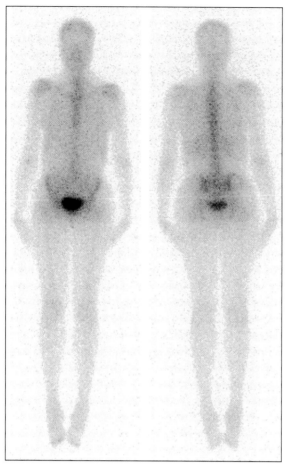

a

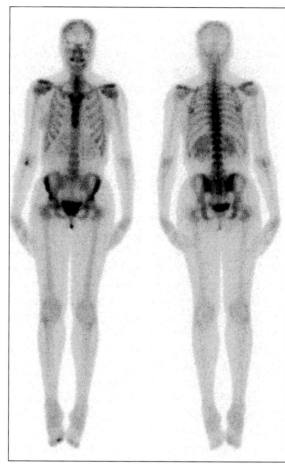

b

Figure 2.110

Patient movement during acquisition, WB. Head movement (arrow) is obvious. The movement in the extremities (thin arrow), which also results in decreased resolution, is less obvious.

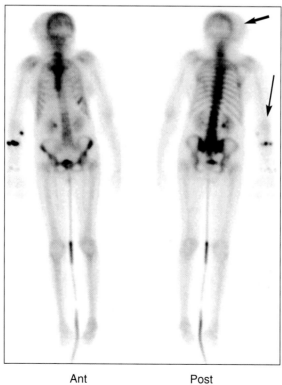

Ant   Post

Pattern recognition

3

With a background knowledge of the appearance of the normal bone scan and the commonly seen variants, we encourage a systematic evaluation of the RNB scan. Abnormal areas of uptake are recognized and related to patient signs and symptoms and correlated with radiographs or other anatomic imaging to make the best possible diagnosis or to provide a differential diagnosis.

Often the distribution of abnormal uptake will have such a recognizable pattern that an experienced observer will regularly be correct in suggesting that a specific diagnosis has a high probability. However, even an expert will be mistaken from time to time. A bone scan should not be considered to be a definitive investigation in most cases, but rather one that provides high sensitivity for lesion detection.

Global pattern recognition

Global pattern recognition consists of those patterns that suggest a specific diagnosis or specific disease category. These include metastasis, trauma, arthritis, Paget's disease, marrow hyperplasia, and metabolic bone disease.

Metastasis

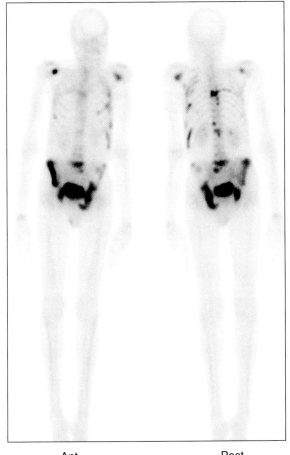

Ant   Post

Figure 3.1

Metastasis, prostate cancer. WB. Areas of intense abnormal activity in the shoulders, ribs, thoracic spine, lumbar spine, and pelvis.

Teaching point

The widespread osseous metastases occur as multiple lesions throughout the axial and proximal appendicular skeleton.

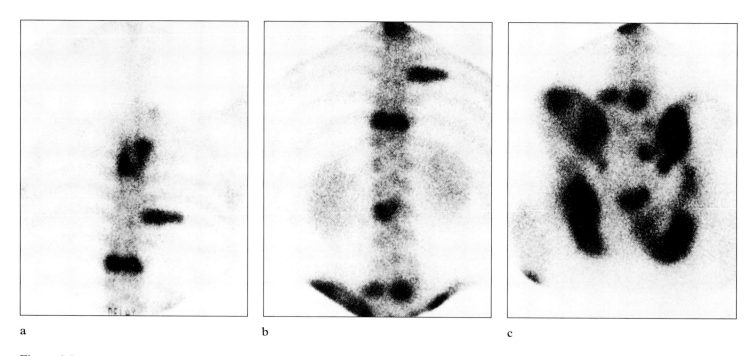

a   b   c

Figure 3.2

Metastasis, breast cancer. Multiple spot images. (**a**) Thoracic spine, posterior. (**b**) Lumbar spine, posterior. (**c**) Pelvis, posterior. Again the random distribution of irregular focal lesions is essentially diagnostic of metastatic involvement of the skeleton.

Figure 3.3

'Superscan of malignancy.' WB. (**a**) Anterior and (**b**) posterior. High uptake of tracer throughout the axial skeleton with the kidneys only faintly visualized. In this patient more focal uptake in the left shoulder would be a clue to the correct diagnosis. (**c**) DS, posterior from another patient with even more homogeneous tracer uptake and less renal visualization.

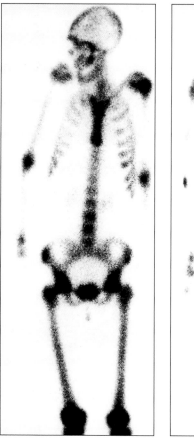
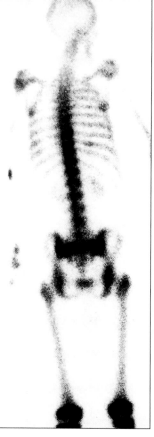
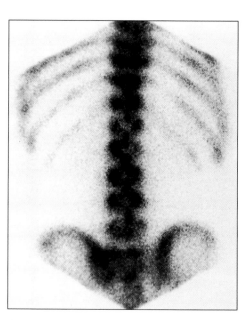

a   b   c

A 'superscan' may be defined as a bone scan where there is increased and relatively uniform tracer uptake throughout the skeleton with high contrast between bone and soft tissue. With standard acquisition parameters renal visualization will be faint or absent, because of increased contrast between bone and kidneys and less tracer being available for urinary tract excretion.

Table 3.1 The 'superscan'

Causes	Helpful features
Malignancy	Irregularity or tracer uptake
	Focal lesions
	Often skull and long bones poorly visualized
Hyperparathyroidism	Metabolic features
	Hypercalcemia
Osteomalacia	Metabolic features
	Psuedofractures
Delayed imaging in normal subject	Usually requires more than a 6-hour delay

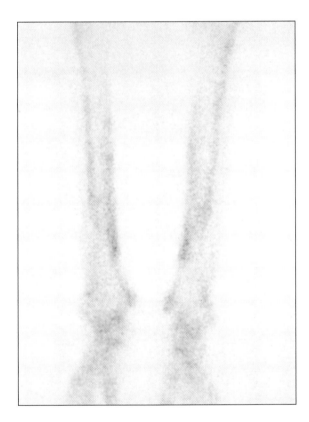

Figure 3.4

Hypertrophic osteoarthropathy. DS, legs. Linear increased tracer associated with the cortical margins. This has been called the 'tramline' or parallel stripe sign.

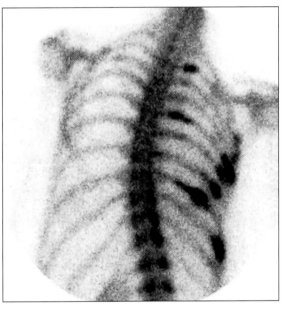

a

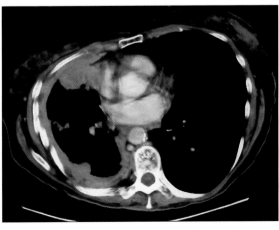

b

Figure 3.5

Direct extension to ribs from pleural mesothelioma. **(a)** DS, posterior. Multiple rib lesions which involve longer segments than typically occur with simple fractures. **(b)** CT, pleural thickening and chest wall invasion on the right. (Compare with Figure 3.6.)

Trauma

Figure 3.6

Rib fractures. (a) and **(b)** DS. Two different patients. The intense round uptake in short segments of rib in a linear pattern one above the other in adjacent ribs is typical of fracture. (Compare with Figure 3.5.)

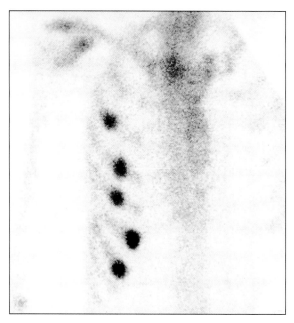

a

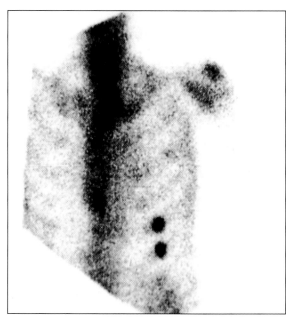

b

Characteristic patterns of fractures

- Rib fractures: involve short focal lesions in multiple adjacent ribs.
- Pelvic fractures: usually involve at least two sites of the bony pelvic ring.
- Vertebrae, osteoporotic: appear as bands of increased uptake extending horizontally across the vertebral bodies. Adjacent vertebral body endplates often involved.
- Mid-foot, fracture dislocations: can involve all the tarsometatarsal joints.

Teaching point

A linear pattern of 'clustered' focal rib lesions 2 cm or less in length are characteristics of fractures, while lesions involving longer segments of rib are suspicious for malignancy.

Figure 3.7 opposite

Vertebral body and rib fractures. (a) WB. Linear T8 vertebral body activity appears on posterior view to involve the lower half of the vertebra with a more superior lateral focus on the left. The intervertebral disk space is still visualized as a photon deficiency beneath the increased activity (arrow). Some minimal increased activity on the anterior view in the region of the sternum, round activity associated with rib fractures, and activity in the pelvis which on 'squat' view was confirmed to be bladder (arrow). **(b)** SPECT, 3-D volumetric projection. The activity is confirmed to be present in the vertebral body; the faint activity at the angle of Louis in the sternum (arrow) is normal. **(c)** SPECT, triangulation display. On the sagittal images the activity involving the vertebral body is somewhat wedge shaped. This accounts for the apparent localization to the lower half of the vertebral body on planar imaging. **(d)** SPECT, triangulation view, magnified. The anterior wedging (arrow) is even better seen.

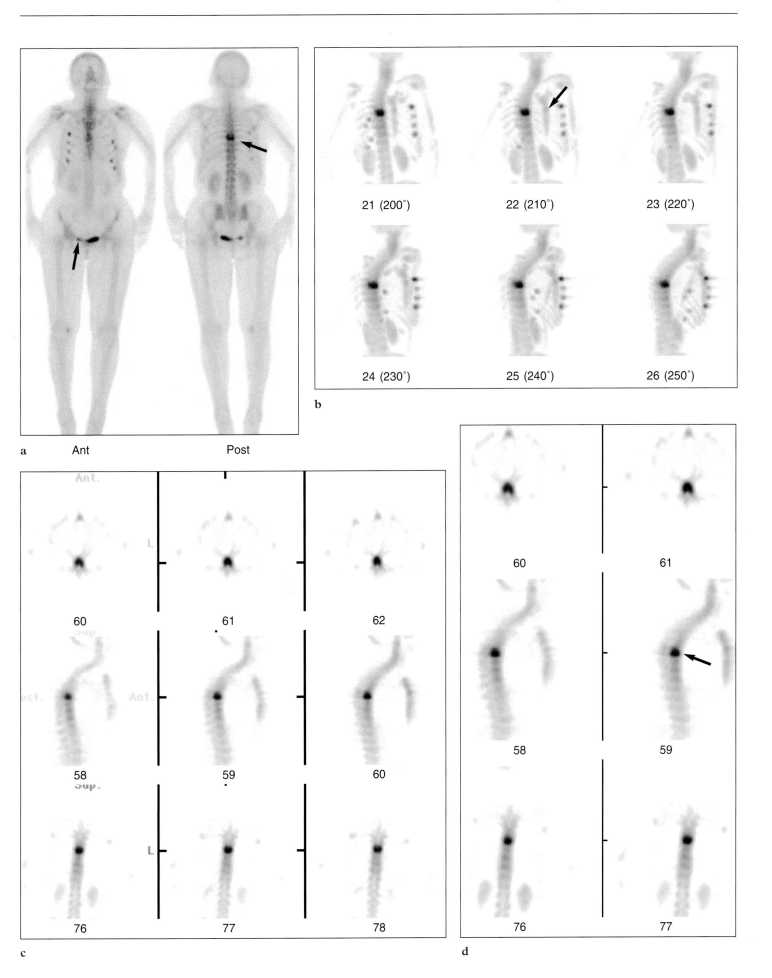

a   Ant   Post

b

21 (200°)   22 (210°)   23 (220°)

24 (230°)   25 (240°)   26 (250°)

c

60   61   62

58   59   60

76   77   78

d

60   61

58   59

76   77

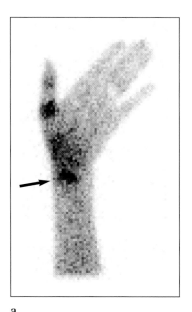

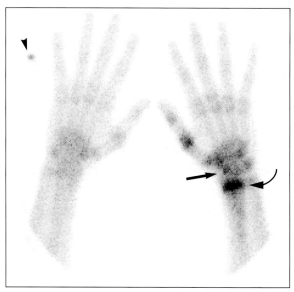

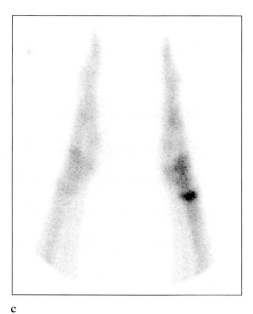

a   b   c

Figure 3.8

Subacute distal radius, impacted fracture. (**a**) BP, ulnar deviation view. A somewhat
horizontally oriented mild-to-moderate increased uptake (relative vascularity) in region of
the distal radius is noted (arrow). There is also some mild increased activity at the first
MCP joint region. (**b**) DS, palmar view. The moderate increased activity involves the distal
radius almost up to the articular surface. The radial carpal joint can be appreciated as a
photon deficiency (arrow) with more of the intensity just proximal to the distal articular
surface. Note also the radial ulnar joint (curved arrow), and the hot right marker
(arrowhead) to identify the right side of body. (**c**) DS, lateral view. The right side marker
is also seen on this view.

Teaching point

Right-sided body markers are important in
all cases, but especially so in views of the
distal extremities when the hands can be
placed on the collimator from different
orientations, and the dorsal and palmar
views can look similar.

Bone marrow

Figure 3.9

**Bone marrow
hyperplasia** in 23-year-
old with sickle-cell
disease. DS. (**a**) Chest,
anterior. (**b**) Pelvis,
anterior. (**c**) Knees,
anterior. Symmetrically
increased tracer uptake at
the ends of long bones.

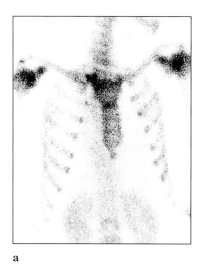

a

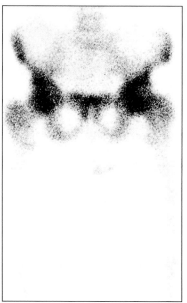

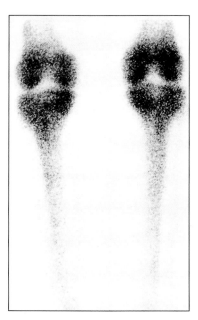

b   c

Arthritis

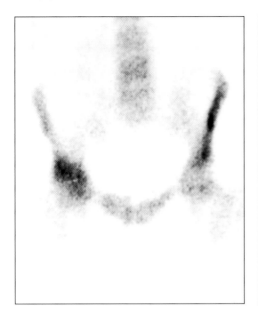

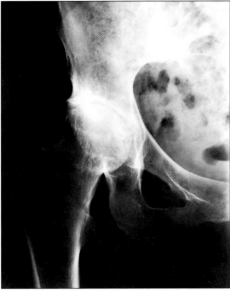

a   b

Figure 3.10

Osteoarthritis right hip. (**a**) DS, pelvis, anterior. Increased tracer in the region of the superior lateral (SL) hip joint. (**b**) X-ray right hip, AP: joint narrowing, subchondral sclerosis, and osteophyte formation. The activity that is greatest at the SL aspect of the joint reflects the weight-bearing forces at this location.

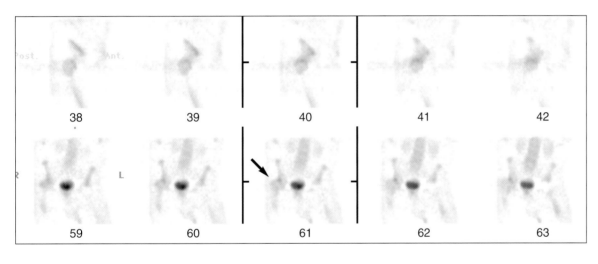

Figure 3.11

Right hip osteoarthritis in another patient. SPECT, triangulation display. Especially on the coronal images the activity at the SL acetabulum is well localized (arrow). The acetabulum is also nicely viewed on sagittal images which help localize the anterior to posterior portions.

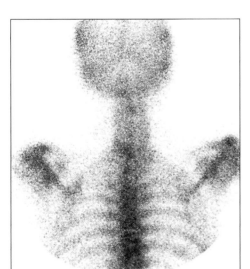

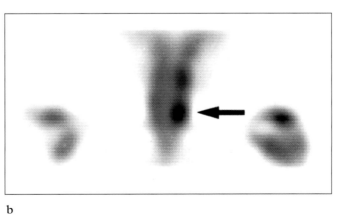

a   b

Figure 3.12

Osteoarthritis left sided C6–C7 Luschka joint. (**a**) DS, posterior. The faint activity on the left side corresponded to the region of patient pain. (**b**) SPECT, coronal. Selected image. The focal asymmetric increased uptake is more convincingly demonstrated on the SPECT image.

Figure 3.13

Osteoarthritis, basal joint, first and second metacarpal base. DS, palmar view. The largest area of focal uptake is in the right first carpometacarpal joint (long straight arrow) also called the basal joint. A similar but much, much less intense area of tracer uptake is noted on the left basal joint (arrowhead). There is also some mild activity between the bases of the first and second metacarpals (short straight arrow) and some mild activity at the third distal interphalangeal joint (curved arrow).

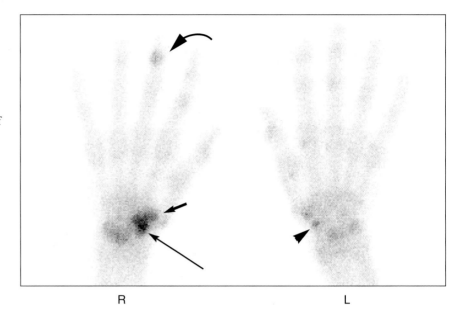

R   L

Figure 3.14

Osteoarthritis, knee, lateral compartment. (**a**) WB. Mild-to-moderate increased uptake in both the distal femoral and proximal tibial surfaces at the lateral compartment. Very subtle genu valgus orientation at the knee. Other areas of degenerative change including the right sternoclavicular joint (curved arrow), the basal joint (long arrow), interphalangeal joints (short straight arrow), and activity at the medial femoral calcar (thicker straight arrow). Photon deficiency of the left hip prosthesis. (**b**) DS, anterior. The lateral compartment activity on the right is more easily seen. (**c**) DS, lateral view, focal activity on both sides of the joint space obliterates it.

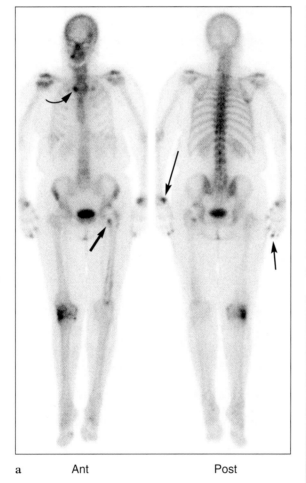

a   Ant   Post

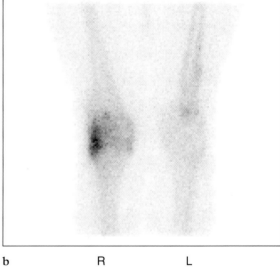

b   R   L

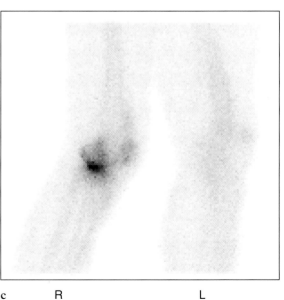

c   R   L

Metabolic bone disease

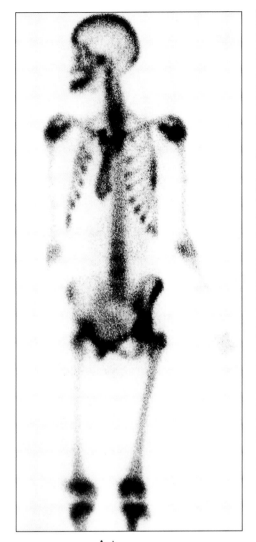

Ant

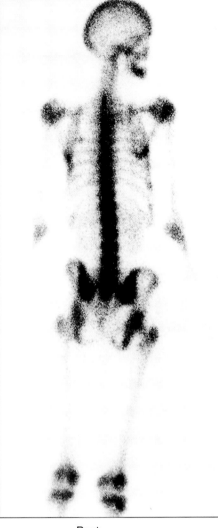

Post

Figure 3.15

Osteomalacia in a 21-year-old woman with anorexia nervosa. WB. Strikingly increased tracer uptake present throughout the skeleton, with high contrast between bone and soft tissue. The renal activity is not visualized. High uptake of tracer in the calvaria and mandible, beading of the costochondral junctions, and a 'tie' sternum are also present. Higher uptake at the ends of the long bones is somewhat unusual.

Metabolic features present on bone scan

1. High tracer uptake in axial skeleton
2. High tracer uptake in long bones
3. High tracer uptake in periarticular areas
4. Faint or absent kidney images
5. Prominent calvaria and mandible
6. 'Beading' of the costochondral junctions
7. 'Tie' sternum

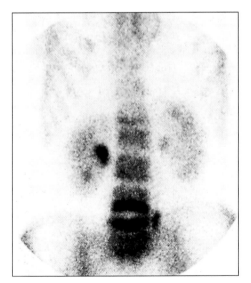

a

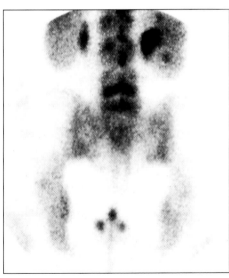

b

Figure 3.16

Osteoporotic compression fractures, lumbar vertebrae. (**a**) DS, thoracic and lumbar spine, anterior. (**b**) Lumbar spine and pelvis, posterior. Linear areas of increased tracer suggest endplate fractures. Varying intensity of uptake is most common with osteoporotic compression fractures. The X-ray (not shown) showed advanced osteoporosis and multiple lumbar vertebral body fractures, some of which did not show increased tracer uptake, suggesting that they were much older than the acute fractures causing the patient's pain.

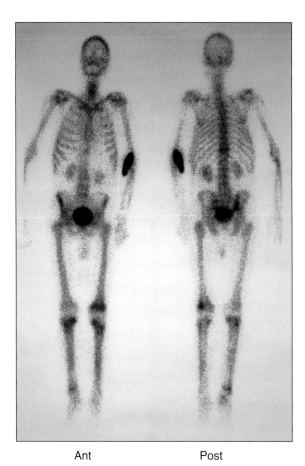

Ant   Post

Figure 3.17

Hypercalcemia associated with secondary hyperparathyroidism, in a patient with chronic renal failure. WB. Prominent calvaria, mandible, and other facial bone activity present a striking appearance. The hypercalcemic pattern is nonspecific.

Paget's disease

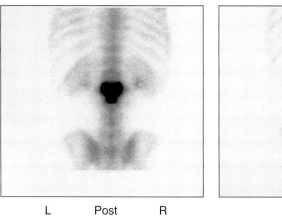

L   Post   R

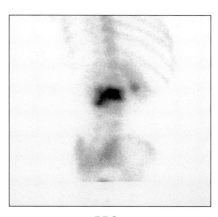

LPO

Figure 3.18

Paget's disease. DS, multiple views. Activity involving the entire vertebrae including body, transverse processes, and facets. This is a very typical appearance which allows a diagnosis to be made even when the involvement, as in this case, is monostotic.

RPO

Teaching point

Paget's disease of the tibia or other long bone is characterized by extension from the diaphysis distally. The bones involved with Paget's disease appear expanded.

Figure 3.19

Paget's disease, proximal tibia. (**a**) DS, legs, anterior view. Intense increased tracer extending distally from the proximal diaphysis. The bone is expanded and bowed, and the activity tapers toward the distal end. (**b**) X-ray. The prominent trabecular pattern is noted.

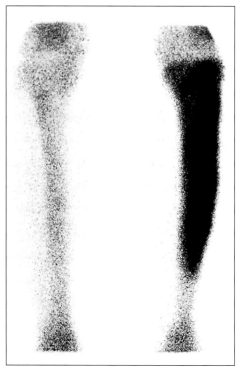

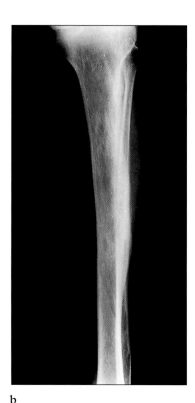

a   b

Focal pattern recognition

One of the most useful approaches to RNBI evaluation and differential diagnosis is to first determine where the lesion is located before deciding what its etiology may be.

This section will illustrate a variety of visual localization clues, as well as some patient positioning suggestions for data acquisition, designed to image or identify a particular region or individual bone. Techniques to isolate foci of abnormal uptake include patient positioning in relation to a stationary camera detector, rotating or angling the detector, SPECT imaging with routine processing, oblique angle reconstruction of SPECT images, and movie-mode viewing of 3-D, volume-rendered, reprojection images.

Correlation with anatomic images – plain radiographs, CT, and MR – is very often helpful. When making such comparisons it is important to be certain that views are similar. For example, a true lateral ankle and foot radionuclide image instead of a slight oblique, which is commonly acquired when the patient is in the supine position, is needed to compare with a true lateral X-ray.

Hand and wrist

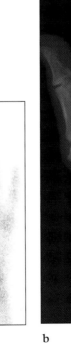
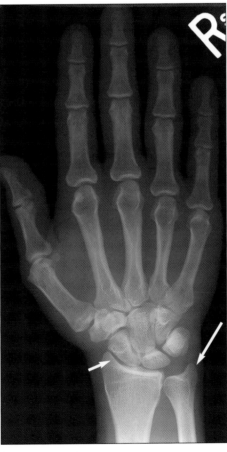

a

b

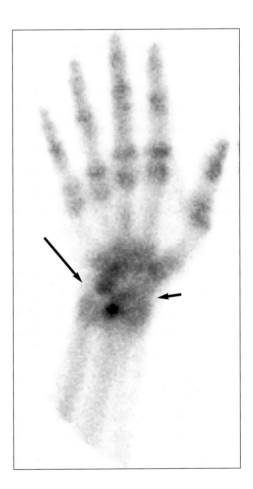

Figure 3.20

(a) Radial styloid. DS, palmar view. Obtained with patient sitting in front of camera with hands and forearms placed with palms on the detector. The edge of the radial styloid (arrow) is noted in relation to the proximal carpal row which is offset slightly to the ulnar side. **(b)** X-ray, hand and wrist, PA view. Used for comparison. Radial styloid (short arrow), ulnar styloid (longer arrow).

Figure 3.21

Lunate, AVN. DS. The epicenter of intense abnormal lunate uptake is just distal to the medial-most portion of the distal radius, and as appreciated on the comparison radiograph (Figure 3.20b) the lunate extends across the radial ulnar joint region. The ulnar styloid is also seen (longer arrow).

Figure 3.22

Ulnar styloid. DS, hand and wrist, dorsal view. The ulnar styloid (arrow) is often better seen on the dorsal view. Minimal focal increased tracer on the ulnar side of the lunate at the lunate trapezium joint.

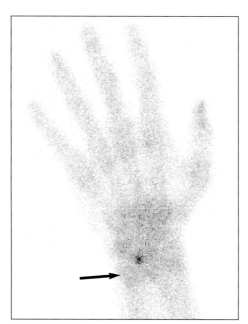

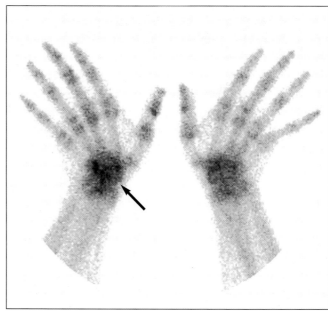

Figure 3.23

Scaphoid, ulnar deviation view. DS, palmar-ulnar deviation views. Even though in the normal patient individual carpal bones are often not identified, the location of the scaphoid (arrow) in relation to the distal radius can be identified.

Elbow

Figure 3.24

Trapezoid. DS, palmar view. Note the relationship of the increased uptake in the trapezoid to the base of the second and third metacarpals. Although the individual normal carpal bones cannot be seen, the radial styloid (short arrow) helps to localize the proximal carpal row (brackets) with the abnormal focus located in the area of the distal carpal row.

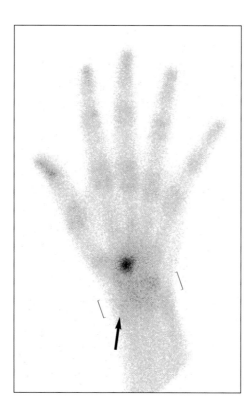

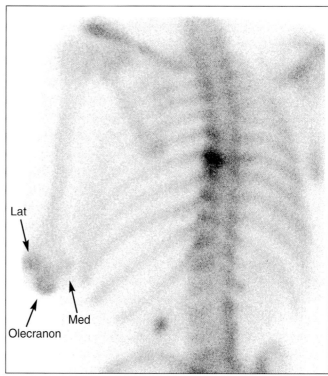

Figure 3.25

Medial and lateral epicondyles. WB, selected portion. The flexed elbow view can be used to isolate the condyles.

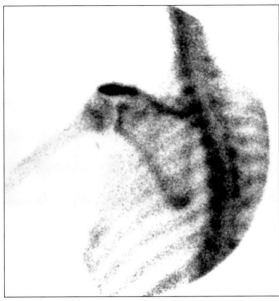

Figure 3.26

Shoulder, 35–55° LPO of the shoulder. Grashey equivalent view. DS. Note the clear definition of the glenohumeral joint. In this patient the remainder of the scapula is also well seen. Overlap of scapular tip and rib gives the appearance of a lesion with abnormal increased uptake. (Compare with Figure 3.27.)

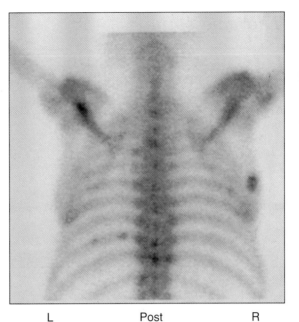

L   Post   R

Figure 3.27

Scapular. DS, posterior, arms up. Movement of scapula away from ribs localizes focus of increased tracer accumulation to the lateral scapula.

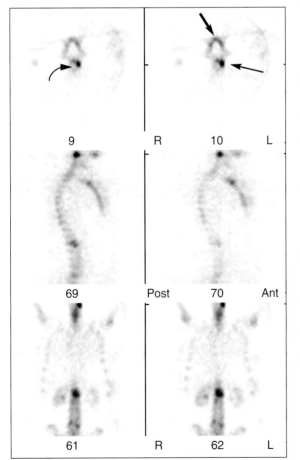

a

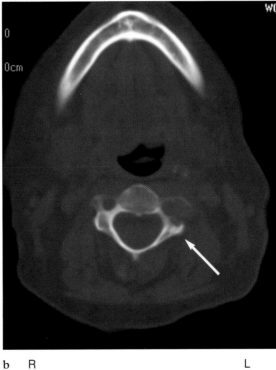

b   R   L

Figure 3.28

Lateral mass activity, C4. **(a)** SPECT, triangulation display. The mandible is seen anteriorly (thick arrow). The less intense vertebral body and right lateral masses contrast with the intense uptake in left lateral mass (thin arrow). The relatively large spinal canal at this level is seen as a photon deficiency (curved arrow). The lateral location is also appreciated on the coronal images. **(b)** CT. A not quite comparable transaxial section; nevertheless shows some subtle asymmetry with sclerosis on the left (arrow). The relative sizes of the vertebral body, lateral masses, and posterior elements, and the spinal canal at this cervical level, can be appreciated.

Figure 3.32

Facet activity lumbar spine. SPECT. Less smooth image (upper) contrasts with more smooth image (lower). Corresponding reconstruction filters to the right. Bilateral facet activity (arrow). Note separation of this activity from the body. (Compare with Figure 3.31.)

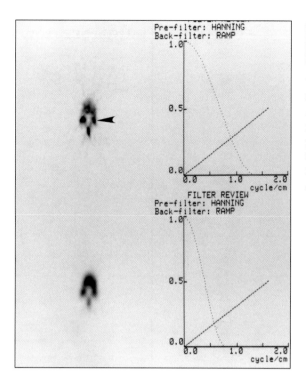

Teaching point

The choice of reconstruction filters is based on many factors including the count density of the data acquired, patient anatomy, and the preference of the interpreting physician. Less smoothed images usually provide better anatomic detail while more smoothed images will often help identify an abnormal focus of increased uptake.

Pelvis and hip

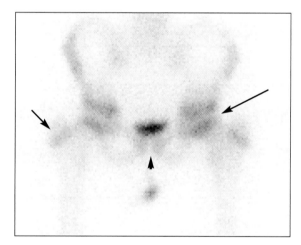

a

Figure 3.33

Slipped capital femoral epiphysis on left. (a) WB, anterior, selected section. The obliquely oriented activity associated with the left proximal femoral epiphysis (long arrow) is slightly broader and more intense than the right side. Note the activity associated with the greater trochanter apophysis (short arrow) and the photon deficiency associated with the symphysis cartilage (arrowhead), both of which are normal. (b) SPECT, triangulation display, transaxial and coronal views. The asymmetry in the proximal femoral epiphyses with more activity on the left (long arrow) is more obvious than on the planar image. The acetabular activity superiorly (curved arrow) and the epiphyseal activity inferiorly surround the less metabolically active femoral head.

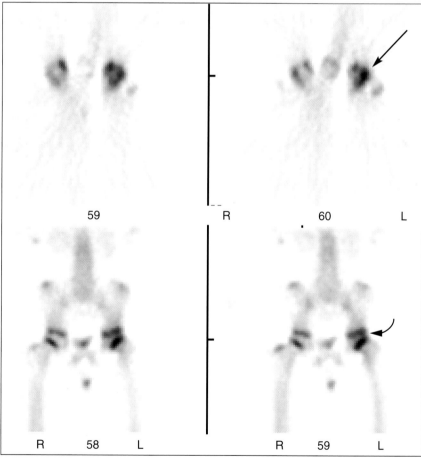

b

Knee

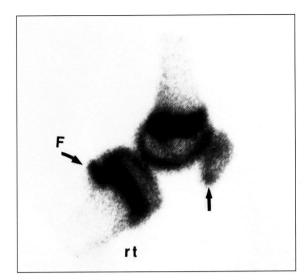

Figure 3.34

Inferior pole patella, healing avulsion fracture. Thirteen year old. DS, lateral view. Converging collimator. Minimal increased tracer accumulation inferior pole (arrow). The intense activity associated with the distal femoral, proximal tibial, and proximal fibular (F) physes reflects active growth.

Ankle and foot

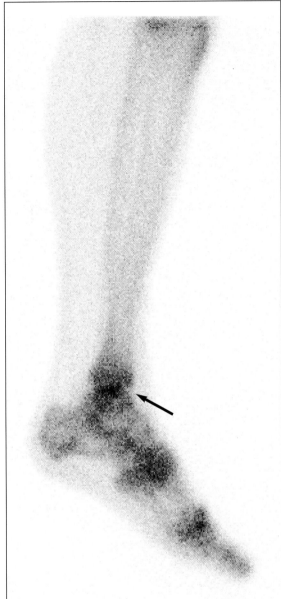

Figure 3.35

Tibiotalar joint, minimal arthritis. DS, true lateral. This true lateral can be exactly compared with a true lateral radiograph. The tibiotalar joint (arrow) appreciated as a subtle photon deficiency is highlighted inferiorly by some minimal increased tracer uptake in the dome of the talus.

Trauma 4

Trauma to the musculoskeletal system accounts for the majority of visits to many emergency departments, family physicians, and internal medicine and pediatric specialists. Acute fractures are usually, but not always, diagnosed clinically and confirmed with plain radiographs. Similarly, certain acute soft tissue injuries, such as cruciate ligament or meniscal tears, are diagnosed by MR imaging. When the etiology of pain of potentially osseous origin in the acute, subacute, or chronic situation remains uncertain, RNBI should be considered. The deposition of tracer in sites of increased bone turnover associated with repair of anatomically small lesions, which may be the focus of pain, is the underlying rationale for radionuclide imaging. The use of WB imaging allows detection of more distant foci of abnormal uptake which may represent the source of referred pain. Especially when the three-phase technique and SPECT imaging supplement the delayed WB images, even if a specific diagnosis cannot be made, anatomic localization and physiologic characterization of a lesion's perfusion, vascular, and metabolic activity can be provided to the clinician for use in diagnosis and management. Overall, most traumatic lesions can usually be detected and in many cases a specific diagnosis established.

Fractures

Fractures are the result of forces exceeding the ability of bone to deform without disruption of the mineral matrix. RNBI depicts the physiology of fracture healing. Stages in fracture healing are as follows:

(1) Inflammatory phase (includes hematoma formation, osteocyte death at fracture, vasodilatation, edema, and acute inflammatory cells).
(2) Reparative phase (includes vascular dilatation of the affected limb, new vessel proliferation, mesenchymal cell proliferation, change from acid to alkaline pH, and collagen production).
(3) Remodeling phase (includes trabecular formation along lines of stress (Wolff's law)).

Fracture subgroups include:

(1) *Frank fracture*
Obvious disruption of normal bone architecture. Orthopedic characteristics, some of which include site, complete, incomplete, alignment, configuration, position of fragments, open and closed, should be reviewed and understood so that the nuclear medicine imager can effectively communicate with the referring physician.
(2) *Occult fracture*
True fractures where the physical examination and initial plain radiographs are not diagnostic.
(3) *Fatigue or stress fracture*
Occur as the result of abnormal repetitive stress in normal bone.
(4) *Insufficiency fracture*
Occurs as a result of repetitive normal stress applied to bone that lacks the elastic resilience or strength of normal bone.
(5) *Avulsion fracture*
The separation of small amounts of bone or cartilage to which tendons are attached.

Skull

Figure 4.1

Postcraniotomy. (**a**) DS, posterior and (**b**) right lateral. Relatively photon deficient bone flap surrounded by rim of minimally intense increased activity associated with reactive bone (arrow).

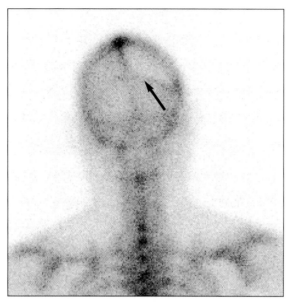

a

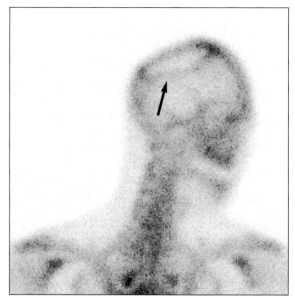

b

Teaching point

Postcraniotomy lesions have varying intensities of activity from normal to moderately intense. They are usually incidental findings.

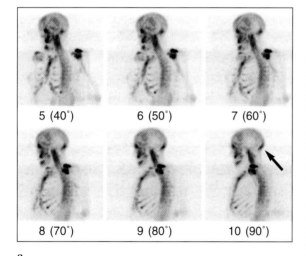

5 (40°)   6 (50°)   7 (60°)

8 (70°)   9 (80°)   10 (90°)

a

Figure 4.2

Postoccipital craniotomy. (**a**) 3-D, volume-rendered, reprojection images. Selected views from 40° to 90°. Note variations in intensity of uptake in lateral skull with a more focal posterior increase (arrow) adjacent to the larger of the photon-deficient regions. (**b**) SPECT, triangulation display. The posterior activity slightly to the right of the mid-line is seen on all three planes. It represents reactive bone.

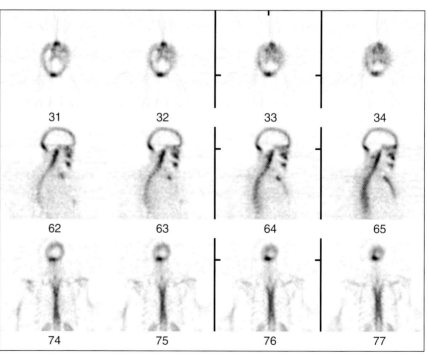

31   32   33   34

62   63   64   65

74   75   76   77

b

Shoulder and arm

A fracture along the anterior–inferior rim of the glenoid may occur in association with recurrent dislocations of the shoulder. These are called Bankart's fractures after the surgeons who described them. The Hill–Sachs lesion, also associated with shoulder dislocation, is a compression fracture of the posterior lateral aspect of the humeral head caused when the dislocated head impacts on the glenoid rim.

Teaching point

The 30–45° posterior oblique view (radiographically termed a Grashey view) places the glenohumeral joint in profile allowing visualization and separation of activity associated with the glenoid and/or the humeral head.

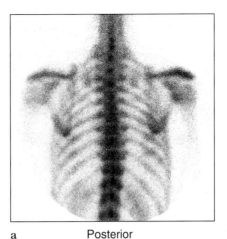

a   Posterior

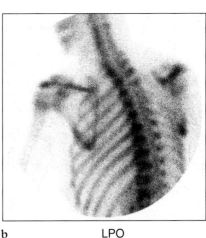

b   LPO

Figure 4.3

Bankart's fracture, right scapula. Three months post trauma. DS. Focal mild-to-moderately intense uptake. Inferior rim of glenoid (arrow) best seen on RPO view.

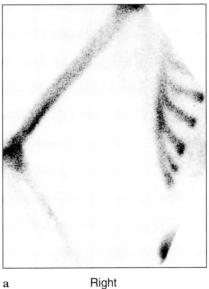

c   RPO

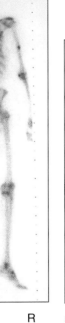

R   Ant   L   L   Post   R

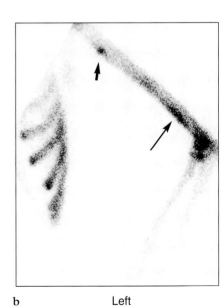

a   Right   b   Left

Figure 4.4

Right humerus stress fracture and left hip subcapital fracture. Patient using walker for three weeks. WB. Focus of abnormal tracer accumulation associated with proximal humeral shaft is relatively nonspecific. It is not as fusiform in shape as seen in typical lower extremity stress fractures.

Figure 4.5

Stress fracture and nonspecific cortical hypertrophy, left humerus. 24-year-old weight lifter. DS. The focal, moderately intense, increased tracer uptake in the medial aspect of the upper third of the humerus (short arrow) contrasts with the linear uptake of varying intensity in the lower third (thin arrow), which is more typical of a periosteal reaction.

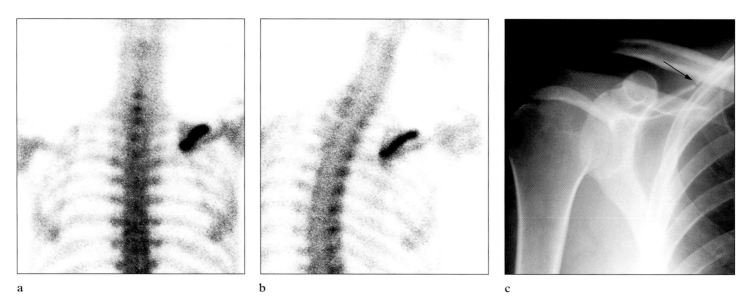

a   b   c

Figure 4.6

Scapular fracture. A 25-year-old male jogger, who was running with weights in both hands. Bone scan views: **(a)** upper posterior thoracic spine, and **(b)** RPO. **(c)** X-ray of the right shoulder. There is a linear intense area of increased tracer uptake extending obliquely across the right scapula. The X-ray confirms the presence of a fracture (arrow).

Hand and wrist

Figure 4.7

Acute scaphoid stress fracture. (a) RNA. Focal, moderately intense, increased perfusion to the right scaphoid. (b) BP, palmar. Focal increased relative vascularity. (c) DS, ulnar deviation (top image) and palmar (bottom image). Intense activity confined to the scaphoid. Note relationship to the distal radius. (d) MR, T1 coronal. The scaphoid has lost the normal brighter marrow signal associated with normal fat. This image demonstrates the anatomic relationships in the wrist.

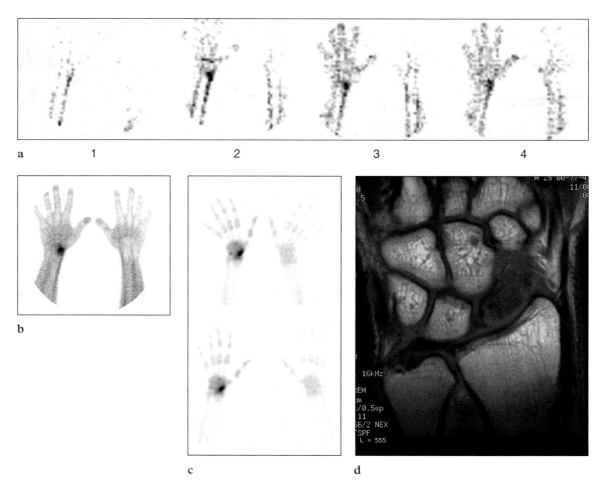

a   1   2   3   4

b

c   d

Nonunion has been defined as that point in time after which spontaneous healing can no longer be expected to occur. When a photon-deficient separation of activity between the edges or ends of bone can be seen, this is termed atrophic nonunion. When there is only a single focus of increased activity encompassing both sides of a fracture site, the term reactive nonunion has been used.

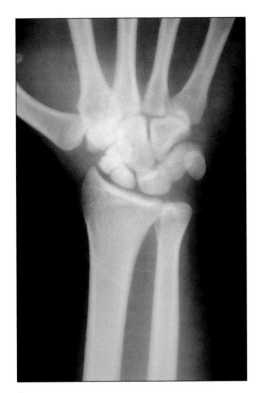

a

Figure 4.8

Acute right scaphoid and nonunion left scaphoid fracture. (a) X-ray, left hand. The fracture line through the midportion of the scaphoid is evident. (b) RNA, five seconds per frame, palmar view. (Top row) Minimal, poorly defined increased perfusion to region of right scaphoid. No increased perfusion to left scaphoid. BP images demonstrate mild increased uptake (relative vascularity) in right scaphoid. (Bottom row) Minimally intense, focal, increased tracer left scaphoid. (c) DS, converging collimator, palmar views. Intense uptake in acute fracture of right scaphoid. Focal increased tracer of moderate intensity in left scaphoid. Even with this magnification technique the fracture line is not resolved.

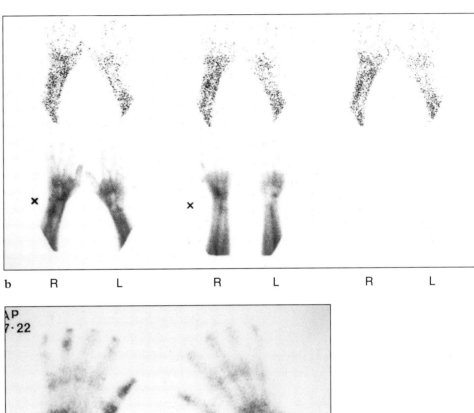

Teaching point

Abnormal tracer uptake associated with fracture nonunion is thought to represent increased metabolic activity associated with nonspecific stress change. More or less abnormal movement occurs at sites of nonunion, which also receive more or less abnormal biomechanical stresses. As a result there may be more or less relative vascularity on BP images and more or less increased metabolic activity on delayed images. Activity is usually more focal than associated with acute healing fractures.

Figure 4.9

Healing scaphoid fracture. DS. As healing progresses activity becomes less intense, more focal, and better defined.

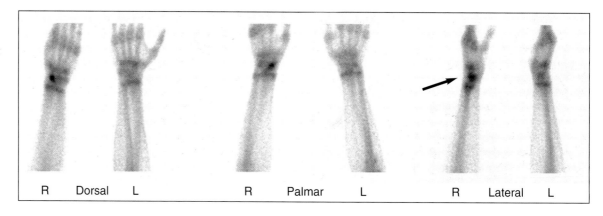

R   Dorsal   L   R   Palmar   L   R   Lateral   L

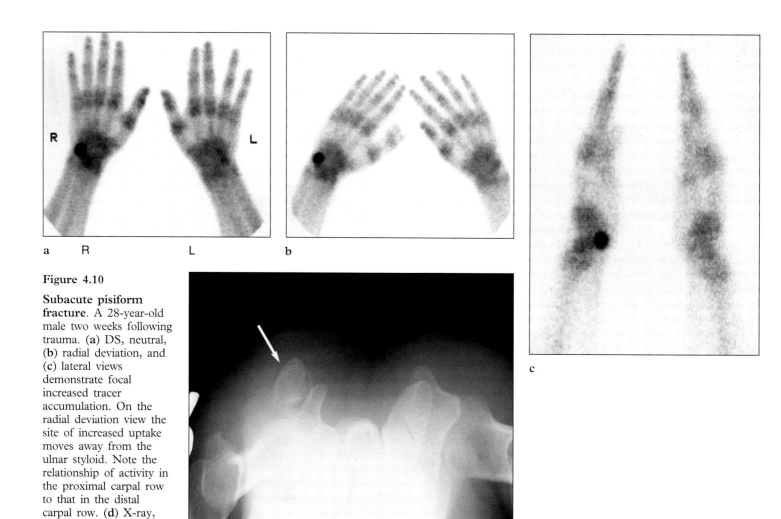

a   R   L   b   c

Figure 4.10

Subacute pisiform fracture. A 28-year-old male two weeks following trauma. (a) DS, neutral, (b) radial deviation, and (c) lateral views demonstrate focal increased tracer accumulation. On the radial deviation view the site of increased uptake moves away from the ulnar styloid. Note the relationship of activity in the proximal carpal row to that in the distal carpal row. (d) X-ray, carpal tunnel view. Fracture identified.

d

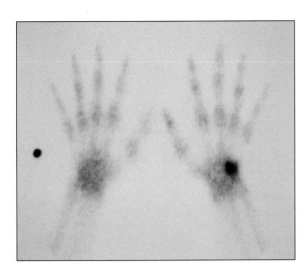

Figure 4.11

Subacute hook of hamate fracture. DS. Focal increased uptake in distal carpal row on ulnar-most side. In acute fracture the abnormal increased activity is often larger than the bone itself secondary to the intense tracer uptake. Computer subtraction will usually help in localizing the epicenter of activity.

Chest and sternum

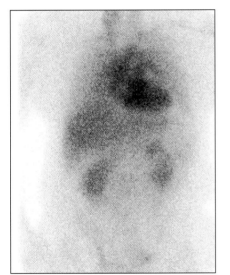

a

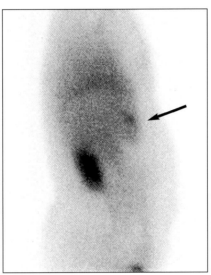

b

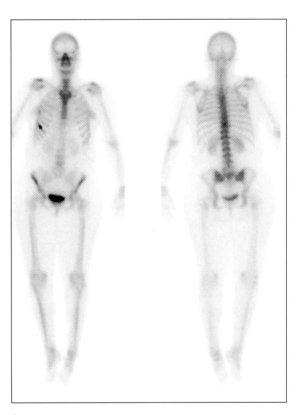

c

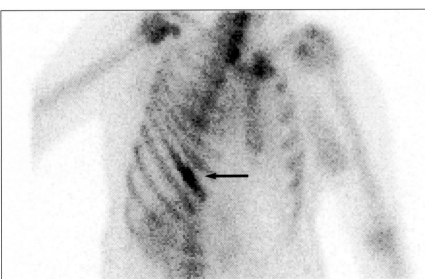

d

Figure 4.12

Strain (cough) fracture, right seventh anterior rib. (a) BP, anterior. No abnormal tracer identified. Heart, great vessels, liver, and kidneys are well seen. (b) BP, right lateral. Focus of round mild-to-moderately intense increased activity identified anteriorly (arrow). (c) WB. Lesion in area of patient's pain is monostotic. (d) DS, chest, RAO. Although somewhat elongated, better definition of the lesion with the focal, fusiform center typical of stress-type fracture identified (arrow).

Figure 4.13

Subacute rib fractures. Four months status after a motor vehicle crash with resuscitation. T8 fracture. WB. Intense rounded areas of abnormal increased tracer uptake in a linear pattern one rib above the other is typical for trauma. In this case the bilaterality does suggest a resuscitation attempt. We have seen this similar pattern in patients who have had fractures secondary to hitting the steering wheel. Intense activity T8 vertebrae better defined on SPECT views (see Figure 4.21).

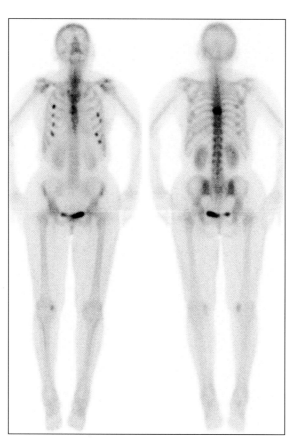

Ant   Post

Teaching point

The increased tracer uptake associated with healing fractures slowly normalizes over time and in over 90% of patients returns to normal in two years, with the minimum time for normalization being approximately six months. Nonaligned fractures in adults may never become scintigraphically normal as stress remodeling continues. The speed at which normalization occurs relates not only to the size of the fracture but also the amount of movement versus immobilization during healing.

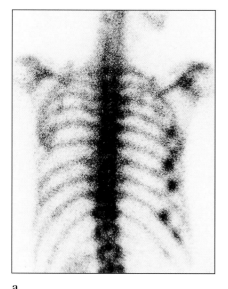

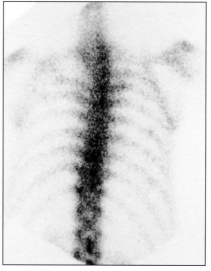

a   b

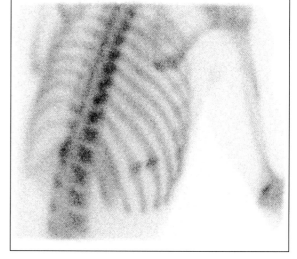

Figure 4.14

Healed rib fractures. (a) DS. Original study (left). (b) Eleven months post-trauma (right). On original scan, multiple focal abnormalities in a linear pattern in the right posterior ribs. This scan appearance is diagnostic of traumatic fractures. On repeat study, there is almost complete resolution, indicating healing.

Figure 4.15

Almost completely healed rib fractures. DS, RPO view. The posterior oblique views often demonstrate an appearance exactly resembling the callous seen on the radiograph.

Cervical spine

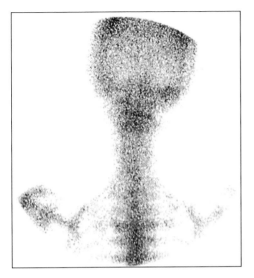

a

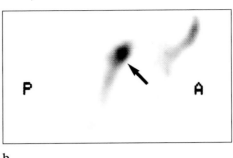

b

Figure 4.16

Acute odontoid fracture. A 26-year-old woman with neck and back pain following an automobile accident. No convincing abnormality is seen on the posterior planar bone scan (**a**). The mid-line sagittal SPECT image (**b**) shows increased activity in the upper cervical spine (arrow). The open-mouth X-ray (**c**) reveals a fracture of the odontoid process (arrows).

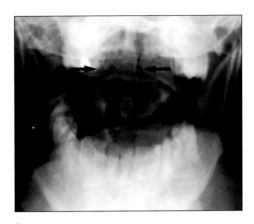

c

Thoracic spine

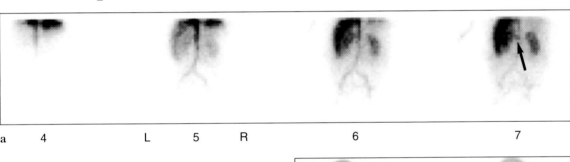

a   4   L   5   R   6   7

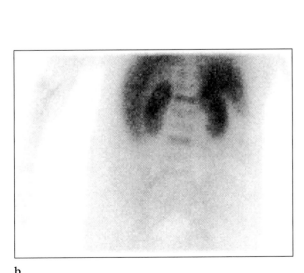

b

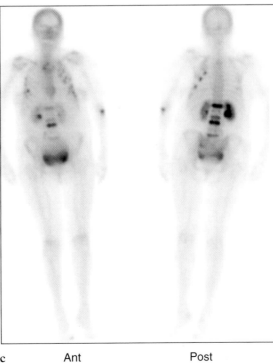

c   Ant   Post

Figure 4.17

Acute compression fractures, thoracic and lumbar spine. (a) RNA, five seconds per frame, posterior. Visualization of lower abdominal aorta, iliac vessels, kidneys, and spine is normal. Faint horizontal areas of increased relative vascularity at the level of the upper pole of the right kidney and lower pole (arrows to upper lesion). (b) BP, posterior. Linear areas of increased relative vascularity which are of varying intensity suggest that fractures may be of varying ages. (c) WB. Rib, spine, and pelvic fractures are identified. Note the linear activity of the abnormal lower thoracic and lumbar vertebrae. This pattern is typical for fracture. Pattern of traumatic right rib fractures also seen.

Lumbar spine

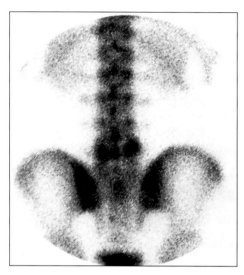

a

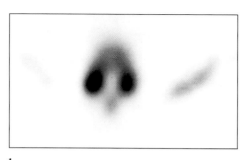

b

Figure 4.18

Bilateral L4 pars interarticularis stress fractures. This 20-year-old American football player complained of increasingly severe low back pain. X-rays, including oblique views, were normal. The posterior planar bone scan (a) shows increased tracer uptake over both the left and right sides of L4. This abnormality is better localized on the transaxial SPECT image through the L4 vertebra (b). The patient gave up vigorous sports, and the low back pain disappeared.

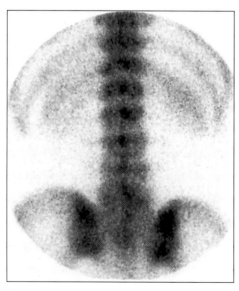

a

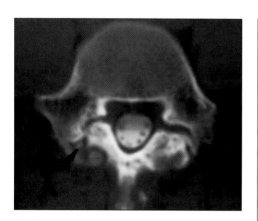

b

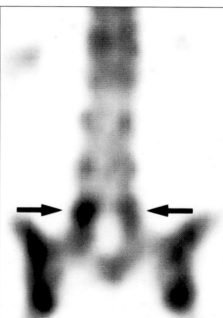

c

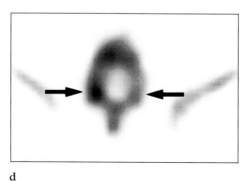

d

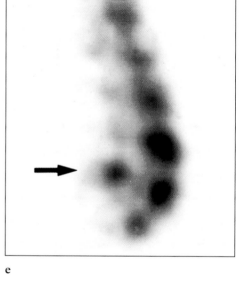

e

Figure 4.19

Bilateral pars stress. A 33-year-old man with low back and right leg pain. The CT scan (a) shows bilateral L5 spondylolysis (arrows) along with an L4–L5 herniated disk on other CT images that were taken. The planar bone scan (b) is normal. The coronal (c), L5 transaxial (d), and sagittal right-of-mid-line (e) SPECT bone scans show increased tracer uptake in the region of the pars interarticularis (arrows), which is more pronounced on the right than on the left. The patient was treated with diskectomy and L4-to-S1 fusion, with good postoperative pain relief.

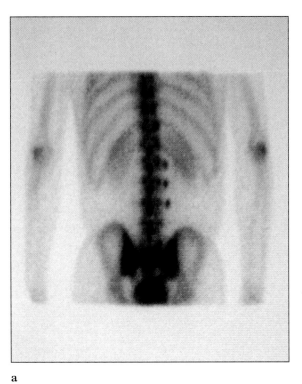

a

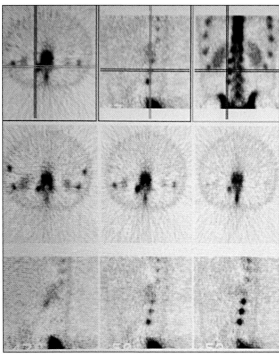

b

Figure 4.20

Acute transverse process fractures. Deceleration injury. **(a)** DS, posterior. Foci of increased tracer L2–L3 transverse processes on right. **(b)** SPECT, triangulation display. The locations of the transverse processes are well seen on all three planes.

59   60   61   62   63

59   60   61   62   63

75   76   77   78   79

Figure 4.21

Subacute compression fracture, thoracic spine. SPECT, triangulation display. This SPECT sequence is for the same patient seen in Figure 4.13. Note the activity confined to the vertebral body, which has a wedge shape with the wedge pointing anteriorly (arrow).

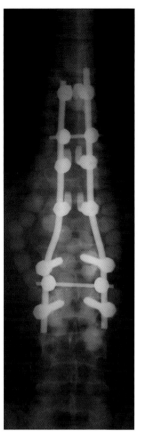

a

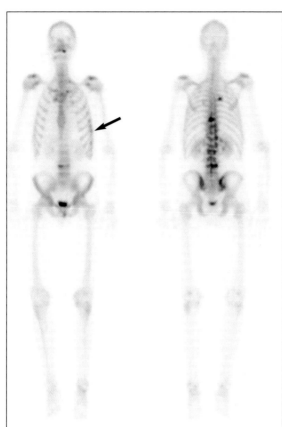

b

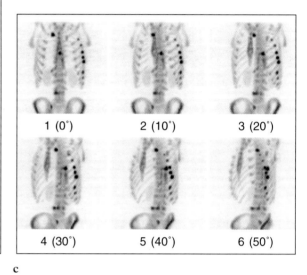

| 1 (0°) | 2 (10°) | 3 (20°) |
| 4 (30°) | 5 (40°) | 6 (50°) |

c

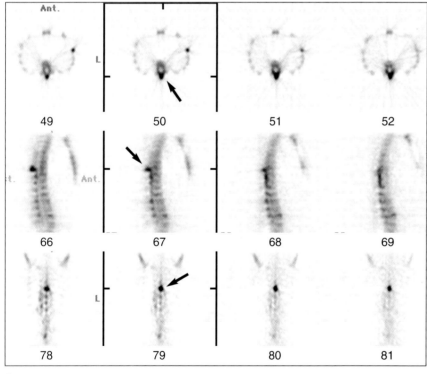

Ant.

49	50	51	52
66	67	68	69
78	79	80	81

d

Figure 4.22

Multiple fractures. Scan performed one year after fall from scaffold with surgical fixation. (a) X-ray. Spine with fixation devices in place. (b) WB. Multiple foci of abnormal increased tracer seen throughout the thoracolumbar spine have varying configurations and intensity. On anterior view left lateral rib fractures may be suspected (arrow). (c) 3-D reprojection images. Rib fractures are well defined including many not suspected from planar WB study. Location of abnormal activity throughout the spine better defined. (d) SPECT, sections through spinous process fracture are seen on all three planes as focus of increased tracer (arrow). (e) SPECT, through plane of right anterior corner fracture of L4 (arrow). (f) SPECT, through plane of right transverse process fracture. Fracture appears as focus of intense increased tracer (arrow). Note that the sagittal plane in the central box is to the right of the mid-line with the transverse process fracture seen on planes even more to the right and the vertebral body seen on the section to the left of the mid-line (right side of image).

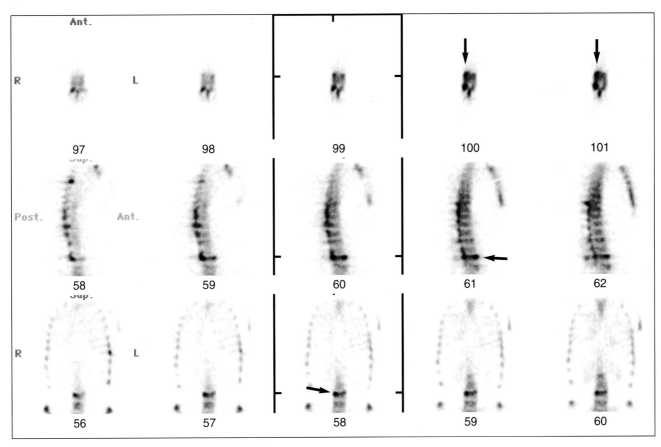

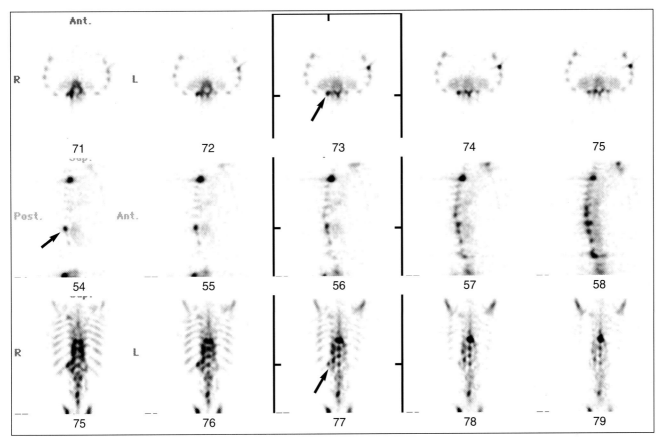

Pelvis and hips

Figure 4.23

Insufficiency fractures, hips and spine. Steroid therapy for severe COPD. **(a)** WB. Intense activity in the left femoral neck is the insufficiency fracture found when the patient presented with pain. Another small focus of mild increase tracer in the right hip seen on anterior view (arrow) and appreciated in retrospect after SPECT study. **(b)** BP, posterior. Mild, focal, poorly marginated, increased uptake (relative vascularity) in left hip region (arrow). **(c)** 3-D reprojection images. The focus of activity in the right hip is now suspected. Spine lesions also seen. **(d)** SPECT, coronal slices. The left hip, spine, and now the right hip insufficiency fractures are identified.

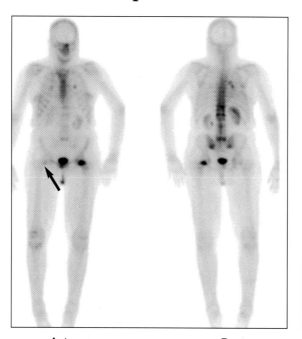

a   Ant   Post

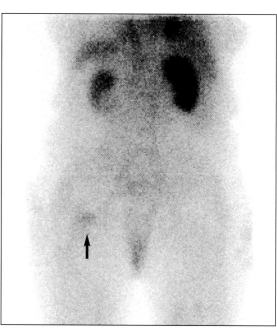

b

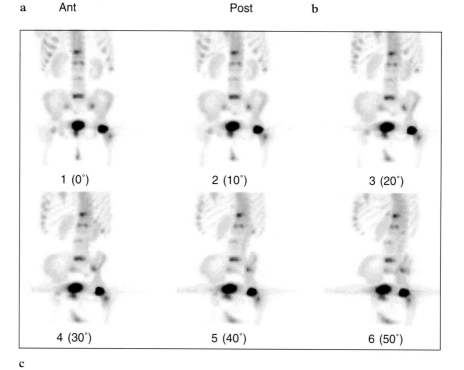

1 (0°)   2 (10°)   3 (20°)

4 (30°)   5 (40°)   6 (50°)

c

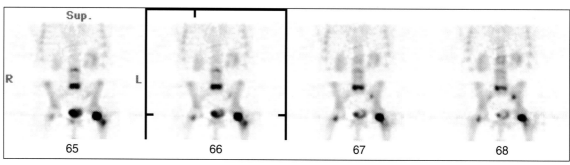

65   66   67   68

d

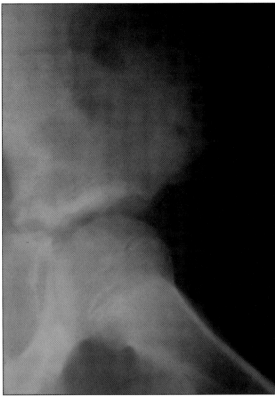

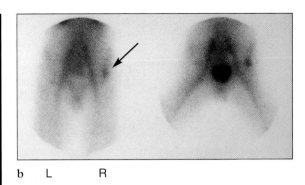

b L R

a

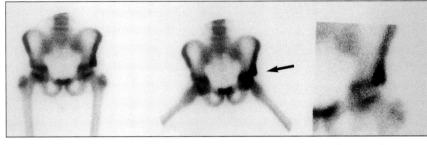

c R L   R L   Mag C+

Figure 4.24

Avulsion fracture. Rectus femoris at anterior inferior iliac crest. **(a)** X-ray, AP. Irregularity of anterior inferior crest. **(b)** BP images, anterior and frog leg lateral. Focus of moderately intense increased vascularity on left (arrow). **(c)** DS, anterior, frog leg, and magnified anterior. Asymmetric, moderately well-defined, moderately intense increase at left crest (arrow).

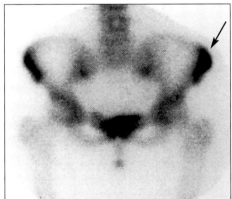

a

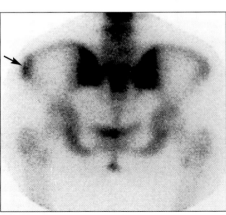

b

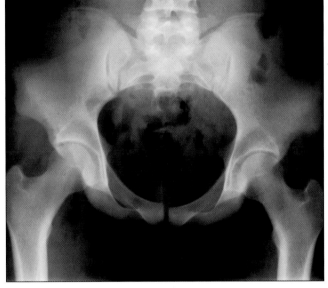

c

Figure 4.25

Avulsion fracture. A 60-year-old female runner, who had complained for several months of left anterior hip pain. Bone scan views: (a) anterior pelvis and (b) posterior pelvis. (c) X-ray of pelvis. There is increased tracer uptake in the region of the left anterior iliac crest (arrows). The X-ray shows separation of the apophysis, which is typical of a traction injury.

Figure 4.26

Acute subcapital hip fracture. An 84-year-old female. (**a**) RNA, anterior, five seconds per frame. Increased perfusion to left hip region, oriented somewhat obliquely (arrow) probably represents medial circumflex or possibly lateral circumflex femoral artery perfusion. (**b**) BP, anterior. Left hip, increased vascularity seen (arrow). (**c**) DS, anterior. Subcapital activity (arrow) is in typical location and orientation for subcapital fracture. (**d**) MR, T1 sagittal. Fracture line (arrow). Minimal displacement.

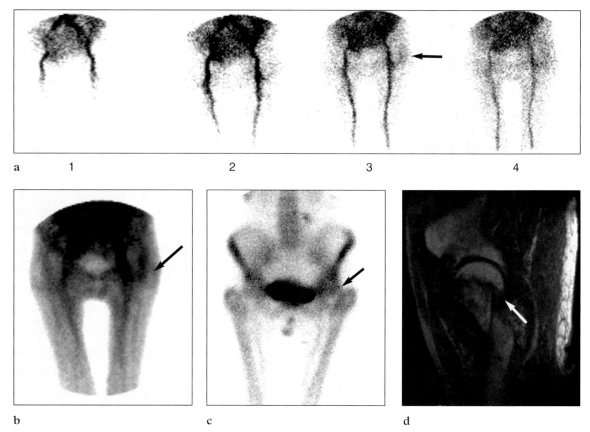

a   1   2   3   4

b   c   d

Teaching point

Radionuclide imaging to detect acute hip fractures can be performed at any time after trauma. Only in an occasional, very elderly patient will the scan be normal. Intensity of activity may be less in the very elderly so that a high index of suspicion must be maintained and any asymmetry viewed with suspicion. The additional value of RNBI is the detection of other lesions accounting for pain in over 40% of patients presenting with possible acute hip fractures.

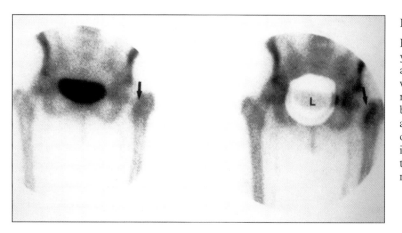

Figure 4.27

Femoral neck fracture. A 72-year-old female imaged 49 hours after injury. Delayed images without (on left) and with (on right) lead shield (L) placed over bladder to decrease bladder counts and scatter. Anterior views. Center of abnormal activity at fracture site is more medial (arrows), even though there is some increase in main intertrochanteric region.

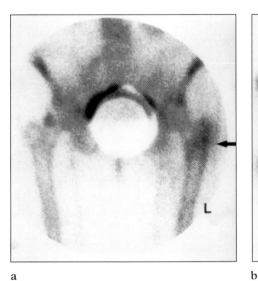 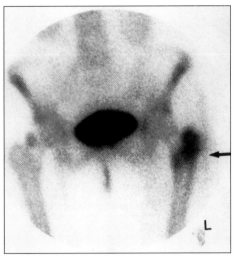

a   b

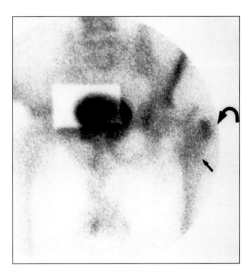

Figure 4.28

Intertrochanteric fracture, left hip. Increased certainty on follow-up examination. A 78-year-old female. DS. Anterior views. (**a**) Initial examination 17 hours after injury. Delayed image. Left (L). Grade 1/3 increased activity throughout intertrochanteric area (arrow). (**b**) Follow-up examination four days after injury. DS. Grade 2/3 intertrochanteric activity (arrow). Activity lateral to right femoral neck was of uncertain significance.

Figure 4.29

Greater trochanter fracture. An 81-year-old male, imaged 71 hours after injury. DS. Anterior view. Focally increased activity centered at greater trochanter (curved arrow), grade 2/3. Increased activity in intertrochanteric region is present but much less intense (straight arrow).

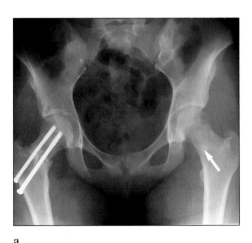 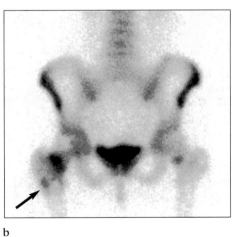

a   b

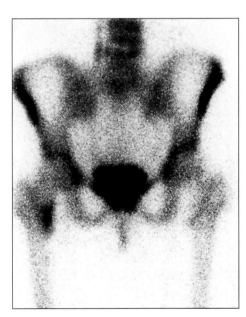

Figure 4.30

Old right femoral neck fracture with AVN and acute left neck stress fracture. (a) X-ray, pelvis. Nonunited neck fracture with fixation screws in place. Subtle sclerosis, possible fracture line and medial neck periostitis on left (arrow). (b) DS, anterior. On the right the intense activity associated with the neck fracture and the less intense activity associated with the head of the most inferior screw (arrow), and the photon deficiency associated with the head region. On the left the focus of increased tracer in the medial neck is seen representing the stress fracture lesion.

Figure 4.31

Stress fracture. A 32-year-old jogger with right hip pain and normal X-rays. The bone scan view of the anterior pelvis shows a focus of increased tracer uptake in the right calcar femorale. This patient had a femoral stress fracture.

Figure 4.32

Pelvic fracture. A 76-year-old man with continued left-sided pelvic and hip pain 6 days after a fall. As the patient was unable to adequately empty his bladder, tracer activity within the bladder meant that the pelvis could not be satisfactorily evaluated. A posterior bone scan of the pelvis with a lead shield over the bladder (**a**) shows no abnormality. A 'squat' view of the pelvis could not be obtained due to the patient's pain. However, a posterior bone scan view the next day (**b**) when bladder activity had cleared shows the left-sided pelvic fractures.

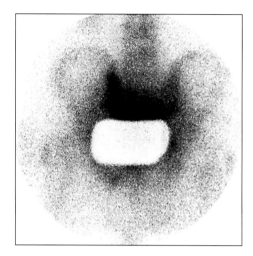

a

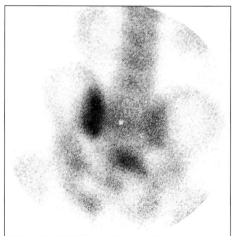

b

Teaching points

Prior to skeletal imaging, a patient should empty the bladder, as retained activity may lead to difficulties in scan interpretation.

It is not possible to exclude abnormality in the pelvis unless the bladder is empty. If the bladder obscures the pelvic bones, the patient should be catheterized or a 24-hour delayed view obtained.

The scintigraphic pattern of insufficiency fractures of the pelvis is described as a Honda or butterfly sign in which the vertical portions represent the sacral alae and the horizontal portion the sacral body. Variants are common in which some involve only the body of the sacrum and others only the alae, or more extensive fractures that involve other bones in the pelvis.

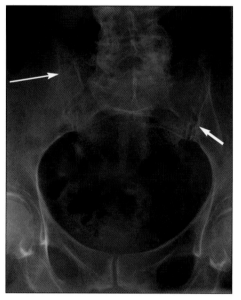

a   R   L

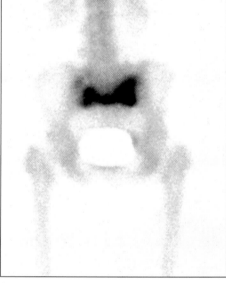

b

Figure 4.33

Sacral fracture. (**a**) X-ray, pelvis, AP. Asymmetry of the SI joints is noted with irregularity and suggested fracture on the right (long arrow) and possible separation on the left (short arrow). (**b**) DS, posterior view. The typical 'butterfly pattern', in this case asymmetrical with more activity on the right, is noted. (**c**) SPECT, coronal plane. Pattern of abnormal activity from front to back is accentuated.

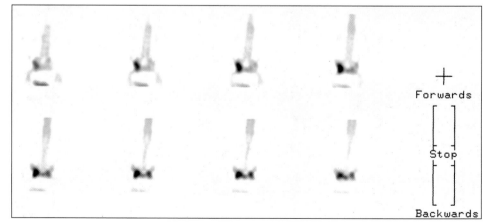

c

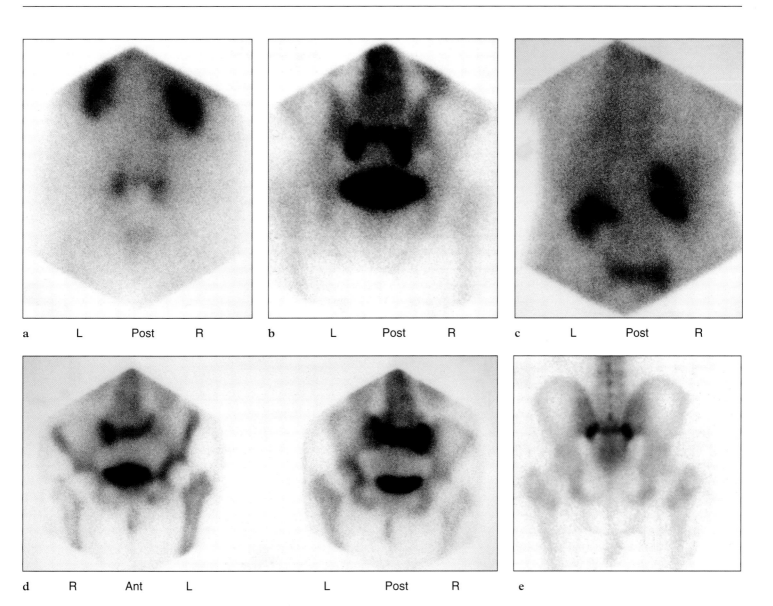

a L Post R

b L Post R

c L Post R

d R Ant L   L Post R   e

Figure 4.34

Sacral fractures, patterns. (**a**) BP, posterior. Subacute fracture demonstrates increased vascularity. (**b**) DS, posterior. Typical H pattern. The sacral alae form the vertical lines and the sacral body the horizontal. Note full bladder. Patients with pain often cannot void. (**c**) Another patient. BP. Asymmetric H also shows increased vascularity. (**d**) DS, anterior (left) and posterior (right). Asymmetric H activity of sacral fracture is seen. Photon deficiencies associated with femoral prosthesis are also noted with possible loosening of acetabular component on the left. (**e**) Another patient. Small, minimal fracture, bilateral.

Femur

Figure 4.35

Stress fracture. A 16-year-old jogger and aerobic dancer. DS, anterior. Focal fusiform increased tracer involving medial femoral cortex.

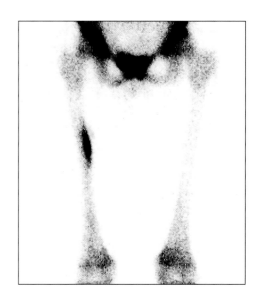

Figure 4.36

Adductor avulsion fracture, right femur. A 27-year-old female runner complaining of chronic right thigh pain. (a) WB. Medially based, somewhat linear, moderately intense uptake in the mid right femur, slightly lower than we usually see for adductor avulsion fractures. (b) BP, anterior view. There is no abnormal increased tracer in the region of the thigh. Incidentally noted is uptake in the BP of the vascular uterus (arrow) that is located above the bladder, which is photon deficient. (c) 3-D reprojection images. The medial eccentric appearance of the lesion is appreciated. There is a suggestion (arrow) that the distal portion is slightly more lateral than the cortex. The normal RNA and BP (not shown), along with some cortical thickening seen on the radiograph (not shown) favor the end stages of the healing process. A stress fracture of the medial cortex could not be completely excluded.

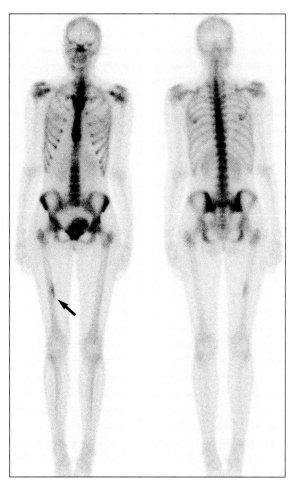

a

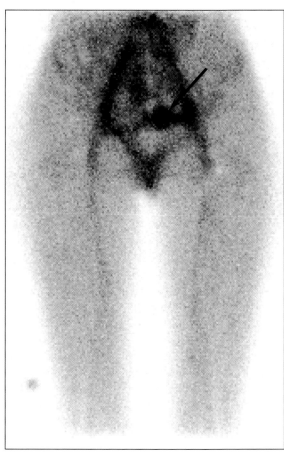

b

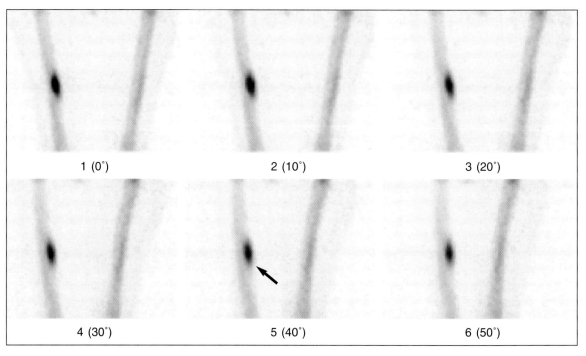

| 1 (0°) | 2 (10°) | 3 (20°) |
| 4 (30°) | 5 (40°) | 6 (50°) |

c

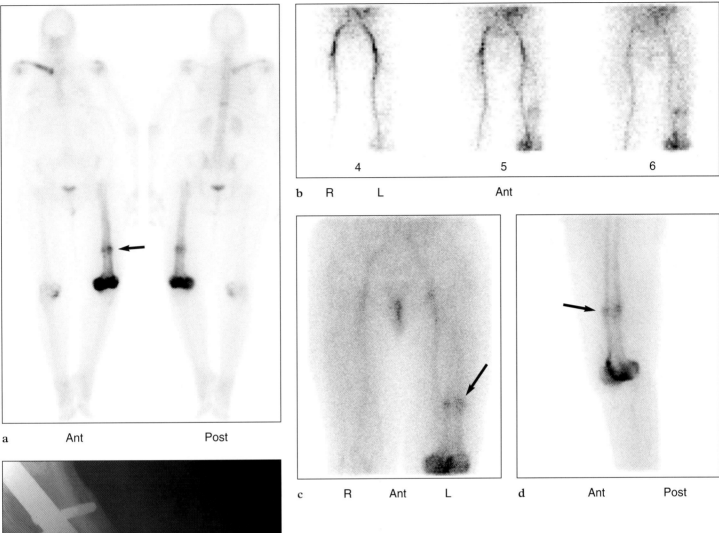

Figure 4.37

Pathologic fracture, pagetoid bone. (a) WB. Pagetoid changes in left femur especially distally and right clavicle. Fracture in distal third (arrow). (b) RNA. The increased perfusion to the distal-most part of the femur seen on the bottom of the image represents the increased vascularity of the pagetoid bone. The more focal, increased vascularity relatively minimal of the healing fracture in the distal third is identified. (c) BP, anterior. Increased vascularity in the same areas as the RNA. (d) DS, left knee, lateral. The photon deficiency in the central marrow cavity associated with the metallic rod that is in place is suggested. The activity of the fracture (arrow) is noted. (e) X-ray mid-femur, anterior. The incompletely healed fracture is identified (arrow) as is the increased sclerosis of the bone and the metallic rod centrally.

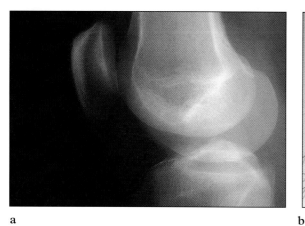

a

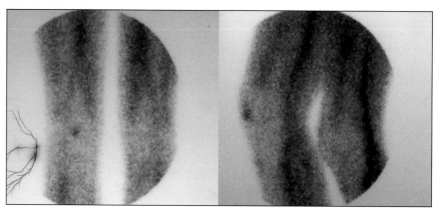

b

Figure 4.38

Patellar avulsion, inferior pole. Subacute versus old fracture with nonunion. (a) X-ray, knee, lateral. The inferior pole patellar fragment. (b) BP, anterior and lateral. Well-defined focus of mild increased uptake (relative vascularity), seen on orthogonal views, allows localization. (c) DS, anterior, right lateral and right medial. The well-defined focus of increased tracer is identified.

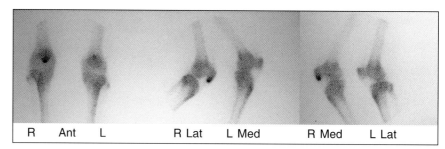

c

Teaching point

Scintigraphic uptake about the patella is often non-specific. Inferior pole uptake in an adult is often a patellar tendonitis associated with injury to the quadriceps mechanism, while in children quadriceps mechanism injury often results in damage and radiotracer uptake at the tibial tuberosity. Abnormal uptake on scan confirms the presence of increased vascular and/or metabolic activity, which provides the clinician with objective evidence of a location for the etiology of the patient's pain.

Figure 4.39 a and b

Multitrauma patient. Nonunion patellar fracture, interosseous membrane tear and calcification, right radius and right anterior rib fracture. Patient evaluated for continuing pain. (a) X-ray, knee, AP. Multiple patellar fragments (arrow). (b) WB. The injection site is identified in the left wrist (IS). Foci of activity associated with healing right rib, right radius, and patella noted. Faint soft tissue activity along the lateral aspect of the right lower leg (arrow) is associated with chronic inflammation. The etiology is uncertain. More medial minimally intense mid-leg activity.

continued

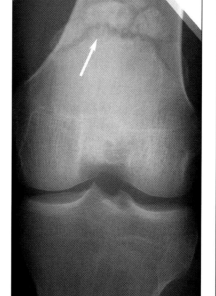

a

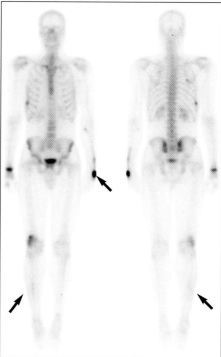

b   Ant   Post

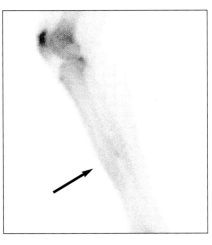

c

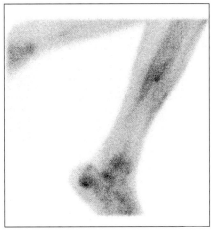

d

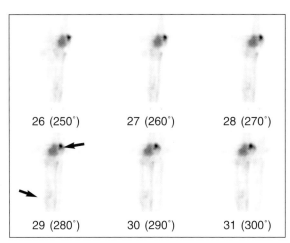

26 (250°)   27 (260°)   28 (270°)

29 (280°)   30 (290°)   31 (300°)

e

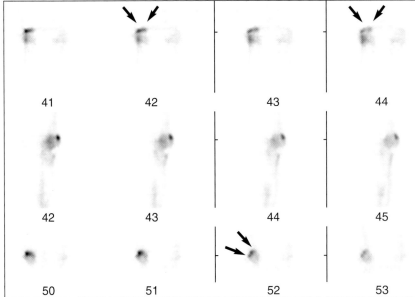

41   42   43   44

42   43   44   45

50   51   52   53

f

Figure 4.39 c–h

(c) DS, right medial knee and leg. Moderately intense activity associated with upper pole of patella. Faint mid-leg activity, not well defined, is noted (arrow). (d) DS, right leg and ankle, lateral view. The mid-leg activity is better defined and is located between the posterior tibial cortex and fibula. (e) 3-D reprojection images. The abnormal activity is better seen between the tibia and fibula (arrow). Superior patellar pole activity also better defined (arrow). (f) SPECT, sections through superior pole of patella. Note that on the transaxial and coronal images two separate fragments with increased metabolic activity are identified (arrows). (g) SPECT, sections through right mid-leg uptake. Especially on the transaxial image the activity (large arrow) is seen between the more anterior medial tibia and the PL fibula. (h) CT, bone window, correlates with the transaxial SPECT in (g). PL = posterior lateral.

TIB

Interosseous membrane calcification

FIB

102   103   104   105

45   46   47   48

64   65   66   67

g

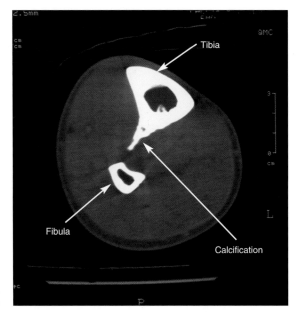

Tibia

Fibula

Calcification

h

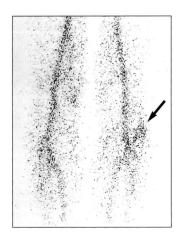 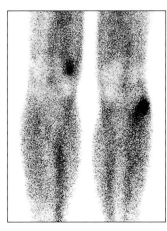 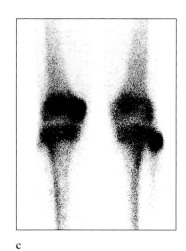 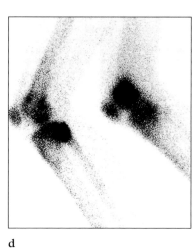

a   b   c   d

Figure 4.40

Acute distal medial condyle femur and proximal tibial fractures. A 31-year-old cricket player. Injuries two weeks previously. **(a)** RNA, anterior, selected view. **(b)** BP, anterior. **(c)** DS, anterior and **(d)** DS, lateral. Focal increased perfusion on the RNA and BP images reflect the acute nature of the injury. The intense activity on the delayed images is less well defined on these analog images. Computer subtraction techniques would have identified the epicenter of the lesion. Acute fractures during the first two weeks of healing often have more intense RNA and BP activity than in this case.

Teaching point

As the age of healing fractures increases, activity on delayed images becomes more focal and more specifically localized to the fracture line.

Leg

When the differential diagnosis of pain in the lower leg in an athlete is of uncertain etiology, RNBI can be particularly valuable to diagnose both a specific lesion or to detect a source of pain referred from the pelvis, thigh, or ankle and foot region. Included in the differential diagnosis of lower leg pain are shin splints, stress fractures, compartment syndrome, interosseous membrane tears, and occasionally avulsion fractures.

Figure 4.41

Subacute oblique fibula fracture. **(a)** RNA. Five seconds per view, and **(b)** BP, anterior higher (left image) and lower (right image). No significant early increased arterial perfusion seen on the RNA. Mild focal increased BP activity at lower part calf. **(c)** DS, anterior (left image) and posterior (right image). More intense, focal, increased metabolic activity. Note the lateral location of the fibula. Orthogonal view not obtained. **(d)** X-ray, lateral right leg. Healing fracture with oblique fracture line still seen.

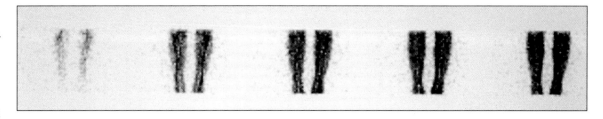

a

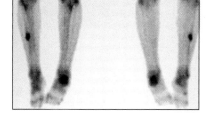 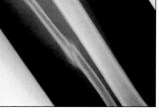

b   c   d

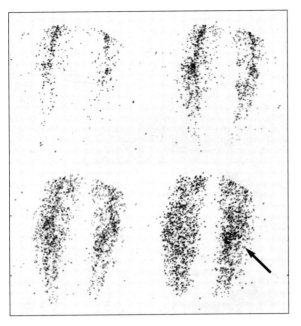

a

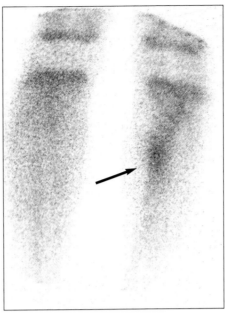

b

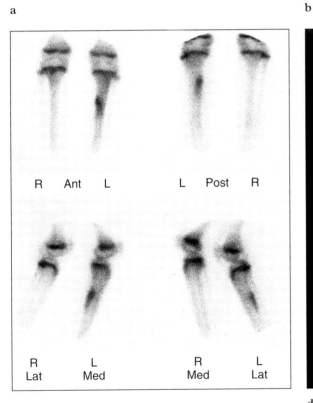

c

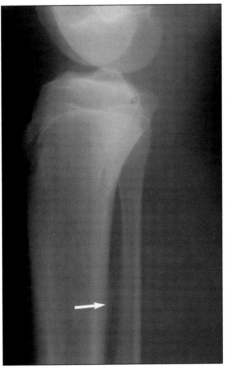

d

Figure 4.42

Two-week-old left tibial stress fracture. Older analogue camera. (a) RNA, two seconds per view. Minimal increased perfusion proximal left tibia (arrow) seen on late arterial/early capillary frame. (b) BP, anterior. Mild-to-moderate increased relative vascularity (arrow). Relative uptake to physeal uptake of both the distal femur and proximal tibia. (c) DS, anterior (top left), posterior (top right), left medial (lower left), and left lateral (lower right). The somewhat fusiform but eccentric uptake is identified. It is clearly not linear. (d) X-ray, leg, lateral. The periosteal reaction (arrow) associated with the fracture appears a little more mature than normally seen with a two-week-old stress fracture.

Teaching point

Acute stress fractures (0–3 weeks) usually have increased perfusion on the RNA, increased uptake (relative vascularity) on BP images, and increased tracer on delayed images. Subacute fractures, up to 10 weeks, usually have increased BP activity and increased delayed activity. Healing fractures over the next several months have normal uptake on RNA and BP images and increasingly well-defined focal uptake on delayed images. Shin splint lesions do not have increased RNA or BP uptake, and have linear uptake, corresponding to periosteal location, on delayed images.

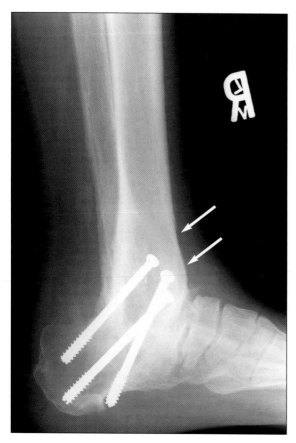

a

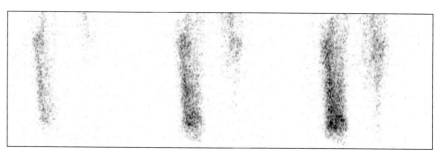

b   Anterior

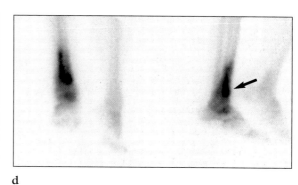

c   d

Figure 4.43

Distal right tibia stress fracture superimposed on previously operated bone.
(a) X-ray, right lateral. Internal fixation screws form tibiotalar calcaneal fusion.
Arrows indicate subtle periosteal changes. (b) RNA, five seconds per image
(anterior). Mild-to-moderate increased perfusion to lateral aspect of right lower leg
extending to the ankle. (c) BP, anterior. Intense increased uptake (relative
vascularity), distal tibia, to the ankle. (d) DS, anterior (left image) and right lateral
(right image). Intense uptake anterolaterally. Although some of the metabolic
activity could be related to continued stress remodeling changes from the five-year-
old fusion, the patient had been asymptomatic until the very recent onset of pain,
swelling, and tenderness.

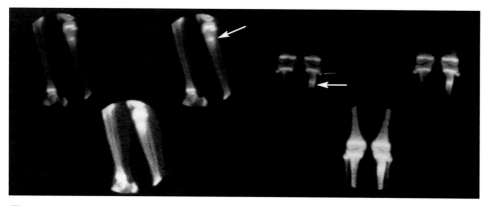

Figure 4.44

Proximal tibial stress fracture in 12-year-old. Triple lens polaroid display. DS, anterior
(right three images) and left lateral and right medial (left three images). Horizontal linear
intense increased activity (arrow) is almost as intense as physeal activity.

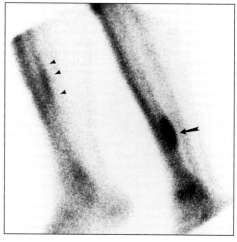

Right medial   Left lateral

Figure 4.45

Stress fracture (left) and skin splint
(**right**, distal third tibia. DS. The very
typical fusiform increased tracer in the
posterior medial tibial cortex is noted
(arrow). On the opposite leg the more linear
increase associated with a shin splint-type
lesion is seen (arrowheads).

Teaching point

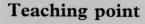

In children the softer cancellous bone of the most proximal tibia is prone to horizontally
oriented stress fractures, which are of the compression type.

Ankle and foot

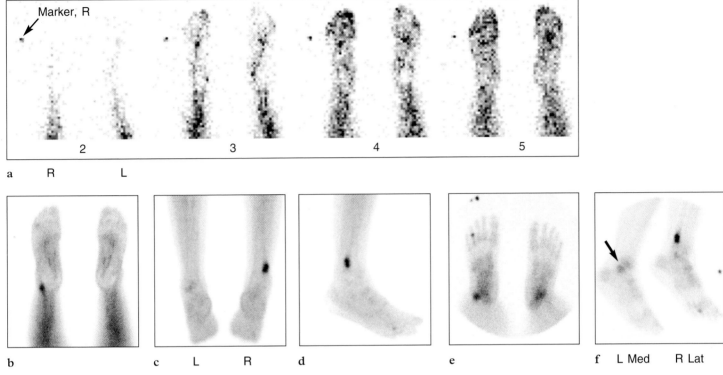

Figure 4.46

Insufficiency fracture fibula; AVN, left talus; stress fracture, fourth proximal phalanx. End-stage renal disease, long-term steroid use. (**a**) RNA, plantar. Five seconds per frame. Selected images. No significant increased perfusion to the area of the distal fibula or bones of the foot. A marker (arrow) is used to indicate the right side. (**b**) BP, plantar. Moderately intense, focal, increased vascularity of distal fibular shaft. Note its projection on this plantar view. (**c**) BP, posterior and (**d**) BP, right lateral. These demonstrate focal increased vascularity of the distal fibula. (**e**) DS, plantar view. The projection of the distal fibula on the plantar view (arrow). The minimal activity at the proximal aspect of the fourth proximal phalanx represents the healing stress fracture (correlative radiograph not shown). (**f**) DS, right lateral, and left medial. The fibula stress fracture is noted as the area of greatest intensity on this image. The healing proximal phalangeal stress fracture is also noted on the right, while activity of osteonecrosis of the talus is seen well on the left. (**g**) SPECT, coronal image through the right fibular fracture also includes the dome of the left talus which has moderately increased tracer, representing the revascularization phase. This is also seen on the sagittal image through this bone (arrow). Slightly superior and anterior is the supra-adjacent distal tibia which also has some minimal activity present.

Figure 4.47

Insufficiency fracture, distal left tibia. An 80-year-old female with severe osteoporosis evaluated for low back pain. Incidental significant degenerative changes, lumbosacral spine. (**a**) WB. Moderately intense, abnormal uptake, distal left tibia. (**b**) DS, ankle, left lateral. Higher-resolution image shows linear configuration of abnormal distal tibial uptake. Correlative X-ray (not shown) demonstrated linear sclerosis in this area.

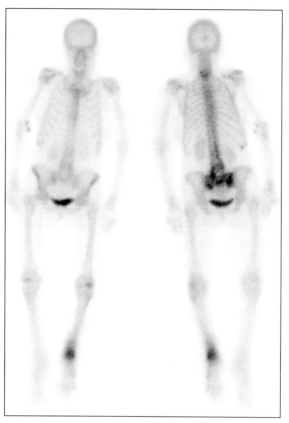

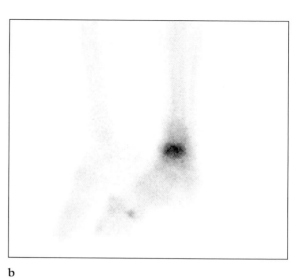

b

a   Ant   Post

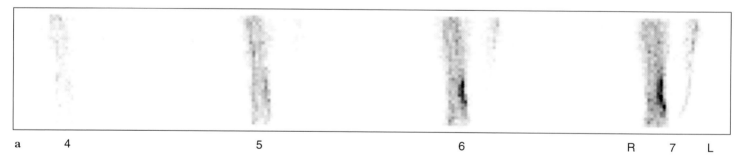

a   4   5   6   R   7   L

Figure 4.48 a–c

Medial malleolar lesion. Avulsion fracture versus periostitis. (**a**) RNA, anterior. Five seconds per frame. Mild, focal, somewhat linear increased perfusion to distal medial right lower leg just above the ankle. (**b**) BP, anterior. The right leg is larger than the left with diffuse relatively increased uptake (vascularity), more focal in the region of the medial malleolus. (**c**) DS, anterior. Moderately increased activity localized to the medial malleolus. Orthogonal view (not shown) could not localize further.

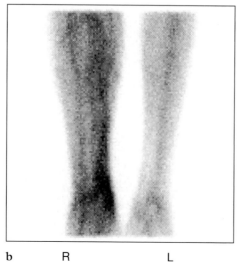

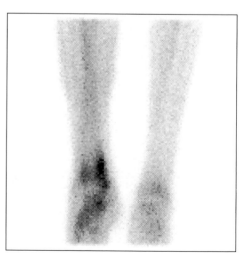

continued

b   R   L   c

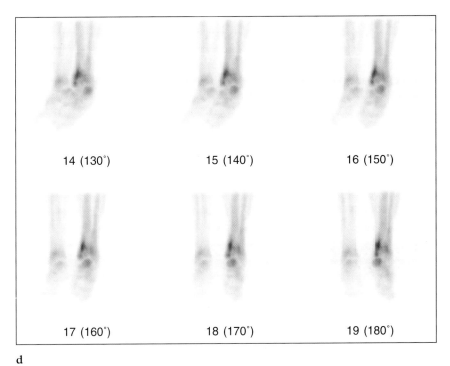

14 (130°)   15 (140°)   16 (150°)

17 (160°)   18 (170°)   19 (180°)

d

Figure 4.48 d–e

(**d**) 3-D reprojection images. Focal activity associated with the medial malleolus. (**e**) SPECT, sections through mid medial malleolus. Coronal image demonstrates medial location of abnormal activity which is also well appreciated on the transaxial view (arrow).

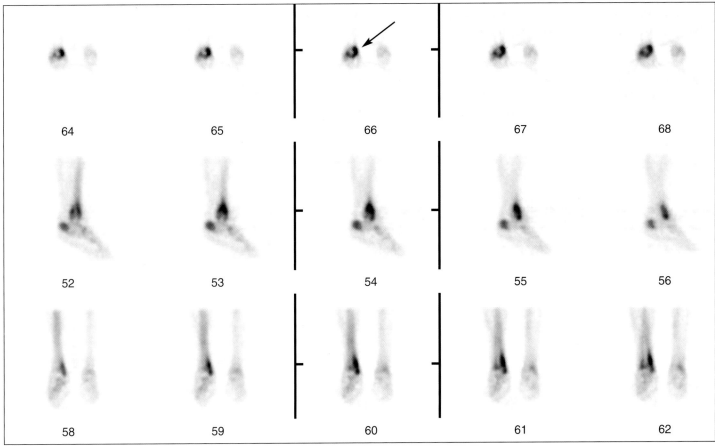

e

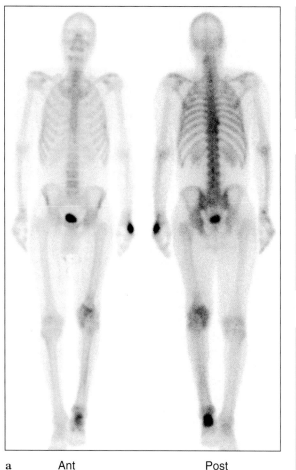

a　　　　Ant　　　　　　　　Post

Fractures of the calcaneous probably have several etiologic factors, since some are oriented horizontally and others are oriented vertically to the long axis of the calcaneous.

Teaching point

On RNAs of the feet, definition of individual vessels or even precise anatomic localization is often difficult or impossible because of the low count data. This results from the low percentage of blood flow reaching the distal extremity and the loss of the bolus injection effect at this distal location.

Value of true lateral projections. Often in an attempt to obtain corresponding views of both the right and left side, the true anatomic position of the images is compromised. When detail is required, the extremity of interest can be imaged separately, allowing positional considerations to emphasize that single extremity.

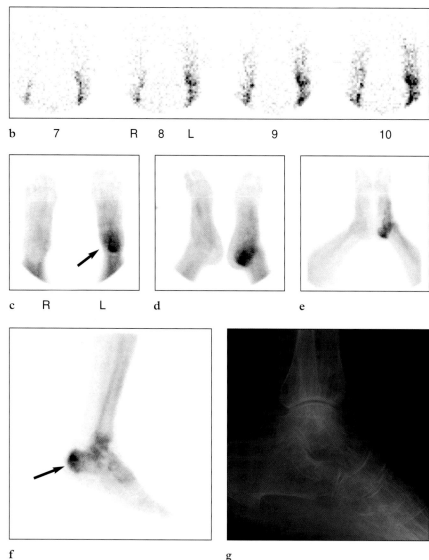

b　　7　　　　R　8　L　　　　9　　　　10

c　　R　　　L　　d　　　　　　e

f　　　　　　　　　　　g

Figure 4.49

Calcaneal stress fracture. Status after remote femoral fracture with leg shortening. (**a**) WB. The short left extremity with nonspecific, poorly defined, left knee uptake. Intense hind foot uptake most marked on posterior view. (**b**) RNA. Plantar view, five seconds per frame. Asymmetric perfusion with mild increase to left hind foot region. (**c**) BP, plantar. Mild-to-moderate increased activity (relative vascularity), left hind foot. More activity is present posteriorly (arrow). (**d**) BP, lateral oblique. Activity localized to calcaneous. Note that these are not true lateral views. (**e**) DS, lateral oblique. Similar to the BP (**d**), activity is localized to the calcaneous, particularly the posterior portion. (**f**) DS, lateral, true anatomic position. In this image the horizontal orientation of the uptake, most typical of a stress fracture, is now easily identified. (**g**) X-ray. Sclerosis of healing fracture.

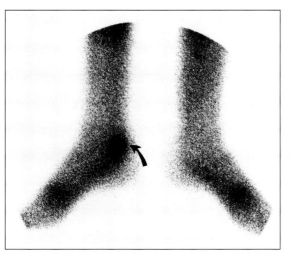

a

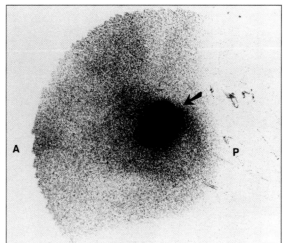

b

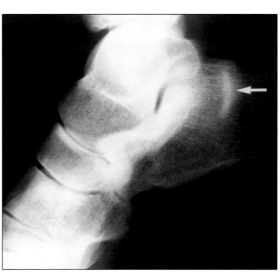

c

Figure 4.50

Vertical calcaneal stress fracture. (a) BP, oblique lateral. Moderately focal, increased activity, posterior calcaneous (curved arrow). (b) DS, magnified lateral view. Intense focal activity in mid-portion of calcaneous (arrow) corresponds to vertical sclerosis seen on radiograph (c). With computer subtraction, even in this relatively acute stage with activity extending beyond the fracture line, the epicenter would be better defined. (c) X-ray, lateral. The vertically oriented fracture line (arrow).

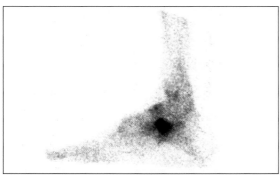

L Lat

Figure 4.51

Anterior process calcaneal fracture. DS, lateral. Intense activity can be localized to the anterior portion of the calcaneous. These fractures are subtle. Patients are usually imaged in the subacute setting, after the pain of a 'routine ankle sprain' fails to resolve as expected.

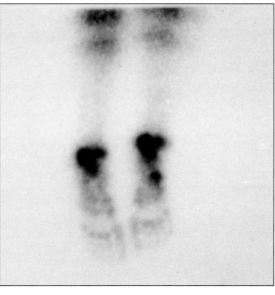

Plantar

Figure 4.52

Subacute cuboid fracture, 'toddler's fracture'. DS, plantar. The abnormal increased tracer in the right foot can be localized in relation to the calcaneous and distal tarsal row. (Patient image courtesy of DP Dalzell and ST Auringer, Winston-Salem, NC.)

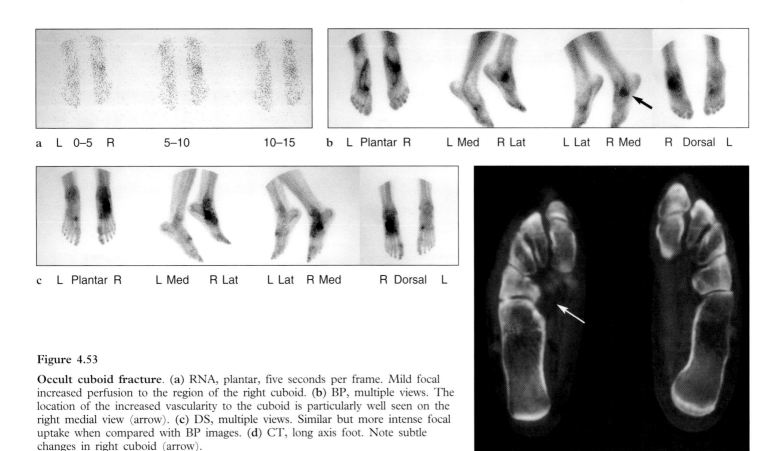

a   L 0–5 R   5–10   10–15   b   L Plantar R   L Med   R Lat   L Lat   R Med   R Dorsal L

c   L Plantar R   L Med   R Lat   L Lat   R Med   R Dorsal L

d

Figure 4.53

Occult cuboid fracture. (a) RNA, plantar, five seconds per frame. Mild focal increased perfusion to the region of the right cuboid. (b) BP, multiple views. The location of the increased vascularity to the cuboid is particularly well seen on the right medial view (arrow). (c) DS, multiple views. Similar but more intense focal uptake when compared with BP images. (d) CT, long axis foot. Note subtle changes in right cuboid (arrow).

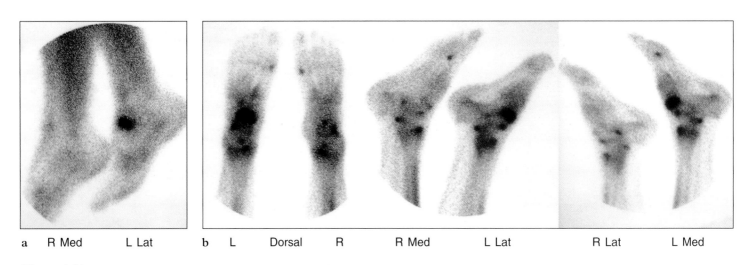

a   R Med   L Lat   b   L   Dorsal   R   R Med   L Lat   R Lat   L Med

Figure 4.54

Navicular stress fracture. (a) BP, lateral. Moderate increased activity (relative vascularity) is in the very typical shape for the navicular. (b) DS. The typical shape of navicular uptake is again seen. Note the other areas of less intense uptake in the ankle and the foot, which are associated with nonspecific stress remodeling changes secondary to the changes in walking that occur because of the pain of the subacute fracture.

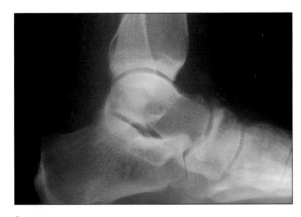

a

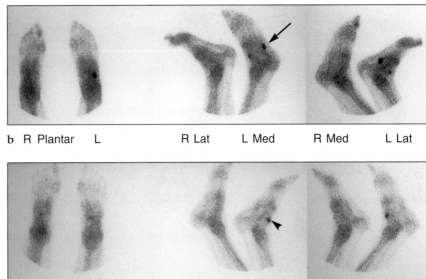

b   R Plantar   L   R Lat   L Med   R Med   L Lat

c   R   Plantar   L   R Med   L Lat   R Lat   L Med

Teaching point

Focal uptake associated with accessory ossicles is not specific for fracture. Scintigraphic differential diagnosis includes acute or subacute fracture, non-union of an older fracture, stress remodeling changes associated with an avulsed or separated ossicle, or even 'bone bruising'. History and correlative anatomic imaging are required for further differential diagnosis. The scintigraphic abnormality does provide objective evidence of active metabolism and presumably an association with the patient's pain.

Figure 4.55

Fracture os peroneum. (a) X-ray, lateral. The os peroneum associated with the inferior aspect of the cuboid is irregular. (b) DS, presurgery. Focal, moderately increased metabolic activity, associated with the os peroneum (arrow), provides objective evidence that this ossicle is the site of patient's pain. (c) DS, postoperative. The os peroneum has been removed. Note the continued activity associated with the small spur at the proximal superior aspect of the navicular (arrowhead).

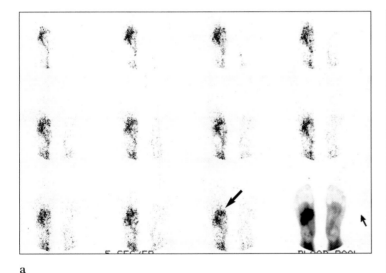

a

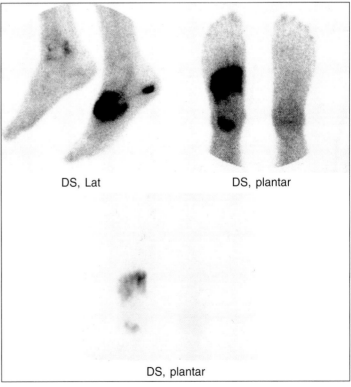

DS, Lat   DS, plantar

DS, plantar

b

Figure 4.56

Tarsometatarsal fracture dislocation (Lisfranc's injury). (a) RNA and BP, plantar. The focal increased perfusion extending horizontally across the MTP joint (arrow) suggests the epicenter of abnormality. The BP image (bottom right) has such intense increased uptake (relative vascularity associated with healing) that the exact area of abnormality is obscured. (b) DS. Lateral (left) image and plantar (middle) image have intense uptake in the entire mid-foot region. The background subtracted plantar view (bottom) image helps localize the site of abnormality and direct further imaging (CT is usually done).

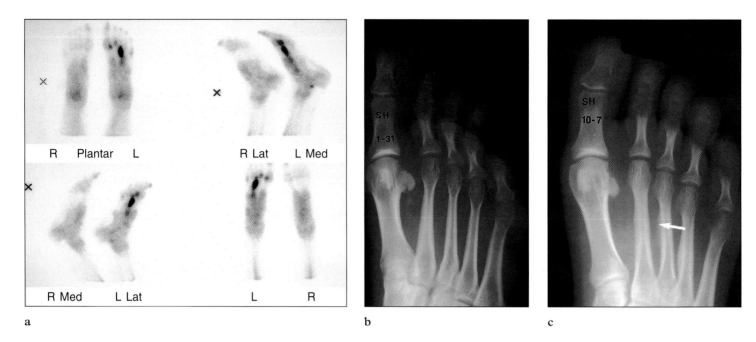

a   b   c

Figure 4.57

Third metatarsal stress fracture. (a) DS, multiple views. The fusiform focus of increased
activity is well defined on all views. (b) X-ray, original. No abnormal periosteal or other osseous
abnormality of the third metatarsal shaft. (c) X-ray, follow-up, ten months post injury. Periosteal
reaction associated with healing is identified (arrow).

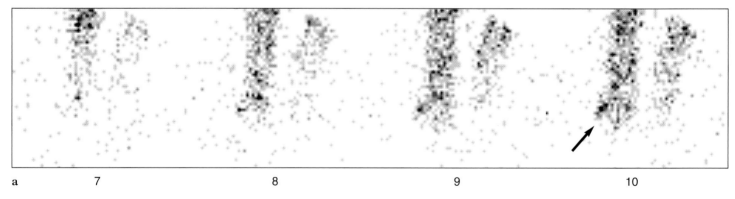

a   7   8   9   10

Figure 4.58

Subacute fracture, base fifth proximal phalanx.
(a) RNA, plantar view, five seconds per frame,
selected images. The minimal asymmetric increased
perfusion to the left foot compared with the right,
with slightly more focal increase in the distal lateral
portion (arrow). RNA in the lower extremity is often
a very low count study. In this case images 7–10
have maximal counts per pixel and total counts of 6
and 471, 5 and 769, 7 and 981, and 8 and 1060,
respectively. (b) BP, plantar view. Moderately intense,
increased relative vascularity in the region of the
distal metatarsal and fifth proximal phalangeal base.
(c) DS, plantar view. The intense activity involving
the base of the fifth proximal phalanx is noted. Note
'washed out' appearance of the foot. This is a normal
variant of delayed foot imaging. No etiology or any
significance has ever been attributed to this pattern.

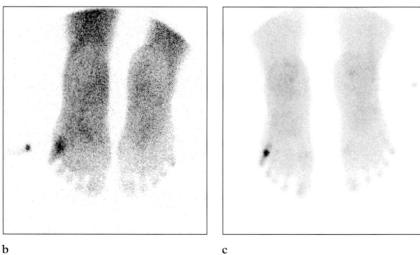

b   c

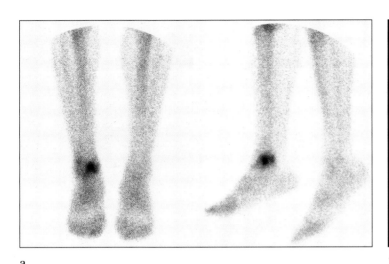

a

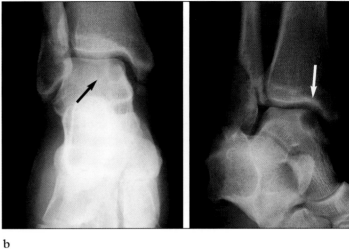

b

Figure 4.59

Transchondral talar dome fracture. (a) DS. Anterior (left image) and right medial (right image). Focus of moderately intense tracer in the medial aspect of the talar dome. (b) X-ray, AP (left image) and oblique (right image) demonstrate subchondral lucency (arrow).

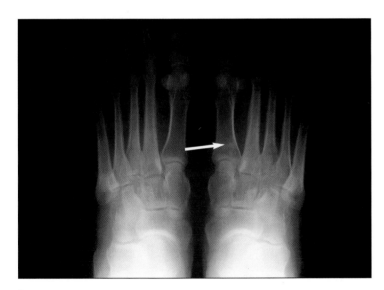

a

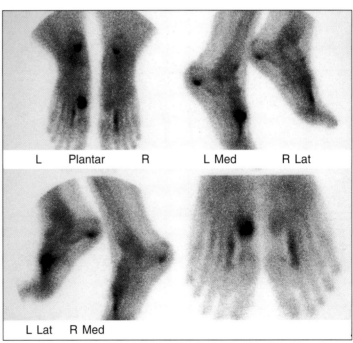

b

Figure 4.60

Fracture, base first metatarsal. (a) X-ray, AP. Note horizontal sclerosis in the proximal metaphyseal diaphyseal portion of the first metatarsal (arrow). Incidental cortical thickening bilateral second metatarsal shafts. (b) DS. Multiple views. The intense abnormal activity in the proximal metatarsal is distal to the first tarsometatarsal joint, and corresponds to the sclerosis on radiograph. Nonspecific increased metabolic activity in both second metatarsal shafts is related to healing of old fractures and/or remodeling secondary to altered biomechanical stress.

Stress lesions

Biomechanical stress lesions are the osseous equivalent of the repetitive stress syndromes, such as the carpal tunnel syndrome, which affect the musculoskeletal system secondary to a wide range of activities. In some cases these lesions may represent enthesiopathies or other more generic-type stress responses of bones and joints. An enthesis is the site of insertion of a tendon, ligament, or articular capsule into bone.

In some cases, the decision to include a lesion in this section rather than in the section on inflammatory lesions was arbitrary. For example, some bursitis lesions have been included here since these are associated with the stress of running sports. On the other hand, pubic symphysitis which is commonly found in runners as well as in patients following genitourinary tract surgery has been included in the section on miscellaneous osseous lesions. RNBI is usually performed in the subacute or chronic setting when pain persists longer than expected following routine trauma or when chronic pain is present with normal radiographs. An abnormal or positive bone scan indicates a possible etiologic relationship between the focus of abnormal increased vascularity and/or metabolism and the patient's signs or symptoms.

Elbow

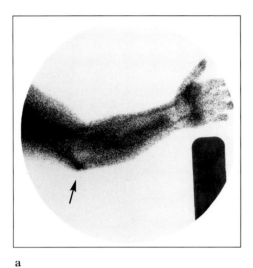

a

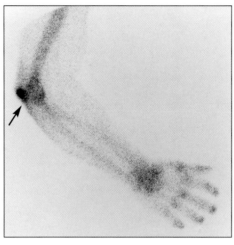

b

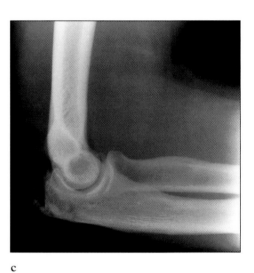

c

Figure 4.61

Triceps tendonitis. (a) BP, focal increased vascularity at the posterosuperior portion of the olecranon (arrow). (b) DS, more focal increased metabolic activity associated with the olecranon (arrow) and the small fragments seen on accompanying radiograph. (c) X-ray, elbow, lateral. Small fragments at the posterior aspect of the olecranon.

Teaching point

When stress-related injuries involving tendinous insertions or attachments are imaged during the subacute and chronic phases, often only focal increased tracer accumulation on delayed images is present, with the RNA and BP images normal.

Figure 4.62

Medial epicondylitis. DS. Focal, well-defined, increased metabolic activity involving the medial epicondyle.

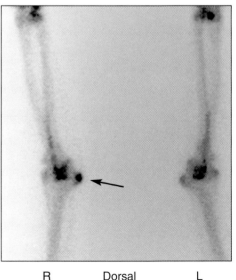

R   Dorsal   L

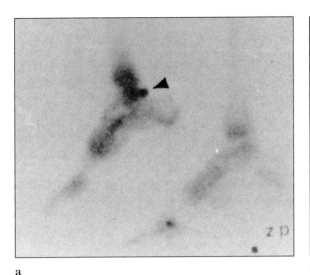

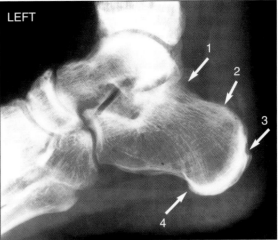

a

b

Figure 4.69

Os trigonum syndrome. (a) DS. Focal increased tracer (arrowhead) at the site of the accessory ossicle. (b) X-ray, lateral. Use this radiograph for anatomic comparison with bone scans for stress lesions in and about the ankle and foot. The region of the os trigonum (arrow 1). The retrocalcaneal or pre-Achilles' bursa (arrow 2). The insertion of the Achilles' tendon (arrow 3). The region of the calcaneal tubercle, the origin of the plantar fascia (arrow 4).

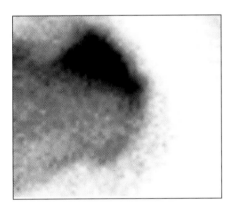

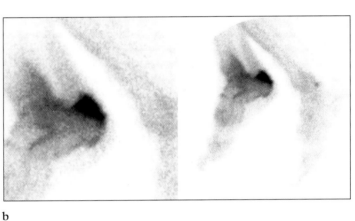

a

b

Figure 4.70

Retrocalcaneal bursitis. (a) BP (top right). There is more increased relative vascularity than usually seen even in acute cases. (b) DS. (right image) and magnified image (left image). The intense activity associated with the retrocalcaneal bursa and subadjacent calcaneous. (See Figure 4.69b.)

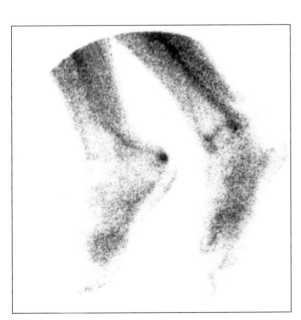

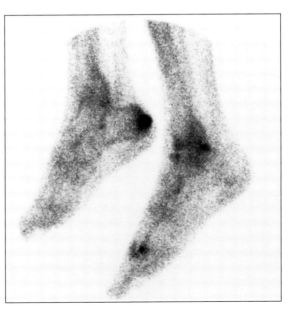

a

b

Figure 4.71

Achilles' tendonitis, subacute. (a) BP. Focal increased tracer uptake (relative vascularity) at the upper third middle third junction of the posterior border of the calcaneous. (b) DS, lateral. Intense focal increased tracer at the insertion of the Achilles' tendon. (See Figure 4.69b.)

Figure 4.72

Plantar fasciitis. Focal increased activity in the area of the calcaneal tubicle (arrow). Although occasionally increased activity can be seen in asymptomatic patients, in the appropriate clinical setting this confirms the diagnosis.

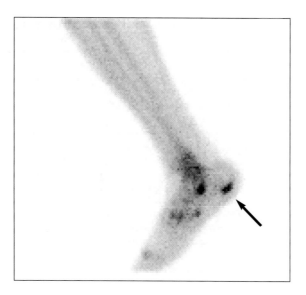

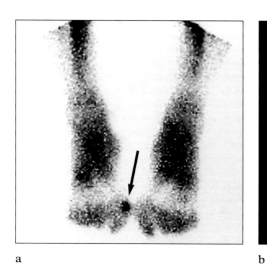

a

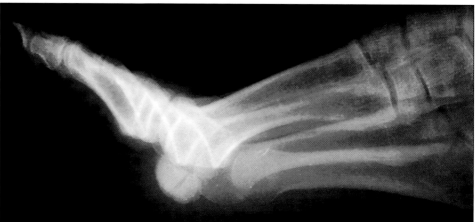

b

Figure 4.73

Sesamoiditis or sesamoid fracture. (a) DS, anterior. Moderately intense, well-defined, round focus of increased tracer associated with the medial-most portion of the first metatarsal head corresponds to the sesamoid (arrow). (b) X-ray, lateral. The sesamoid at the head of the first metatarsal may have a fracture line visualized.

Teaching point

Sesamoid bones are often bipartite. When pain is present, the positive bone scan indicates significant alterations in skeletal metabolism and suggests that this bone may be related to the patient's pain. Differential diagnosis would include a healing fracture, a bone bruise, or other inflammatory, but not infectious, process.

Miscellaneous osseous lesions

Arbitrarily included in this section are traumatic conditions which are associated with increased radiotracer uptake, but which do not easily fit into more specific sections. Most are related to abnormal biomechanical stress, but have more specific etiologies or are named conditions for which objective evidence of their presence in a particular patient is often desired by the clinician.

In the case of unilateral sacralization of L5 – a developmental abnormality – biomechanical stress results in the abnormal uptake. Shin splints, on the other hand, is a well-documented noninfectious periostitis secondary to abnormal movement of the soleus muscle tendon complex.

Hand and wrist

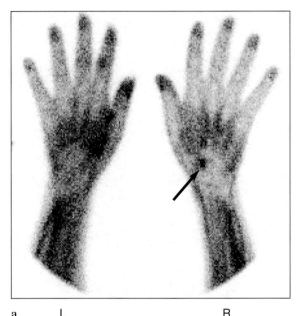

a   L   R

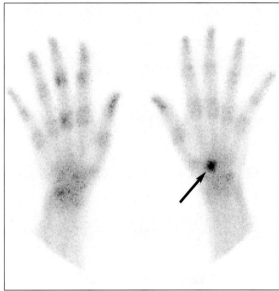

b

Figure 4.74

Trapezoid, bone bruise. (a) BP, palmar. Minimal-to-moderate small focal area of relative increased vascularity in the left wrist (arrow). (b) DS, palmar. More intense focal activity in the trapezoid. Note relationship of focal uptake in the distal carpal row to the base of the second and third metacarpals. (c) DS, ulnar deviation view, and (d). DS, lateral. Additional views aid in anatomic localization.

c

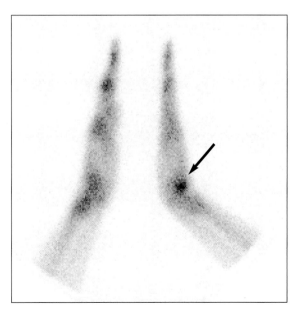

d

Pelvis and hip

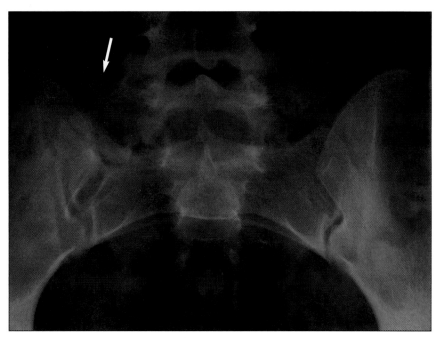

a

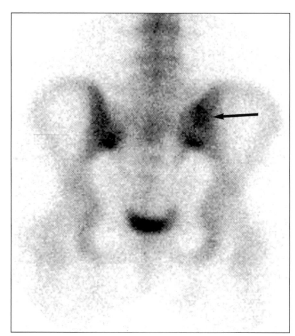

b

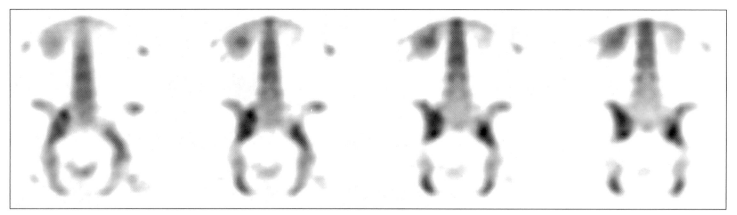

c

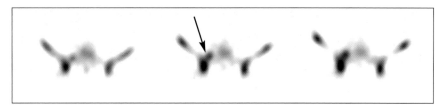

d

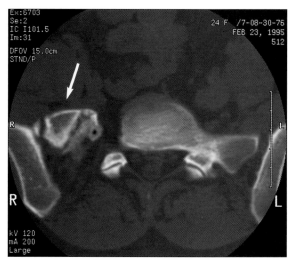

e

Figure 4.75

Unilateral partial sacralization L5. A 25-year-old female with chronic low back pain. (a) X-ray, PA. The asymmetry of the transverse processes of L5 with sacralization on the right (arrow). (b) DS, pelvis, posterior. Mild asymmetry in the SI joint regions with the right wider and with an area of rounded mild increased tracer centrally (arrow). (c) SPECT, coronal and (d) SPECT, transaxial demonstrate the asymmetric focal uptake involving the right lateral transverse process and adjacent ilium. (e) CT. Compare the area of the sacralization (arrow) with the transaxial SPECT in (d).

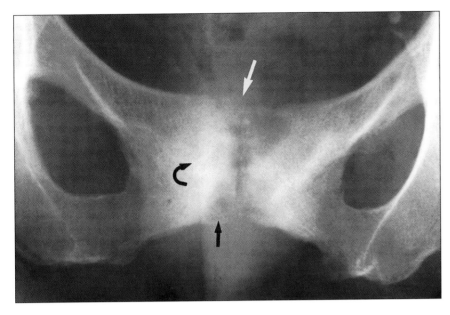

a

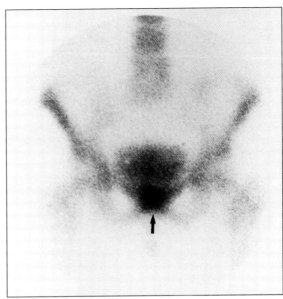

b

Figure 4.76

Pubic symphysitis. (a) X-ray, AP. The normal radiolucency of the cartilage at the symphysis is obliterated. There is loss of cortical margins with apparent periosteal proliferation (straight white arrow), bony sclerosis (curved black arrow), and subchondral erosion (straight arrow). (b) DS, anterior. Increased tracer accumulation at the symphysis with loss of the vertical band of decreased density (arrow) seen when the symphysis is normal (compare with Fig. 2.8c).

Teaching point

An abnormal plain X-ray and pain over the pubis usually confirm this diagnosis. When radiographs are normal or when a radiographic abnormality is thought to be an incidental finding, RNBI provides objective proof of an active process at this location.

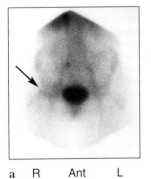

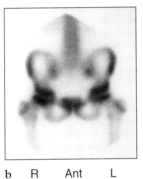

a R   Ant   L

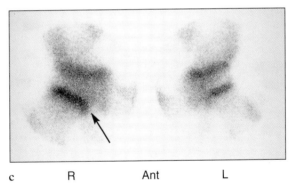

b R   Ant   L   c R   Ant   L

Teaching point

When spot views of comparable body parts are obtained as separate data acquisitions (images), relative intensities can be compared only if images are obtained for similar times. In addition when pin-hole collimation is used similar distances from the end of the collimator to the body part of interest should be maintained.

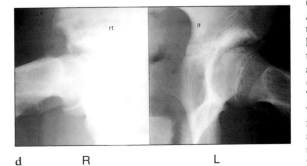

d R   L

Figure 4.77

Slipped capital femoral epiphysis (SCFE). A 14-year-old female complained of mild pain in proximal femur for three months. (a) BP, pelvis, anterior. Very subtle increased tracer accumulation (relative vascularity) in the right proximal femoral epiphysis region (arrow). (b) DS, anterior. Asymmetric increased uptake involving the right hip area compared with the left is seen but anatomic detail is lacking. (c) DS, pin-hole views. The activity associated with the right physis is more intense and thicker and broader than the left side (arrow). (d) X-ray, frog leg lateral. Obtained after the bone scan. The femoral head displaced in relation to the neck is seen on the right.

Knee

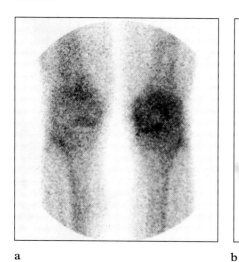

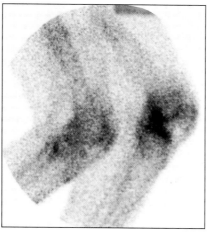

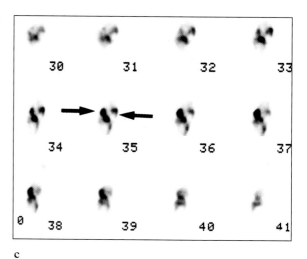

a   b   c

Figure 4.78

Anterior cruciate ligament tear. DS. (a) Anterior and (b) lateral. Diffuse increased activity, left knee. (c) SPECT, sagittal. Review of sequential images is necessary to localize activity to the origin (medial aspect of the lateral femoral condyle) posteriorly and insertion (tibial plateau) anteriorly of the anterior cruciate ligament.

Correlative imaging comment

Acute soft tissue injuries are usually initially evaluated using MR imaging. Knowledge of the scintigraphic appearance in the subacute and chronic stages is important, since these lesions are often found when imaging patients for unexplained pain of potentially osseous origin.

Figure 4.79

Meniscal tear. Patient 1. (a) DS, knee, posterior and (b) SPECT, transaxial, selected image. Increased uptake in the medial compartment of the left knee with greater activity on the tibial side, principally at the joint line. Similar but less intense activity on the right side. SPECT images demonstrate a crescent of increased activity in the tibial plateau predominantly in the posterior two-thirds of the left knee. There is a suggestion of similar activity in the mid-portion on the right. Patient 2. **Medial and lateral meniscal tear.** (c) DS, knee, posterior and (d) SPECT, transaxial, selected images. Similar findings as in patient 1, but with both lateral and medial menisci of the right knee involved.

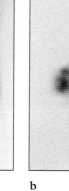

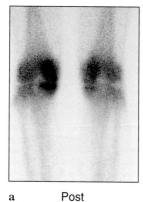

a   Post

b

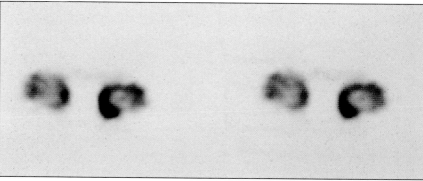

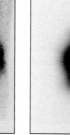

c   Post

d

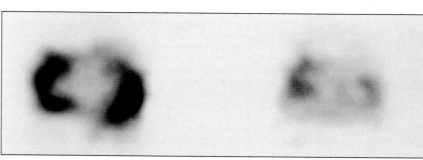

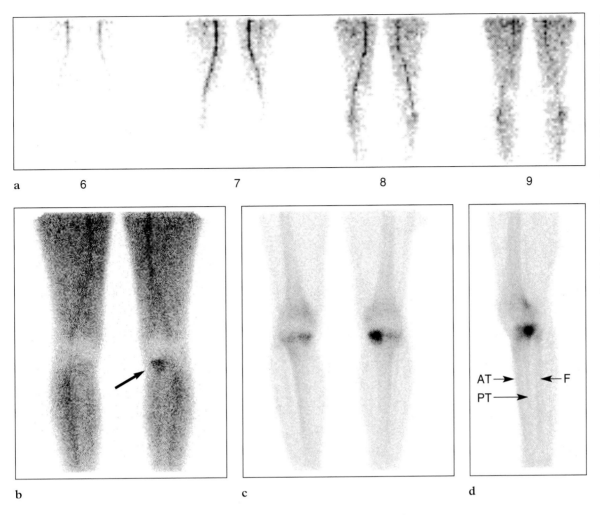

a   6   7   8   9

b   c   d

AT→   ←F
PT→

Figure 4.80

Bone bruise, left knee. (a) RNA, anterior, five seconds per frame. RNA is essentially normal without any increased perfusion. (b) BP, anterior. Mild focal increased tracer accumulation (relative vascularity) in the medial aspect of the left knee (arrow). (c) DS, anterior, and (d) DS, left lateral. Focal tracer accumulation localized in orthogonal projections. On this lateral view, the fibula (F), the anterior tibial cortex (AT), and the posterior tibial cortex (PT) are all seen.

Leg

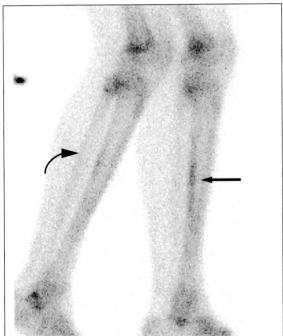

R Lat   L Med

Figure 4.81

Shin splint, left leg. Right lateral and left medial views obtained simultaneously. Mild-to-moderate linear activity associated with the mid-portion of the left posterior tibial cortex (straight arrow). On the right lateral image the anterior and posterior tibial cortices are normal as is the fibula which can be visualized on the lateral (curved arrow).

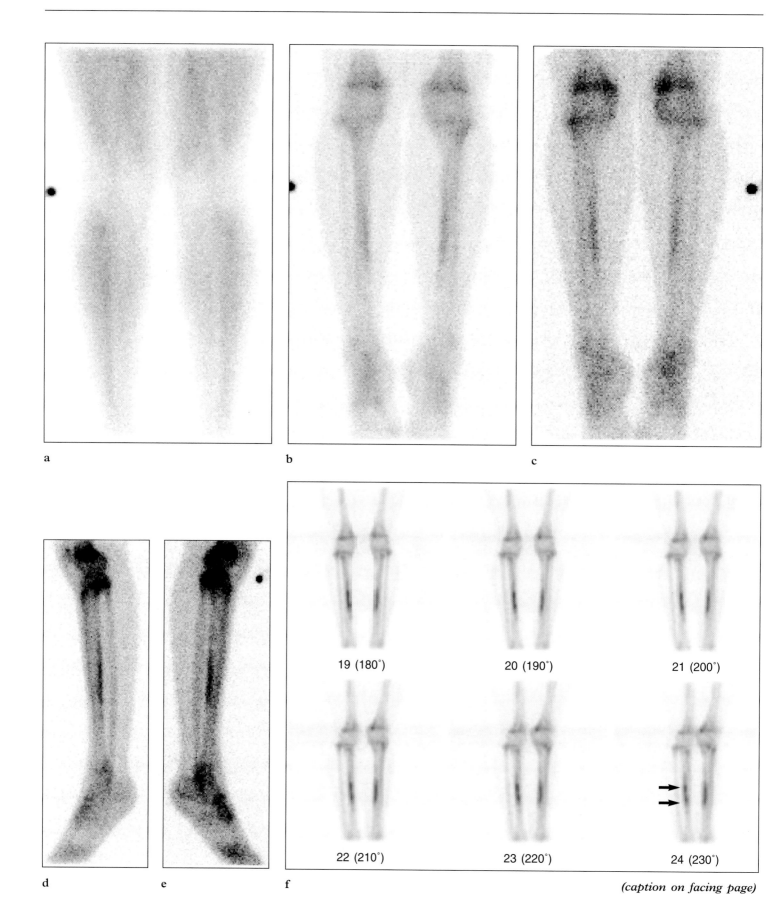

a

b

c

d

e

f

19 (180°)   20 (190°)   21 (200°)

22 (210°)   23 (220°)   24 (230°)

(caption on facing page)

Foot and ankle

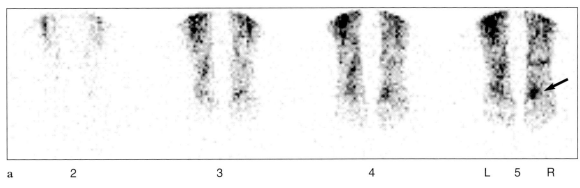

a   2   3   4   L 5 R

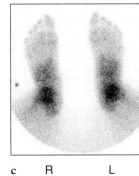

b

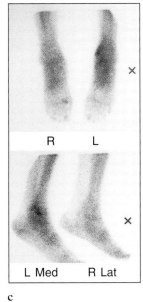

c   R   L

Figure 4.88

Soft tissue bruise over first metatarsal. (a) RNA, plantar, five seconds per view. Mild increased perfusion to the region of the first MTP joint (arrow). (b) BP, plantar. Mild increased tracer uptake (relative vascularity) over the region of the first metatarsal (arrow). (c) DS, plantar. Obtained with feet on detector. No abnormal increased tracer on delayed images.

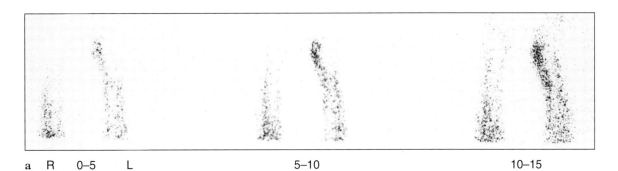

a R   0–5   L   5–10   10–15

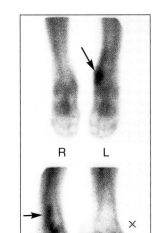

R   L   R   L

L Med   R Lat   L Med   R Lat

b   c

Figure 4.89

Inflammation medial tenosynovial membranes. (a) RNA, anterior. Minimal increased perfusion to the medial aspect of the ankle. (b) BP, anterior (top) and left medial (bottom). Abnormal tracer uptake (relative vascularity) is very superficial as appreciated on anterior images, and has the configuration of the medial tenosynovial membranes on the medial view (arrows). (c) DS. Anterior (top image) and left medial (bottom image). Relative uptake on delayed images less than on the BP images.

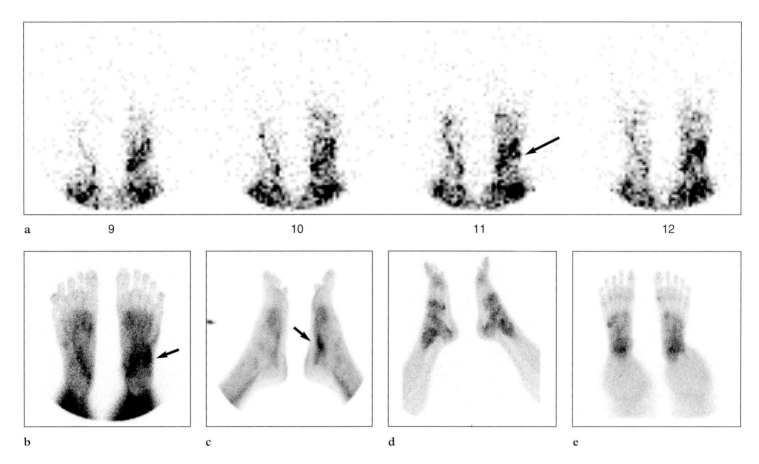

a 9 10 11 12

b c d e

Figure 4.90

Inflamed lateral plantar tendons (peroneal). (a) RNA, plantar.
Five seconds per view. Mild increased perfusion to lateral aspect of
left foot (arrow). (b) BP, plantar. Increased relative vascularity
lateral aspect mid-foot (arrow). (c) BP, left lateral increased relative
vascularity (arrow). (d) DS, lateral and (e) DS, plantar. No
abnormal activity associated with osseous structures.

Heterotopic ossification (HO), after nonsurgical trauma

The deposition of bone tracer as a result of primary soft tissue injury was illustrated in the previous section. In this section the deposition of tracer in association with heterotopic ossification (HO) or heterotopic bone formation will be illustrated. Some authors have used the term myositis ossificans when new bone arises as the result of inflammation in muscle tissue, with HO used for new bone formed in soft parts in the absence of a well-defined cause. This differential is probably artificial. Additional images of heterotopic ossification associated with postoperative trauma will be found in pages 178–183 of this chapter.

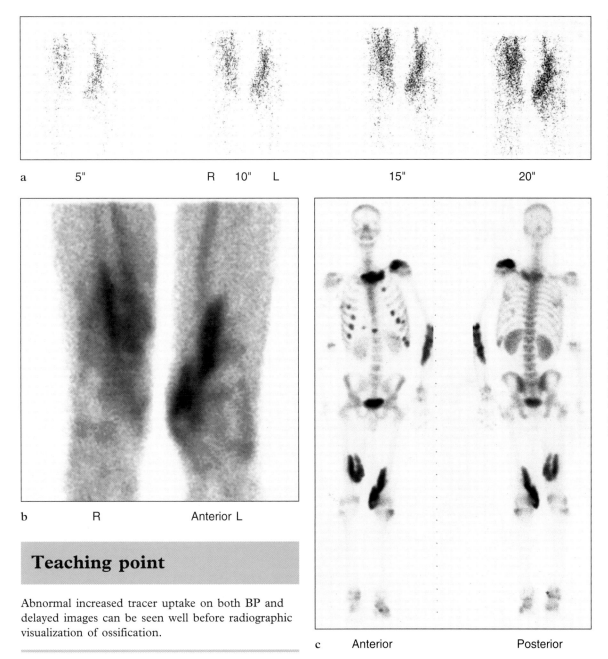

a   5"   R   10"   L   15"   20"

b   R   Anterior L

c   Anterior   Posterior

Figure 4.91

Multifocal heterotopic ossification. Twenty-one days after a motor vehicle crash. Normal X-rays. Complaints of multifocal pain. (a) RNA, knees, anterior, five seconds per view. Mild-to-moderate increased perfusion to the medial aspect of the left knee and more centrally to the region of the right distal thigh. (b) BP, anterior. Intense increased tracer accumulation (relative vascularity). (c) WB. Intense abnormal tracer near left acromio-clavicular joint, sternum, left elbow, medial aspect distal right thigh, and medial aspect distal left thigh. There was fixation of a fracture of the proximal radius. Round areas of tracer uptake associated with rib fractures.

Teaching point

Abnormal increased tracer uptake on both BP and delayed images can be seen well before radiographic visualization of ossification.

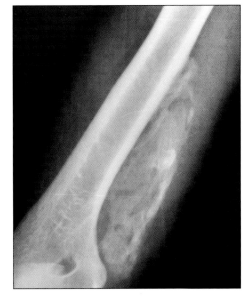

a

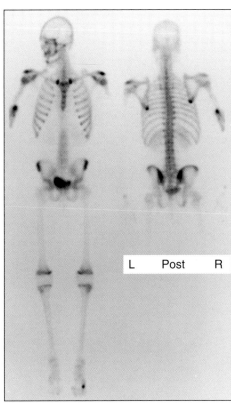

b   R   Ant   L

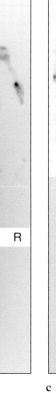

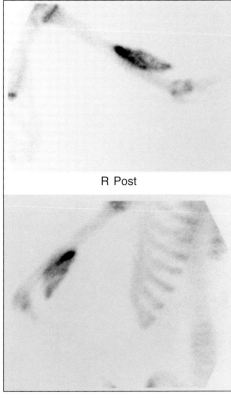

R Post

c   R Ant

Figure 4.92

Heterotopic ossification brachialis muscle. Throwing injury. (a) X-ray, distal humerus. Ossification in the soft tissues. Note the close relationship to the cortex superiorly. (b) WB. The intensity of uptake at the superior aspect of the mass. The entire arm and forearm are not visualized on the WB image. Incidentally note the overlap between the tip of the scapula and the eighth posterior rib on the left, and sixth rib on the right. These are often mistaken for fractures. (c) DS. The abnormal tracer corresponds to the ossified muscle.

Figure 4.93

Heterotopic ossification lateral to left femoral neck at greater trochanter. Twisting injury three years prior to bone scan. (a) RNA. Mild increased perfusion to the left hip region (arrow). (b) DS, anterior. Round intense focus of tracer uptake. (c) X-ray, left hip. Initially interpreted as normal, there is focal increased density corresponding to the region of the abnormal tracer uptake.

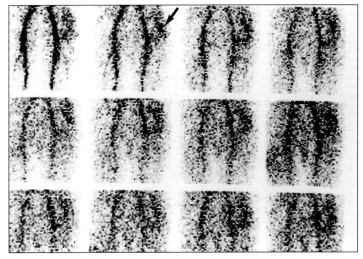

a

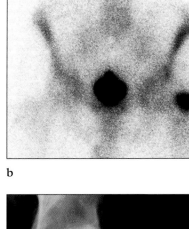

b

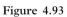

c

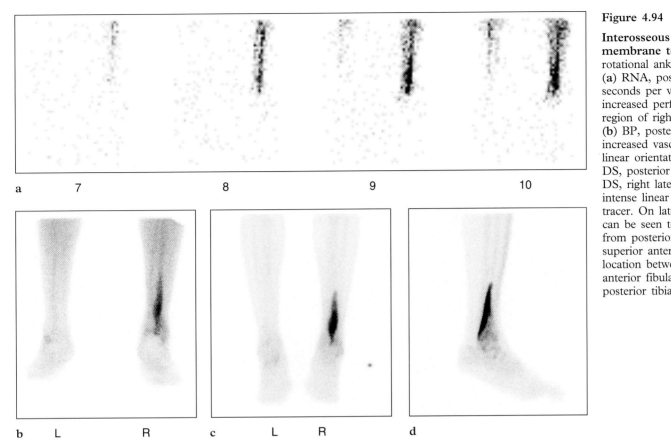

a   7   8   9   10

b   L   R   c   L   R   d

Figure 4.94

Interosseous membrane tear. Acute rotational ankle injury. (a) RNA, posterior, five seconds per view. Intense increased perfusion to region of right lower leg. (b) BP, posterior. Intense increased vascularity in a linear orientation. (c) DS, posterior and (d). DS, right lateral. Very intense linear increased tracer. On lateral view it can be seen to extend from posterior inferior to superior anterior in the location between the anterior fibula and posterior tibial cortex.

Teaching point

If surgical resection of HO is being considered to relieve pain, RNBI is used to determine when active ossification has ceased. Surgery during active ossification is often unsuccessful, with recurrence common.

Post-orthopedic intervention

Radionuclide bone imaging is ideally suited to aid the clinician in patient management after a variety of orthopedic interventions. Many issues and clinical questions relate to physiologic processes which can best be evaluated with three phase and SPECT bone imaging. These include normal and abnormal healing, biomechanical stress after the insertion of hardware or prostheses, graft viability, the presence and maturity of heterotopic ossification, pain of uncertain etiology and the significance of anatomic changes seen on plain radiographs, CT or MR imaging.

Both planar and SPECT radionuclide bone imaging are less affected by the presence of orthopedic hardware than are CT or MR imaging, so that the full range of radionuclide imaging options are available. For the imager to provide an optimal consultation, radionuclide image correlation with available anatomic images, and details of any operative procedures or treatments are necessary.

Hardware

Compression plates

Figure 4.95

Compression plate fixation, radial and ulnar shaft fractures. (a) DS, forearm. Minimal uptake underlying compression plates (seen in **b**) represents mild remodeling change. More focal uptake (long arrows) represents normal healing of screw tracks. (b) X-ray, left forearm. Compression plate with screw fixators. Fracture obscured. Good anatomic position and alignment.

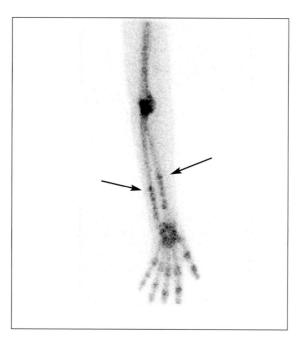

a

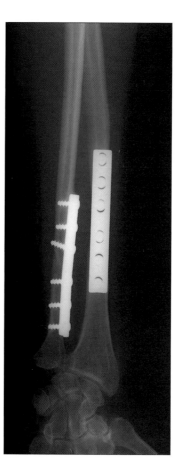

b

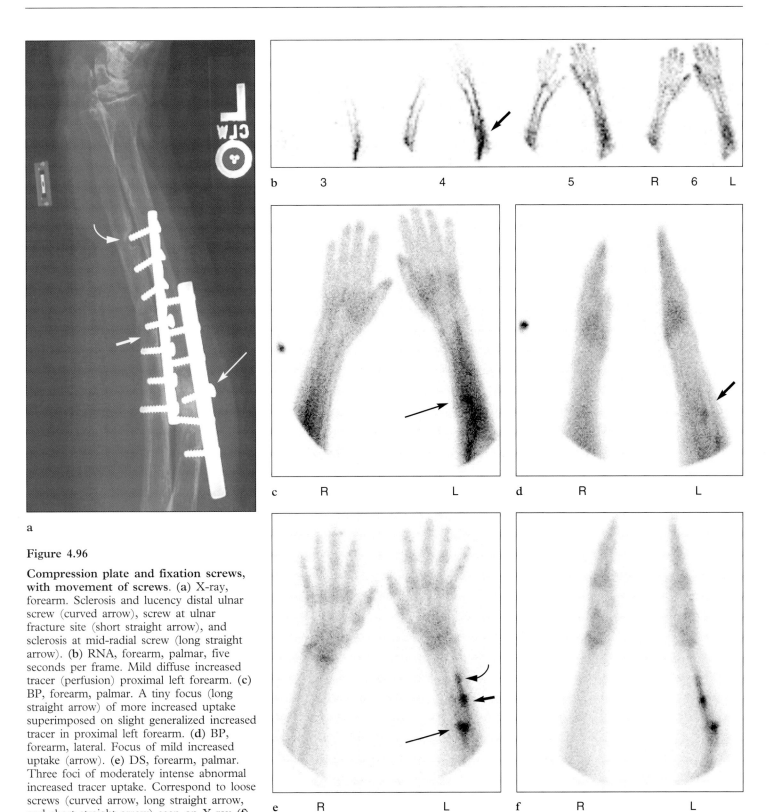

Figure 4.96

Compression plate and fixation screws, with movement of screws. (a) X-ray, forearm. Sclerosis and lucency distal ulnar screw (curved arrow), screw at ulnar fracture site (short straight arrow), and sclerosis at mid-radial screw (long straight arrow). (b) RNA, forearm, palmar, five seconds per frame. Mild diffuse increased tracer (perfusion) proximal left forearm. (c) BP, forearm, palmar. A tiny focus (long straight arrow) of more increased uptake superimposed on slight generalized increased tracer in proximal left forearm. (d) BP, forearm, lateral. Focus of mild increased uptake (arrow). (e) DS, forearm, palmar. Three foci of moderately intense abnormal increased tracer uptake. Correspond to loose screws (curved arrow, long straight arrow, and short straight arrow) seen on X-ray (f). DS, forearm, lateral.

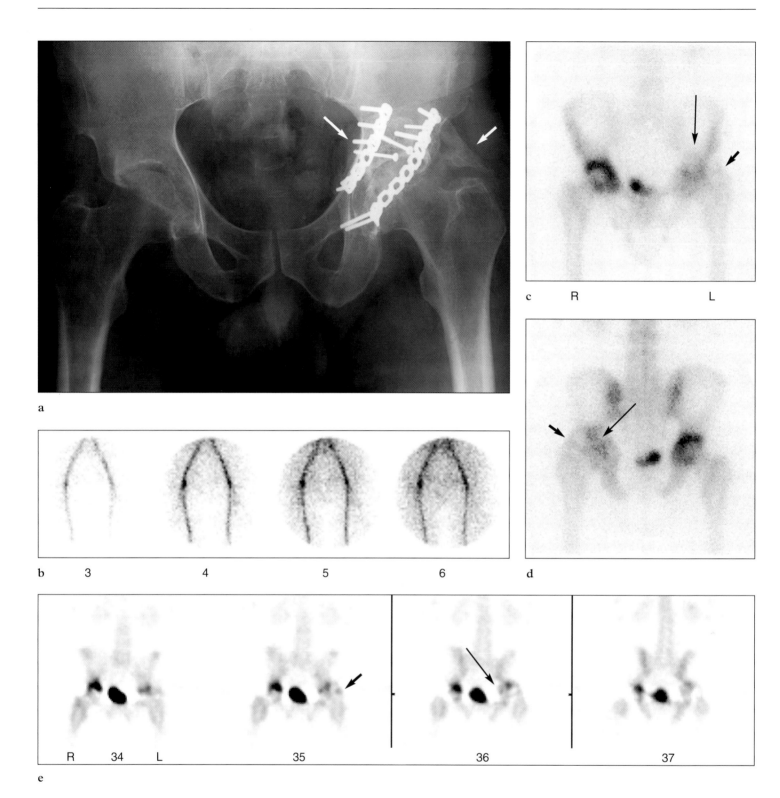

Figure 4.97

Acetabular fracture, compression bands with fixation screws and HO. (a) X-ray, pelvis. Compression bands and compression screws are seen (long straight arrow). Some mature HO (short straight arrow). (b) RNA, pelvis and hips anterior. Five seconds per view. No areas of abnormal increased perfusion. (c) DS, pelvis, anterior and (d) DS, pelvis, posterior demonstrate the mild activity associated with the healed acetabular fractures (long straight arrow).

The minimal, normometabolic activity of the mature HO seen best on the posterior view (short arrow). (e) SP, coronal images. The increased tracer associated with the healed acetabular fracture is seen best on these coronal images (long arrow). The HO is also seen (short arrow). Incidental degenerative change with increased activity at the superior lateral portion of the right acetabulum. The joint narowing at the right hip can also be seen on the radiograph (a).

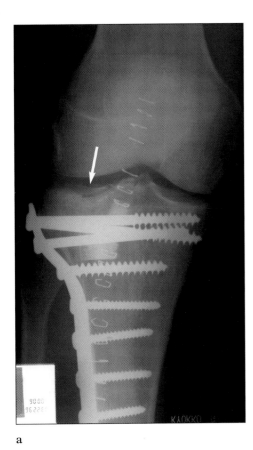

a

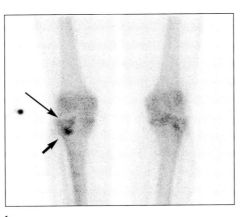

b

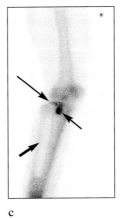

c

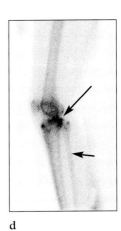

d

Figure 4.98

Tibial plateau fracture with compression plate and fixation screws. (a) X-ray, knee. The side plate and transverse fixation screws are seen as is the residua of the tibial plateau fracture (arrow). **(b)** DS, knee, anterior and **(c)** DS, right knee, lateral view. Minimally intense focal increased tracer at the articular surface represents the tibial plateau fracture (long straight arrow); the more intense but still well-defined activity in the PL tibia below the articular surface (short straight arrow) is associated with one of the upper fixation screws. The photon deficiency of the side plate is seen (thick arrow). Compare with **(d)**. **(d)** DS, left knee lateral. For comparison with **(c)**. Note the anterior and posterior tibial cortices and the more posterior fibula (short arrow). There is some minimal posterior stress remodeling change at the knee joint (long arrow).

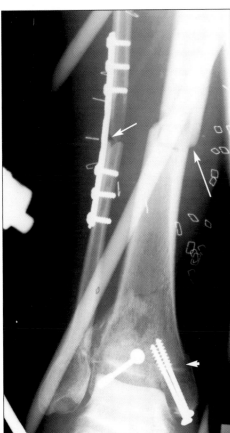

a

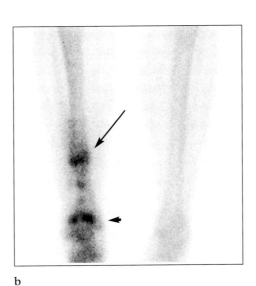

b

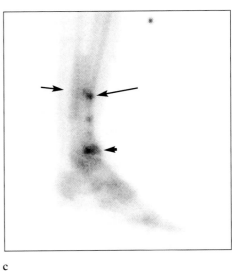

c

Figure 4.99

Healed fibula and tibial fractures with compression plates and fixation screws. (a) X-ray right leg, AP. The fibular compression plate bridges the fracture which is healing without the exuberant callus (short straight arrow). The mid-shaft tibial fracture (long straight arrow) and the screws through the medial malleolar fracture (arrowhead). **(b)** DS, leg and ankle, anterior and **(c)** DS, right lateral. The horizontal healing tibial fracture (long straight arrow) and the malleolar fractures (arrowhead) are seen. Activity beneath the compression plate (short straight arrow) is normal.

Fixators, screws, and cerclage wires

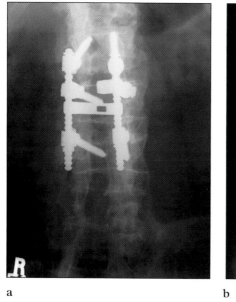

a

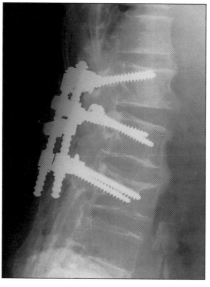

b

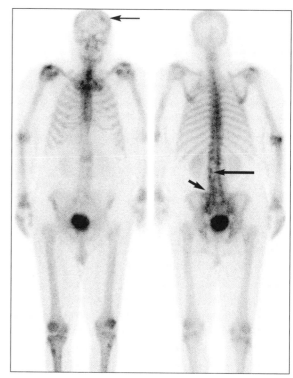

c

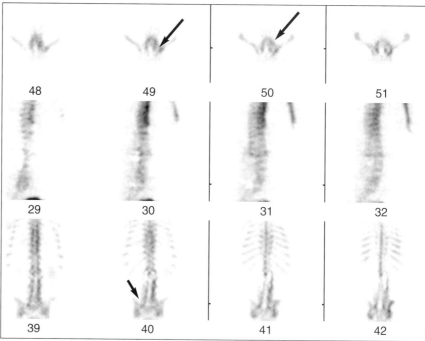

e

Figure 4.100

Extensive laminectomy and spinal fusion with Edward's rods and pedicle screws. (a) X-ray, AP and (b) lateral. The extensive laminectomy with the rods and pedicle screws stabilizing L1 and L3 vertebra. Solid, well-incorporated bone graft from L1 to S1. (c) WB. The photon deficiency associated with the laminectomy (long straight arrow) and the mild increased activity associated with the fusion mass (short straight arrow). Incidental somewhat linear activity in the left skull (thin arrow) is at the site of an old, well-healed, depressed, skull fracture. (d) 3-D volumetric images, selected views from 180° to 230°. The photon deficiency, fusion mass, and minimal focal increased uptake associated with pedicle screws are noted. (e) SPECT, triangulation display. The fusion mass (short straight arrow) and the marked photon deficiencies of the laminectomy are seen. There are, in addition, some stress changes in the upper thoracic spine which are nonspecific. In this case there is no significant increased metabolic activity associated with the fixation screws that have good purchase (i.e. holding tightly without movement).

Teaching point

SPECT imaging can be done even when there is significant metallic hardware present. The results are often surprisingly good.

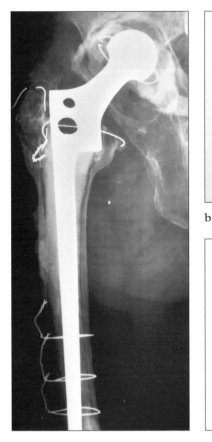

a

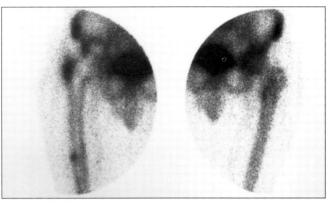

b

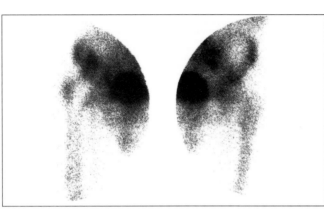

c

Figure 4.101

Total hip arthroplasty, cerclage wire fixation. (a) X-ray, anterior. Tip of the femoral component not seen on this view. Cerclage-type wires around greater and lesser trochanter are broken. They are intact around the distal portion of the femoral stem. (b) DS, anterior, six months following surgery. There is moderate increased activity associated with the healing greater trochanteric fragment. The small focus of increased tracer involving the distal lateral cortex, which was originally thought to represent activity at the tip of the femoral component of the prosthesis, but in retrospect is most likely associated with the upper distal femoral cerclage wire. There is no significant activity associated with the distal two wires. Photon deficiency of the prosthesis is noted. (c) DS, 16 months following surgery. There is less metabolic activity associated with the greater trochanteric fragment and no significant activity associated with the cerclage wires. Compare cerclage wires with those in Figure 4.111. (Study courtesy of Randall Winn, MD and reprinted with permission from *Skeletal Nuclear Medicine*, 1996 Mosby-Yearbook, Inc. Figure 14–16, page 278.)

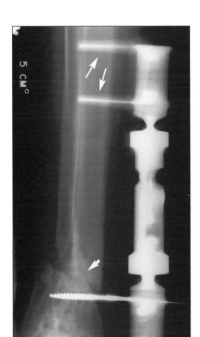

a

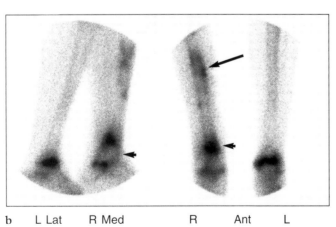

b   L Lat   R Med   R   Ant   L

Figure 4.102

Tibial fracture nonunion, distraction immobilization device with fixation screws. (a) X-ray, AP tomogram, selected image. The external distraction fixation device is noted. Horizontal fixation screws (straight arrow) and an area of nonunited tibial fracture (arrowhead). (b) DS, right medial, left lateral (left image), and anterior (right image). The activity around the screw holes (straight arrow) can be seen during the early and mid-stages of healing. The nonunited fracture (arrowheads) demonstrates reactive nonunion, with increased tracer on both sides of the fracture without visualization of the fracture line as a photon-deficient region.

Rods

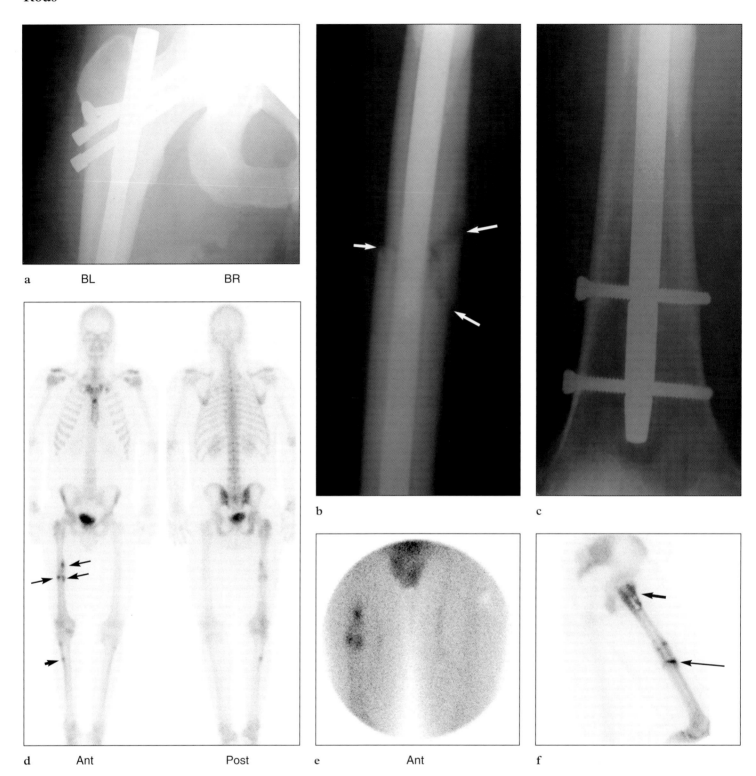

Figure 4.103

Healing femur fracture with intramedullary rod and proximal and distal screw fixation. (a) X-ray, femur, proximal third. (b) Middle third and (c) distal third. The intramedullary rod, screw fixation, and the comminuted fracture (short arrow). (d) WB. The three foci of healing fracture (short arrows). A healing fibular fracture (arrowhead). (e) BP, femur, anterior. The foci of increased tracer uptake (relative vascularity). (f) DS, hip and femur, right lateral. The healing femoral fracture foci are seen (long straight arrow). The photon deficiency of the rod extends into the proximal-most femur. Foci of mild increased uptake associated with the fixation screw in the proximal femur (short arrow) can be normal during the first months of healing and do not necessarily indicate loosening. Note, however, that the distal fixation screws do not show abnormal increased uptake.

Prosthesis

Shoulder

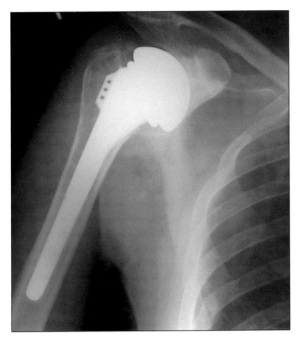

a

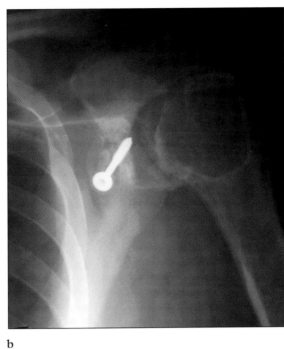

b

Figure 4.104 a–e

Shoulder arthroplasty, right shoulder, and Bankart's procedure left shoulder. Shoulder pain. **(a)** X-ray, right shoulder, AP. The shoulder arthroplasty. **(b)** X-ray, left shoulder, AP. Screw at inferior glenoid associated with Bankart's repair. **(c)** WB. Photon deficiency of head of prosthesis (long arrow). Minimal increased tracer uptake associated with screw in left shoulder (short arrows). **(d)** Biplane RNA. Anterior and **(e)** posterior, five seconds per frame. No area of increased perfusion to the area of the right shoulder (arrow).

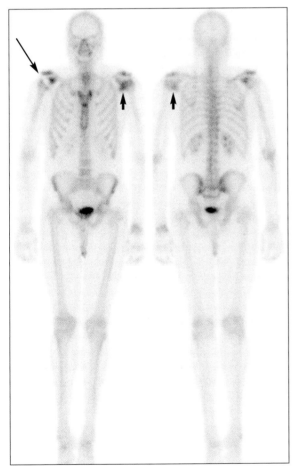

c   Ant   Post

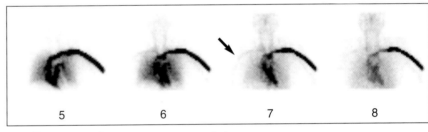

d   R   L   Ant

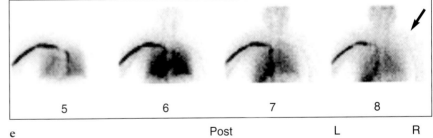

e   Post   L   R

continued

Teaching point

RNA images of the upper extremities and chest can be successfully viewed using window and leveling of digital images.

Figure 4.104 f–k

(**f**) BP, chest and shoulders, anterior, and (**g**) BP, right lateral, and (**h**) BP, left lateral. Photon deficiency associated with the metallic prosthetic head on anterior and lateral view and with the stem on lateral view (arrows) without any surrounding increased uptake (relative vascularity). The left lateral is for comparison. Note the mild increased tracer uptake (relative vascularity) posteriorly (arrowhead). (**i**) DS, right lateral and (**j**) DS, left lateral. On the symptomatic right side there is some mild-to-moderate increased tracer accumulation in the posterior glenoid (arrow). On the less symptomatic left side, abnormal increased tracer involves both the posterior glenoid humeral joint area as well as milder uptake involving other portions of the joint. (**k**) SPECT, triangulation display. Transaxial images through plane of humeral heads, sagittal images through the mid-line. The increased activity associated with the screw fixation on the left is well seen on the coronal images (long thin arrow). The increased glenoid uptake on the right is well seen on the transaxial image (short arrow).

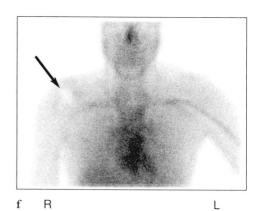

f   R   L

g   h   i   j

63	64	65	66	67
63	64	65	66	67
61	62	63	64	65

k

Hip

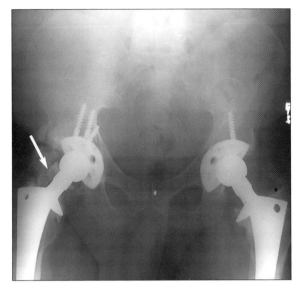

a

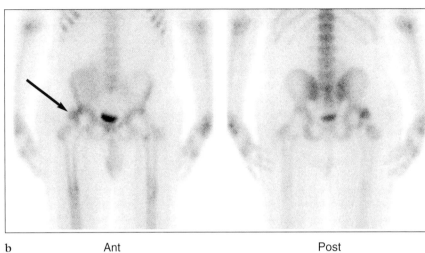

b   Ant   Post

Figure 4.105

Normal bilateral hip prosthesis. A 33-year-old male with renal transplant. Steroid therapy. **(a)** Pelvis, AP. Bilateral total arthroplasty with screw fixation of acetabular components. Bone fragments on the right (arrow). **(b)** WB, mid-portion. The photon deficiencies associated with bilateral prosthesis are noted. There is mild increased metabolic activity associated with the incompletely incorporated bone fragments (arrow).

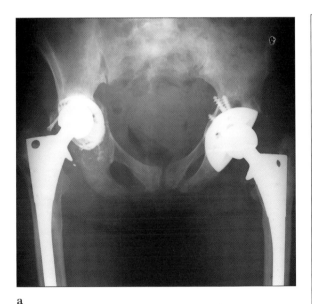

a

Teaching point

The differential diagnosis of patients who present with pain after hip arthroplasty includes: (1) HO, (2) loosening, (3) infection, (4) refracture, and (5) abnormal biomechanics with new focal stress loading or (6) a low tolerance for pain.

Figure 4.106 a and b

Loose acetabular component of left total arthroplasty. Patient with sickle-cell anemia. **(a)** X-ray, pelvis, AP. Bilateral arthroplasty. Note superior lateral acetabular sclerosis on right and lucency on left. Bony changes of anemia. **(b)** WB. Moderately intense, homogeneous, increased tracer uptake in entire acetabulum. Uptake in right proximal humerus associated with repairing infarct. Focal uptake in a small splenic infarct (arrow) seen on posterior view.

b   Ant   Post

continued

Figure 4.106 c–f

(c) RNA, anterior, five seconds per view. No area of increased tracer uptake (perfusion). (d) BP, anterior. No abnormal increased tracer uptake. Photon deficiencies associated with metallic prosthetic heads (arrows). (e) 3-D volumetric display, reprojection images, selected views from 180° to 230°. Homogeneous uptake involving the acetabulum. (f) SPECT, coronal images. The most minimal increased tracer uptake at the interface between the distal tip of the femoral stem component and the femoral cortex (arrows) is normal.

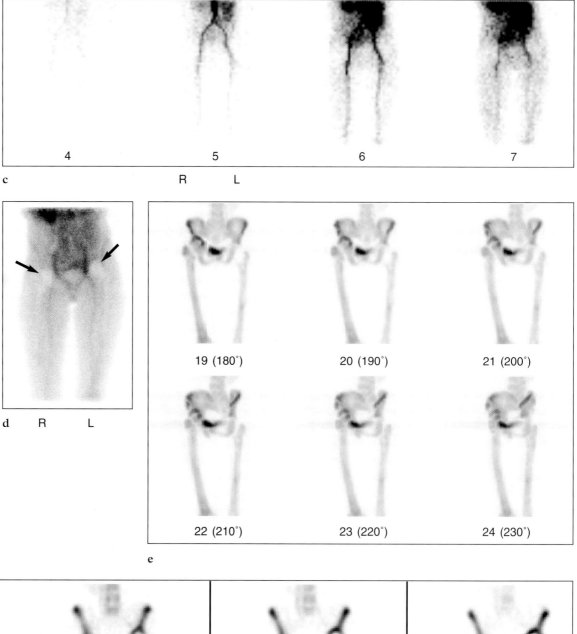

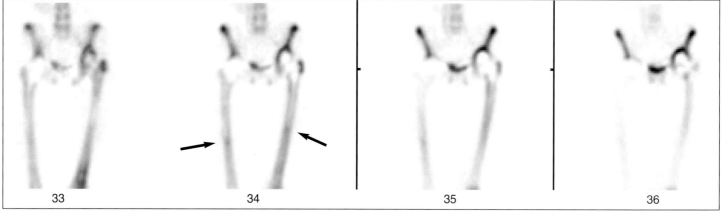

Figure 4.107

Loose femoral component hip arthroplasty. Noncemented, nonporous, coated prosthesis. (**a**) X-ray, cone-down view of distal tip. Focal sclerosis (arrow). (**b**) DS, femur, anterior. Intense focal increased tracer uptake associated with the tip of the prosthesis. Medial cortical uptake proximal to the tip represents abnormal stress-loading response.

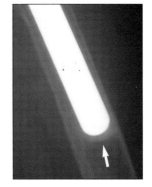

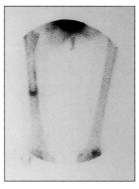

a   b   R   Ant   L

Knee

Figure 4.108 a–c

Total knee arthroplasty, five months prior to bone scan. A 55-year-old female with pain. Final diagnosis was prolonged healing, stress remodeling, suprapatellar inflammation without infection. (**a**) X-ray, knee, anterior and (**b**) lateral. Prominent soft tissue fullness including the suprapatellar bursa. (**c**) WB. Mild-to-moderate activity in both the distal femoral and proximal tibial regions beneath the metallic prosthesis, which appears as a photon deficiency. The area of most marked uptake in the tibia is medial (straight arrow).

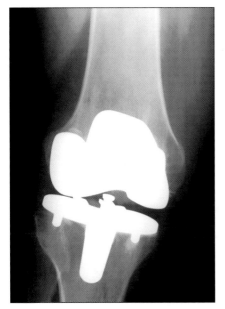

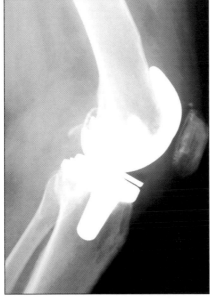

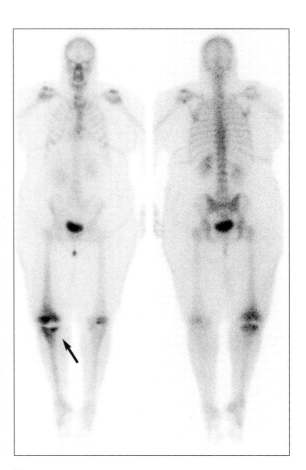

a   b   c

Teaching point

Gallium-67 or other infection-imaging radiopharmaceuticals can be utilized to provide further differential diagnosis between increased tracer uptake secondary to repair only and increased tracer uptake as a response to an infection involving the bone. When the ratio of abnormal bone uptake to normal bone uptake is greater than the ratio of gallium uptake in abnormal bone to gallium uptake in normal bone, then infection is considered much less likely.

continued

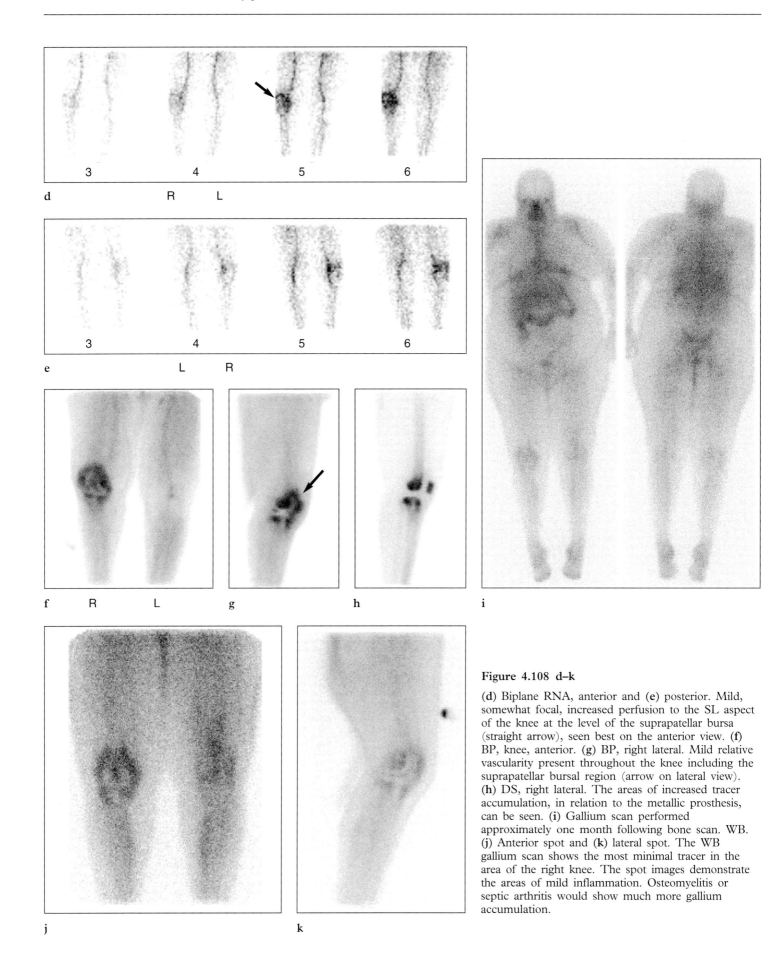

Figure 4.108 d–k

(d) Biplane RNA, anterior and (e) posterior. Mild, somewhat focal, increased perfusion to the SL aspect of the knee at the level of the suprapatellar bursa (straight arrow), seen best on the anterior view. (f) BP, knee, anterior. (g) BP, right lateral. Mild relative vascularity present throughout the knee including the suprapatellar bursal region (arrow on lateral view). (h) DS, right lateral. The areas of increased tracer accumulation, in relation to the metallic prosthesis, can be seen. (i) Gallium scan performed approximately one month following bone scan. WB. (j) Anterior spot and (k) lateral spot. The WB gallium scan shows the most minimal tracer in the area of the right knee. The spot images demonstrate the areas of mild inflammation. Osteomyelitis or septic arthritis would show much more gallium accumulation.

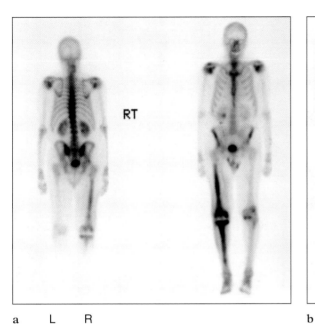

a   L   R

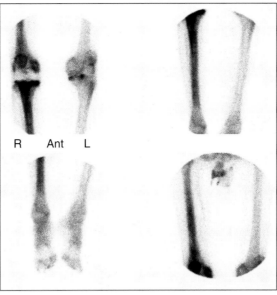

R   Ant   L

b

Figure 4.109

Total knee arthroplasty, normal healing with increased femoral and tibial shaft uptake, secondary to medullary cavity trauma that is associated with insertion of metallic alignment rods during surgery. (a) Initial scan one month following surgery. WB. Increased tracer uptake throughout the femoral and tibial shafts. (b) Follow-up scan 2½ months following initial scan. Patient less symptomatic. Femoral and tibial shaft activity still present but relatively less intense.

Limb salvage surgery

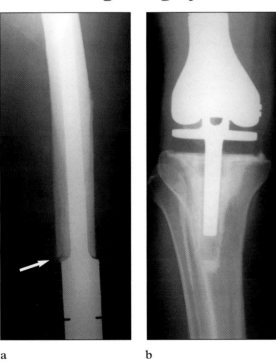

a   b

Teaching point

The operating surgeon should be consulted prior to evaluating postoperative images after complex surgery. Knowledge of the procedure, the use of autograft bone harvested from the medullary canal or elsewhere, and the expected locations of stress loading of the particular prosthesis are as important as knowing the metastatic and recurrence characteristics of the resected tumor.

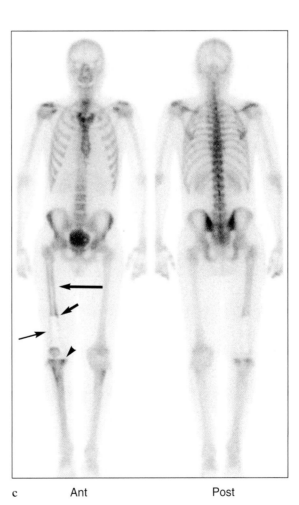

c   Ant   Post

Figure 4.110 a–c

Right femur, malignant fibrous histiocytoma, limb salvage surgery. (a) X-ray, femur and (b) X-ray, knee. Resection of the distal-most femur with insertion of metallic prosthesis. Intramedullary stem is seen entering the native femur proximally (arrow in **a**). A small amount of cancellous autograft is often used at this location. The distal portion of the femoral prosthesis in this case involves total joint replacement. The stem of the tibial component enters the proximal tibia. (c) WB. The photon deficiency associated with resected bone and metal prosthesis (thin arrow), mild-to-moderate cortical activity surrounding the stem within the proximal femur (long arrow), activity associated with incorporating autograft bone (short arrow), and a focus of biomechanical stress medially beneath the tibial component (arrowhead).

continued

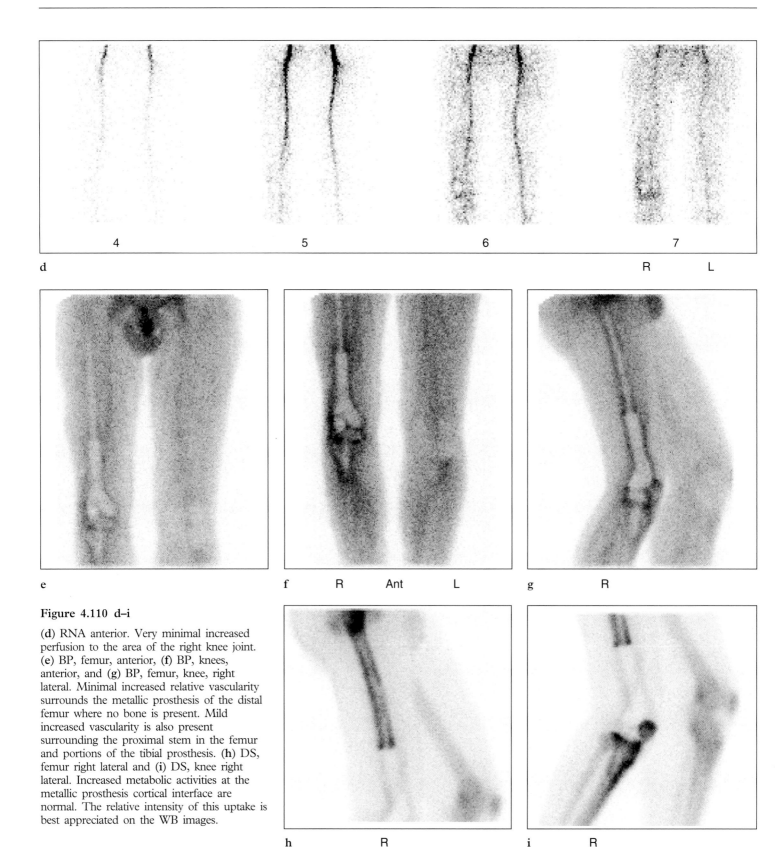

Figure 4.110 d–i

(**d**) RNA anterior. Very minimal increased perfusion to the area of the right knee joint. (**e**) BP, femur, anterior, (**f**) BP, knees, anterior, and (**g**) BP, femur, knee, right lateral. Minimal increased relative vascularity surrounds the metallic prosthesis of the distal femur where no bone is present. Mild increased vascularity is also present surrounding the proximal stem in the femur and portions of the tibial prosthesis. (**h**) DS, femur right lateral and (**i**) DS, knee right lateral. Increased metabolic activities at the metallic prosthesis cortical interface are normal. The relative intensity of this uptake is best appreciated on the WB images.

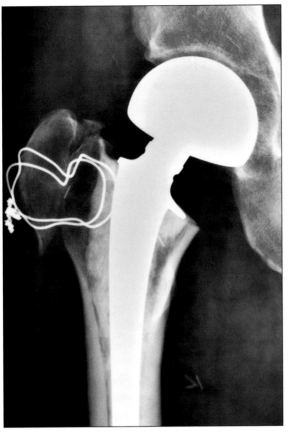

a

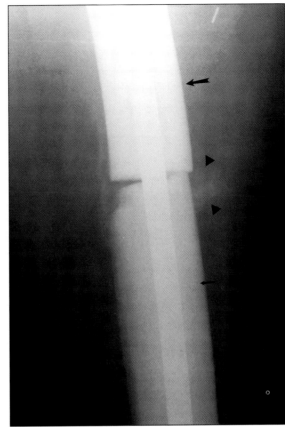

b

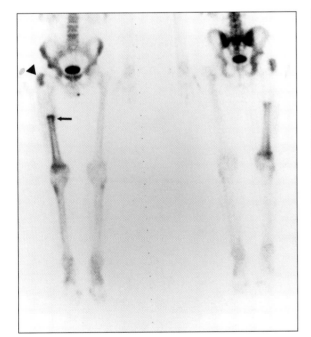

c

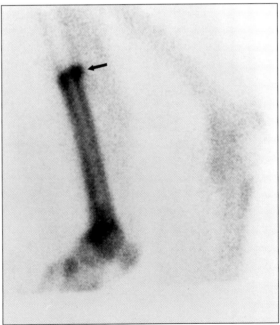

d

Figure 4.111

Femur and hip, chondrosarcoma proximal femur; limb salvage surgery. (a) X-ray, proximal femur and hip. Metallic femoral prosthesis, cerclage wires immobilizing greater trochanteric fragment. (b) X-ray, mid-femur. Intramedullary stem of metallic prosthesis bridges upper proximal allograft (large arrow) and native femur distally (small arrow). A small amount of cancellous autograft is present (arrowheads). (c) WB. Mild-to-moderate activity associated with greater trochanteric fragment (arrowhead), photon deficiency associated with metallic prosthesis and the allograft, minimal increased focal activity associated with the cancellous autograft (arrow), and mild activity associated with the native bone surrounding the metallic stem. (d) DS, lower femur, lateral. The lip of anterior activity associated with the cancellous autograft (arrow) at the junction between the photon-deficient proximal allograft and the distal native bone is normal.

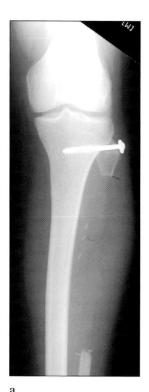

a

Figure 4.112 a–g

Proximal fibula, fibrosarcoma. Limb salvage surgery with resection of fibula only. (a) X-ray, tibia, AP. Lag screw overlies the proximal fibular head entering the proximal tibia. (b) CT, transaxial sections above, and through the lag screw. Lag screw fixes fibular remnant proximally to the tibia. The loss of sharp detail due to metal artifact can be appreciated. (c) WB, mild-to-moderate increased activity at the residual fibular head (arrow) just above the photon deficiency of the resected fibula. (d) RNA, anterior, and (e) RNA, posterior. Very minimal increased uptake, left calf with a minimal amount of focality at the proximal fibula (arrow). (f) BP, posterior. The minimal focal increased uptake at the proximal fibula (arrow). Beneath this uptake is the very slight increased uptake (relative vascularity) associated with the soft tissues at the site of resection. (g) DS, leg, left lateral. The photon deficiency associated with the fibula can be seen with the minimal uptake at the proximal fibula (short arrow) and the most minimal increased activity at the proximal aspect of the distal portion of the native bone (thin arrow). In this slightly obliqued view, the posterior tibial cortex is not optimally visualized at the resection site.

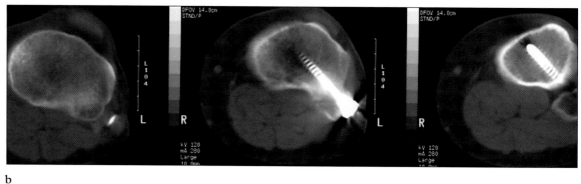

b

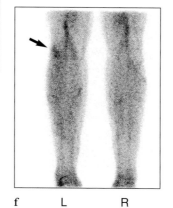

c

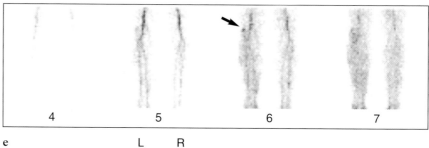

d   R   L

e   L   R

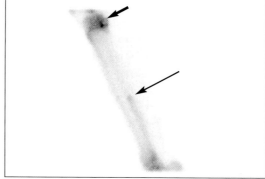

f   L   R   g

continued

Figure 4.112 h

(h) 3-D volumetric reprojection images. Selected views from 180° to 230°. In this view the minimal increased uptake associated with the distal native bone (arrow) can be nicely appreciated. This study demonstrates the ability to perform SPECT imaging when metal is in place. The increased uptake associated with the lag screw is normal healing and decreased on subsequent studies.

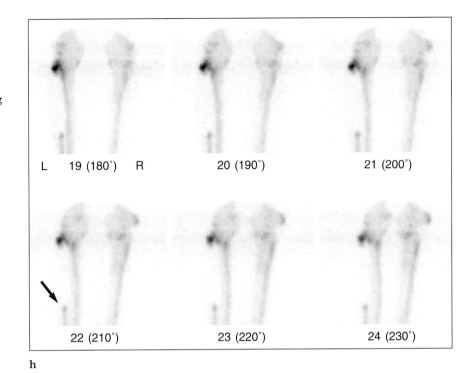

h

Bone replacement

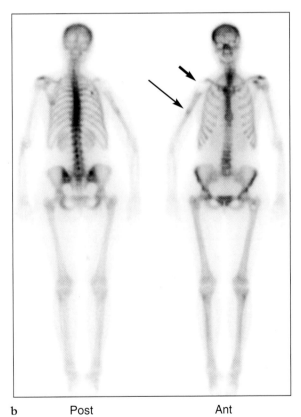

a

b　　Post　　　　　　Ant

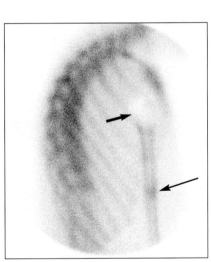

c

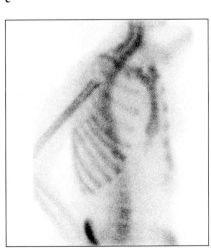

d

Figure 4.113 a–d

Limb salvage surgery with removal of right proximal humerus, right distal clavicle, and right scapula. Right scapular osteosarcoma. Insertion of metallic humeral prosthesis. (a) X-ray, AP. Postoperative. Showing resection and prosthesis replacement. (b) WB. Photon deficiency associated with the absent proximal humerus and metallic prosthesis (arrow). Minimal increased uptake at the tip of the stem of the prosthesis – bone interface (thin arrow). (c) DS, right lateral. Orthogonal view of photon deficiency (arrow) and focal stress (thin arrow). (d) DS, posterior, slight oblique. The absent scapular activity is accentuated.

continued

Figure 4.113 e and f

(e) X-ray, humerus. After removal of prosthesis and insertion of bone fragments. (f) WB. After bone chip insertion. Activity at the tip of the prosthesis, on prior study, has resolved. Mild diffuse activity associated with the mid-right humerus is a post-surgical stress response. It usually takes many months for surgically placed bone chips to become incorporated and to develop normal metabolic activity.

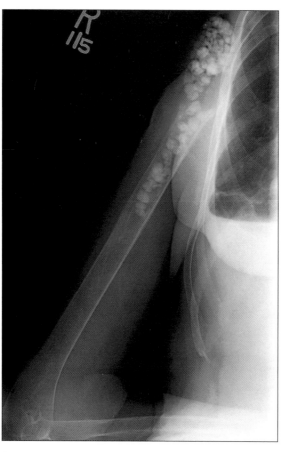

e

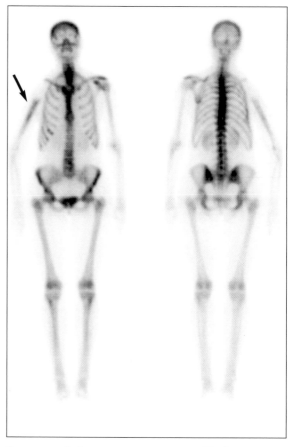

f   Ant   Post

Figure 4.114 a and b

T12 to L2 stabilization after vertebral body resection, allograft placement, with Edward's rods and pedicle screw fixation. Scan six months following surgery. Diagnosis after surgery was aspergillosis osteomyelitis which occurred five months after heart transplantation. (a) X-ray, AP, and (b) X-ray, right lateral. Allograft bone block (arrowheads), rods (long arrows), and screws (short arrows) are seen.

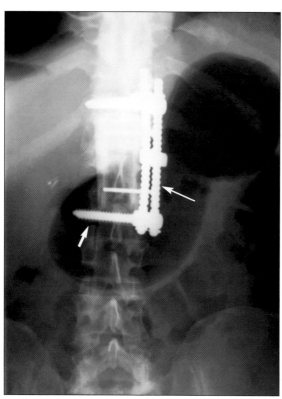

a

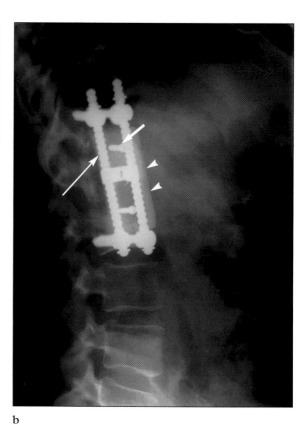

b

continued

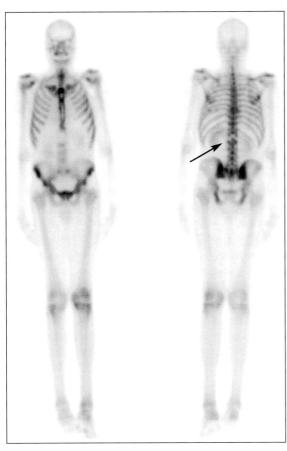

c

Figure 4.114 c and d

(c) WB. Six months after spinal surgery and eight months after dehiscence of median sternotomy site. The photon deficiency associated with the bone block (thin arrow) and healing changes associated with median sternotomy are seen. (d) SPECT, sagittal through the mid-line. Photon deficiency associated with the bone block (short arrow). Minimal increased uptake (long arrow) associated with some stress remodeling changes which are, in turn, associated with the fixation screws.

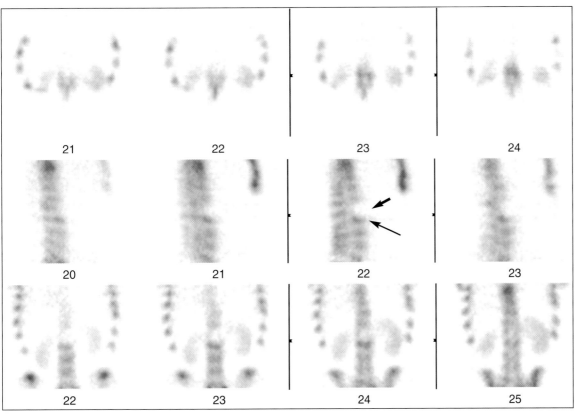

d

Heterotopic ossification

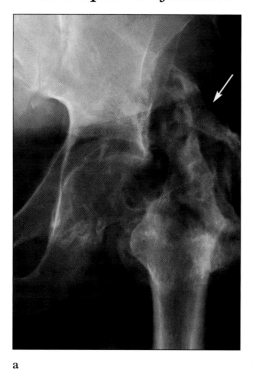

a

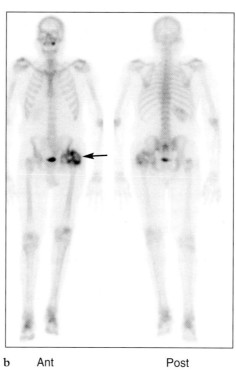

b   Ant   Post

Figure 4.115

Heterotopic ossification, mature, post-girdlestone procedure. (a) X-ray. The mature-appearing heterotopic bone (arrow). **(b)** WB. The increased tracer associated with HO. A focus of slightly more intense uptake (arrow) is a site of greatest biomechanical stress. **(c)** RNA, anterior. There is no increased tracer accumulation (perfusion) to the region of the left hip. Incidental, focal, increased perfusion just overlying and medial to the left iliac artery (arrow) represents perfusion to a transplanted kidney in the left iliac fossa. **(d)** BP, anterior. No increased tracer uptake (relative vascularity) to the left hip region. The transplanted kidney is seen. **(e)** 3-D volumetric reprojection images. Selected views from 0° to 90°. The location of the HO is appreciated. **(f)** 3-D reprojection images, magnified. Selected view from 0° to 50°. With magnification, detail of the greatest metabolic activity (tracer uptake) can be appreciated.

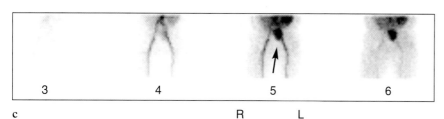

3   4   5   6

c   R   L

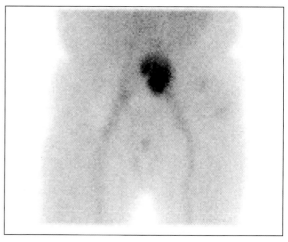

d   R   L

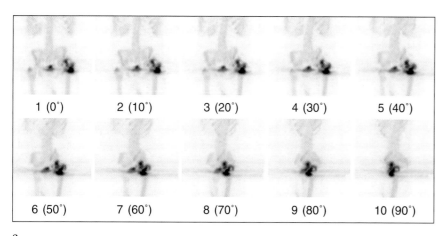

1 (0°)   2 (10°)   3 (20°)   4 (30°)   5 (40°)

6 (50°)   7 (60°)   8 (70°)   9 (80°)   10 (90°)

e

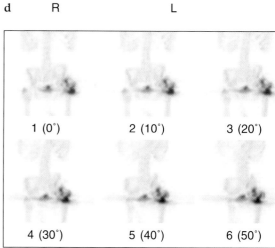

1 (0°)   2 (10°)   3 (20°)

4 (30°)   5 (40°)   6 (50°)

f

Teaching point

RNA and BP images help characterize the rate of metabolic activity present, and help ascertain the stage of a process. When the rate of bone turnover is highest, such as during the early stages of HO formation, the RNA and BP images will be abnormal. As the rate of repair slows down, first the RNA and then the BP images become normal.

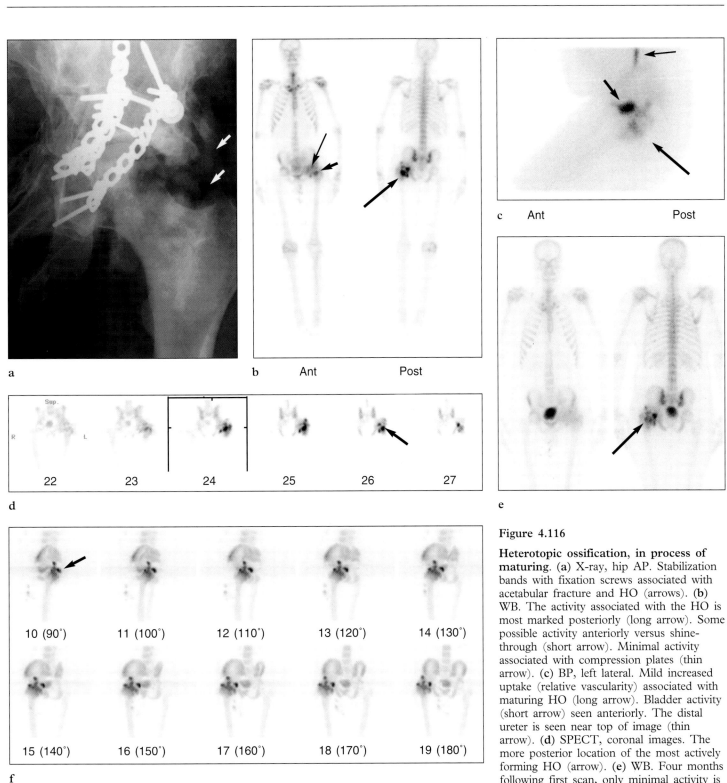

Figure 4.116

Heterotopic ossification, in process of maturing. (**a**) X-ray, hip AP. Stabilization bands with fixation screws associated with acetabular fracture and HO (arrows). (**b**) WB. The activity associated with the HO is most marked posteriorly (long arrow). Some possible activity anteriorly versus shine-through (short arrow). Minimal activity associated with compression plates (thin arrow). (**c**) BP, left lateral. Mild increased uptake (relative vascularity) associated with maturing HO (long arrow). Bladder activity (short arrow) seen anteriorly. The distal ureter is seen near top of image (thin arrow). (**d**) SPECT, coronal images. The more posterior location of the most actively forming HO (arrow). (**e**) WB. Four months following first scan, only minimal activity is now appreciated anteriorly. The most intense posterior focus seen earlier is now much less intense (long arrow). (**f**) 3-D reprojection images, selected views from 90° to 180°. The posterior location of the HO can be appreciated (short arrow). (**g**) SPECT coronal, four months following the initial study. The change from the most actively forming HO on the earlier study is noted (arrow) with interval decrease in metabolic activity.

Figure 4.117

Actively maturing HO.
Healing compound mid-
femur fracture with
internal fixation. (**a**)
RNA, thigh, anterior.
Mild, somewhat focal
(arrow) increased tracer
uptake, lateral aspect
right thigh. (**b**) BP,
thigh, anterior, and (**c**)
BP, thigh, right lateral.
The anterior lateral
location of the increased
tracer uptake (increased
relative vascularity)
(arrow). (**d**) DS, thigh,
anterior. The increased
tracer associated with the
healing fracture can be
appreciated with more
focal lateral activity
(arrow) of the actively
metabolizing HO
identified.

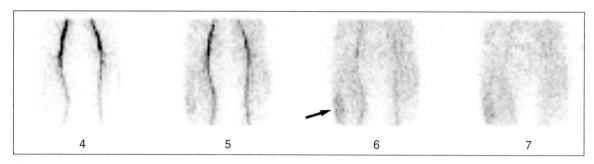

a

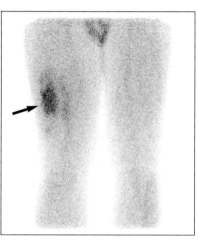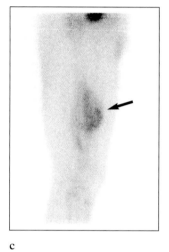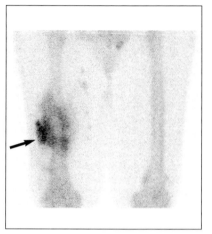

b   c   d

Figure 4.118 a–b

Mature HO, distal
femur. Status after
below-the-knee
amputation. (**a**) X-ray,
anterior, and (**b**) X-ray,
left lateral. Bridging HO
(arrow) between the
distal native fibula and
distal tibia.

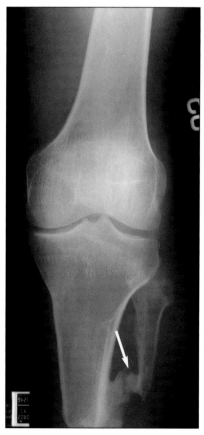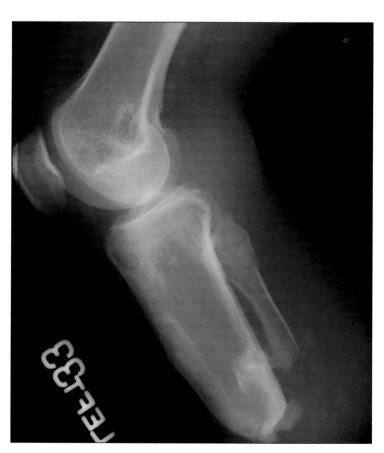

continued   a

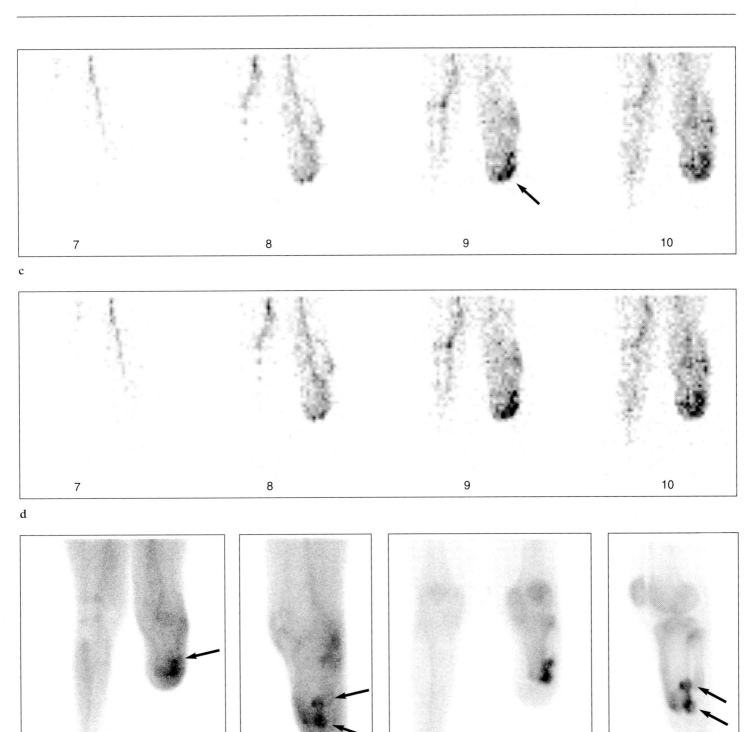

Figure 4.118 c–h

(c) RNA, anterior, and (d) RNA, posterior. Mild increased perfusion to the distal-most aspects of the native leg above the level of the amputation. As appreciated on the anterior view, it is slightly more focal distally and laterally (arrow) where the patient's stump abuts his prosthesis. (e) BP, anterior, and (f) BP, left lateral. There is less increased tracer associated with the surface soft tissues, but some mild-to-moderate, more focal, increased tracer uptake in the area of HO (arrows). (g) DS, anterior, and (h) DS, left lateral. The areas of HO (arrows) demonstrate moderate, very well-defined uptake. The distal fibula is particularly well seen.

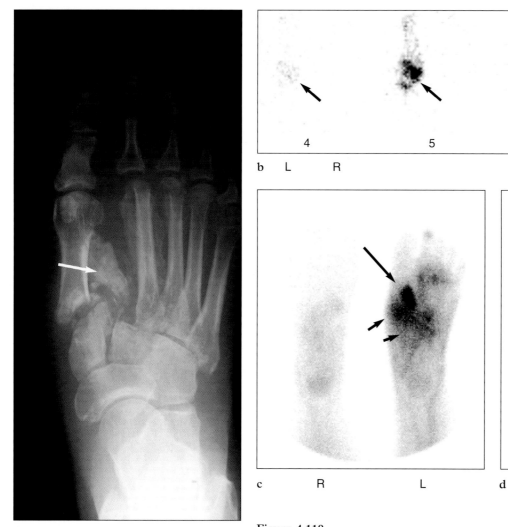

a

b   L   R

4   5   6   7

c   R   L   d   R   L

Figure 4.119

Heterotopic ossification, left foot. Patient with right foot cellulites, Lisfranc's fracture, and underlying diabetes mellitus, being evaluated for osteomyelitis. **(a)** X-ray, AP. Changes at the metatarsal joints with dislocation and neuropathic changes. Exuberant callus surrounds the second and third metatarsal shafts. HO (arrow). **(b)** RNA. Moderate increased perfusion to the area of the left mid-foot. More focal perfusion (arrows) will correspond to the HO seen on BP and delayed images. **(c)** BP, plantar. The intense, but well-defined, focal tracer uptake (arrow) corresponds to the HO. Mild activity at the tarsometatarsal joints (short arrows) associated with some continued inflammation at the site of the Lisfranc fractures and neuropathic changes. **(d)** DS, plantar. The area of greatest uptake is associated with the HO (arrow). Mild increased activity associated with the HO around the second metatarsal shaft.

Teaching point

When there is a need to evaluate relative vascularity in multiple areas, manifested by increased tracer accumulation on the immediate post-injection BP or tissue phase images, then a WB BP should be considered. Because the half-time of tracer movement from the intravascular to the extravascular, extracellular space is 2–3 minutes, a rapid acquisition is required, not only for a WB BP, but for multiple BP images taken by spot technique.

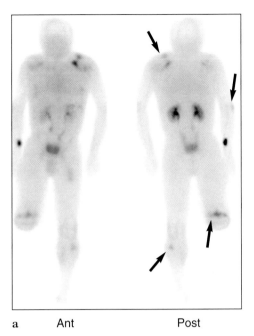
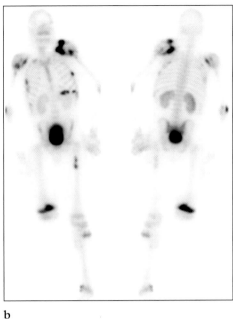

a   Ant   Post   b

Figure 4.120

Multifocal, actively maturing HO. Patient is two weeks status after motor vehicle crash with acute amputation below right knee. Soft tissues normal on X-ray. **(a)** WB BP obtained immediately after injection using WB scanning table with scan speed at 16 cm per minute. Increased relative vascularity around multiple joints (arrows). **(b)** WB. Intense abnormal activity about the shoulder, right elbow, distal femur, and proximal fibula represents actively metabolizing HO. Healing fractures also noted throughout. Prominent renal uptake secondary to multiple blood transfusions.

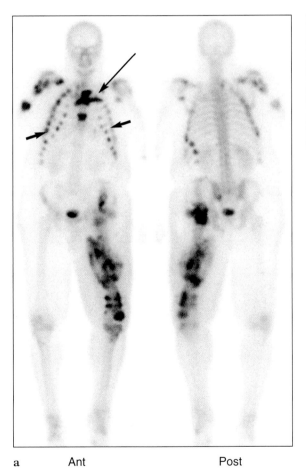

a   Ant   Post

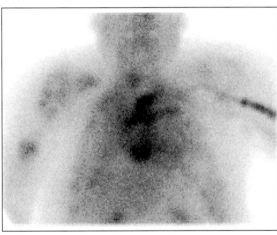

b

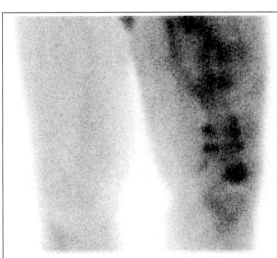

c

Figure 4.121

Heterotopic ossification, multifocal, following motor vehicle crash. **(a)** WB. Multiple areas of HO around the left femur and right shoulder. The typical appearance of sternal (long thin arrow) and rib (short arrows) fractures from a steering wheel injury is apparent. **(b)** BP, chest, anterior, and **(c)** BP, thigh, anterior. BP images demonstrate increased tracer uptake (relative vascularity) associated with actively metabolizing HO. The femur **(c)** is taken after the chest **(b)** and the more intense uptake is partially due to early fixation of tracer.

Postoperative stress

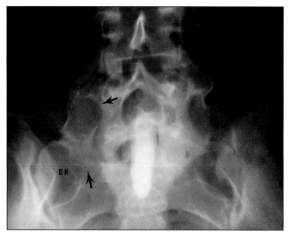

a

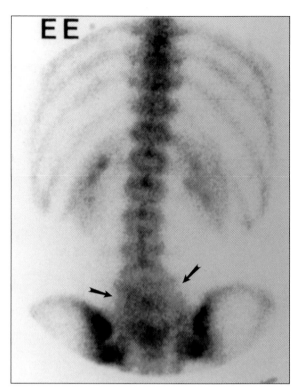

b

Figure 4.122

Lumbosacral laminectomy and fusion. Healed fusion mass. **(a)** X-ray, AP. Bilateral fusion mass best seen on right (arrows). Incidental radio-opaque contrast in the lumbar subarachnoid space. **(b)** DS, posterior. The fusion mass has the same relative tracer uptake as the adjacent normal bone. (Reprinted with permission, *Skeletal Nuclear Medicine*; Collier, Fogelmann and Rosenthal, Mosby-Year Book, Inc., Chicago, 1996. Chapter 13, Figure 13-18.)

Figure 4.123 a and b

Biomechanical stress, four years following spinal fusion of L3 to S1. **(a)** X-ray, lower lumbosacral spine, AP, and **(b)** X-ray, lateral. Fusion mass (thick arrows), osteophytes (short thin arrow), joint narrowing with retrolisthesis (long thin arrow).

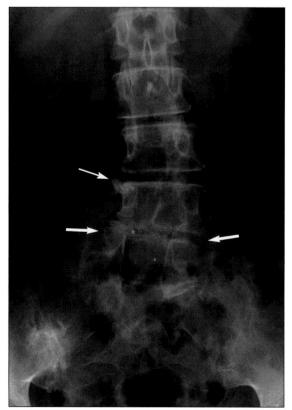

a

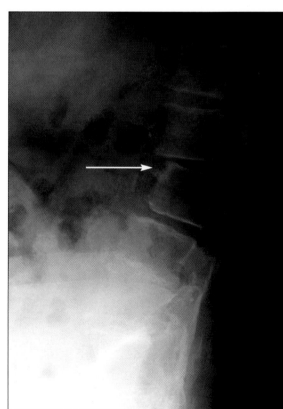

b

continued

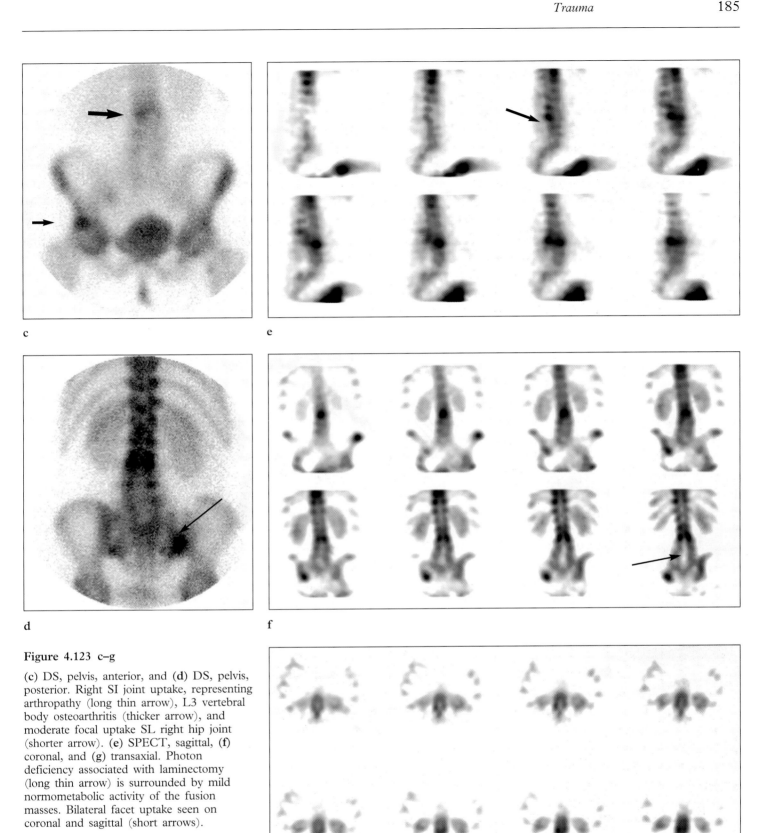

c

d

e

f

g

Figure 4.123 c–g

(c) DS, pelvis, anterior, and (d) DS, pelvis, posterior. Right SI joint uptake, representing arthropathy (long thin arrow), L3 vertebral body osteoarthritis (thicker arrow), and moderate focal uptake SL right hip joint (shorter arrow). (e) SPECT, sagittal, (f) coronal, and (g) transaxial. Photon deficiency associated with laminectomy (long thin arrow) is surrounded by mild normometabolic activity of the fusion masses. Bilateral facet uptake seen on coronal and sagittal (short arrows).

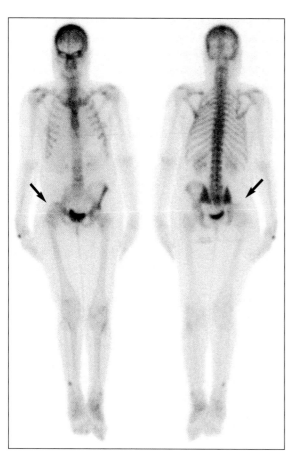

a   Ant   Post

Figure 4.124 a–c

Hemipelvectomy, normal postoperative stress. Chondrosarcoma right ileum. (a) WB. The site of the surgery (arrows). Note the subtle difference in position of the knees as a result of the minor superior luxation of the right femur. (b) 3-D volumetric reprojection images. Selected views from 0° to 50°. Normal postoperative stress at the sacrum (arrow). (c) SPECT, triangulation display. Mild increased tracer uptake at the operative site where the minimal residual ilium meets the sacrum (arrows).

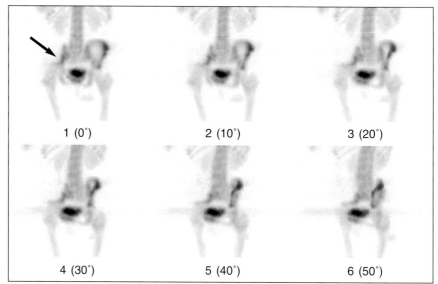

| 1 (0°) | 2 (10°) | 3 (20°) |
| 4 (30°) | 5 (40°) | 6 (50°) |

b

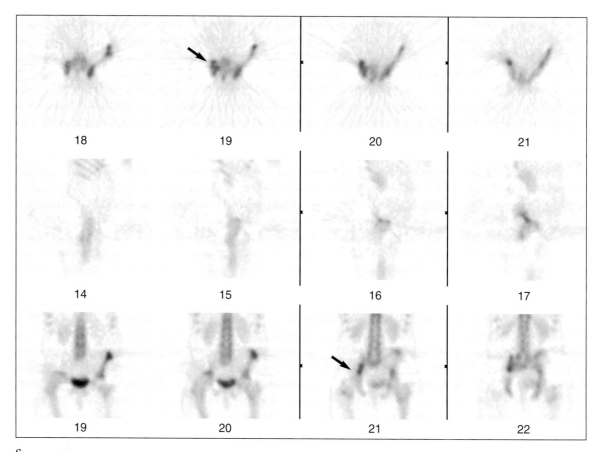

18	19	20	21
14	15	16	17
19	20	21	22

continued

c

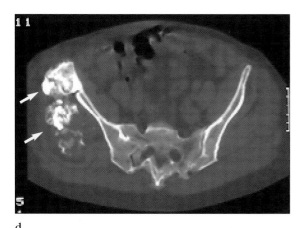

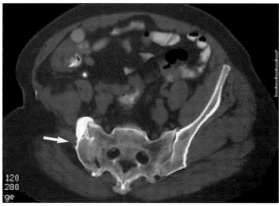

d   e

Figure 4.124 d and e

(**d**) CT, sacrum, preoperative. The chondroid calcification involving the ilium and extending into the soft tissues (arrows). (**e**) CT, postoperative. The sclerosis at the operative site (arrow) can be contrasted to the normal left side.

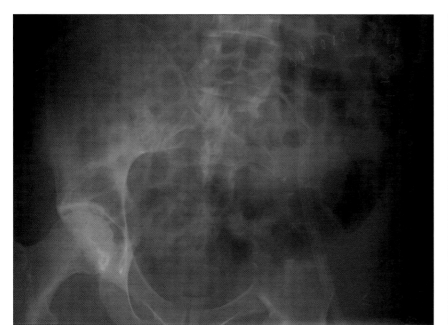

a

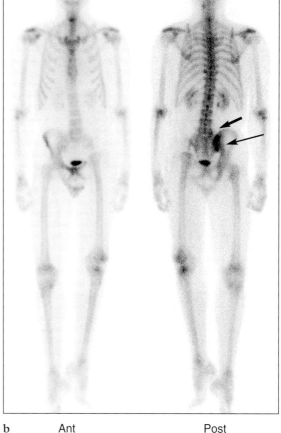

b   Ant   Post

Figure 4.125

Chondrosarcoma, hemipelvectomy. Ipsilateral SI and L5–S1 postoperative degenerative changes. (**a**) X-ray, pelvis, AP. Postoperative left hemipelvectomy. (**b**) WB. Mild-to-moderate, focal, increased tracer uptake at the right S1 joint (long thin arrow on posterior view) and at the lateral aspects of L5–S1 (short arrow). Note the greater discrepancy in relative position of the knees and the mild increased metabolic activity there, all resulting from abnormal postoperative biomechanical stress.

Teaching point

RNBI follow-up after tumor surgery is designed to detect foci of abnormal increased tracer accumulation. Although most will be associated with remodeling secondary to altered biomechanical stress, each abnormal focus must be further investigated with other more anatomic imaging modalities, such as CT or MR, and even then biopsy may still be required for diagnosis.

Normal healing

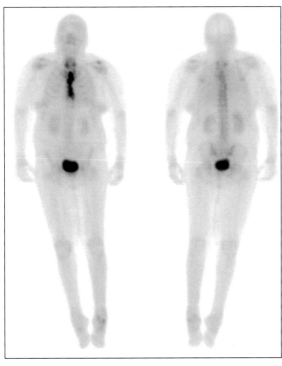

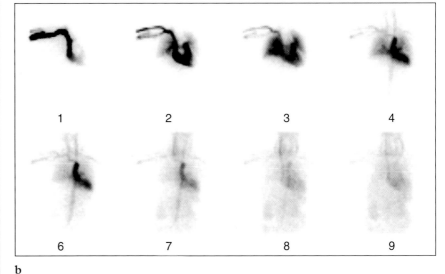

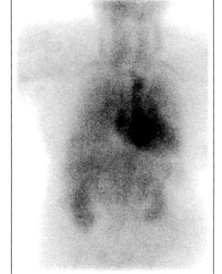

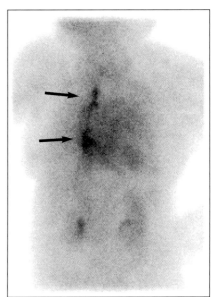

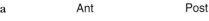

a   Ant   Post

Figure 4.126

Sternum, six months post median sternotomy for
CABG, now complains of pain. Final diagnosis:
normal healing. (**a**) WB. Moderately intense, but
relatively well-marginated, focal, irregular tracer
uptake throughout the sternum. (**b**) RNA, anterior,
five seconds per frame. Normal perfusion through the
heart and great vessels. On later capillary and venous
phase images, there are no areas of abnormal
increased tracer accumulation (no abnormal
perfusion). (**c**) BP, anterior, and (**d**) BP, LAO. The
oblique view is necessary to project the sternum off
the heart and demonstrate the mild-to-moderate
increased tracer uptake (relative vascularity) (arrows).
(**e**) DS, chest, LAO. Compare with BP. Moderate
increased tracer uptake. When BP or tissue phase
images are abnormal, it is difficult and not always
possible to exclude a low-grade infection and
confidently attribute all the activity on delayed images
to normal or delayed healing. In those cases or when
the clinician has a very high index of suspicion for a
postoperative osteomyelitis, then dual imaging with
one of the infection imaging agents such as gallium-
67 or labeled WBCs can be done (see Figures 4.111c
and 4.127).

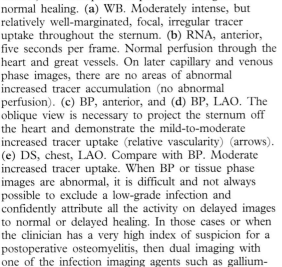

c

d

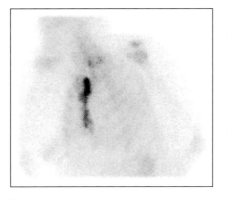

e

Teaching point

The time to complete healing of
operated bone depends on many
general and local factors. General
factors include, for example, health,
age, and diet of the patient. One local
factor is the amount of movement at
the operative site. The act of breathing
puts continued stress on the sternum
and can result in abnormal increased
tracer uptake on delayed images for
many years after surgery.

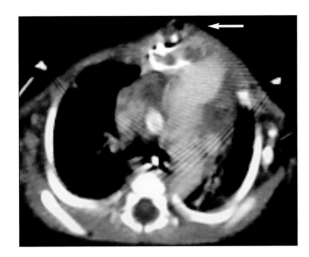

a

Figure 4.127

Sternum, normal healing. One-month-old female, status after Norwood stage I open heart surgery. Parasternal cellulitis. (**a**) CT, chest. Soft tissue fullness with air and metal artifact from sternal wire fixation. Nonspecific findings. Unable to differentiate postoperative changes from possible infection. (**b**) BP, anterior. No abnormal increased uptake (relative vascularity) overlying the chest. (**c**) DS, chest, anterior, and (**d**) DS, chest, RAO. Both images acquired with zoom × 2. Minimal activity about the sternum (arrow) is similar to adjacent bone. (**e**) Gallium, WB, 24-hour, anterior, and (**f**) gallium, WB, 24-hours, RAO. Both images acquired with zoom × 1.3. Minimal activity in sternum (arrow) is similar to other bone.

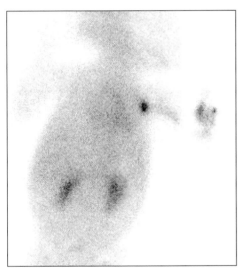

b

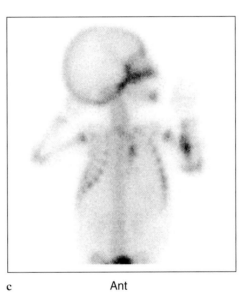

c   Ant

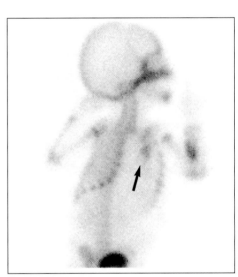

d

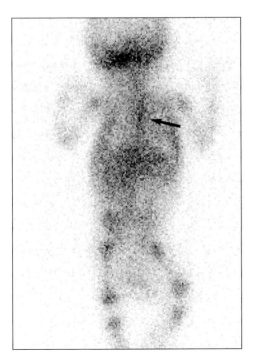

e

f

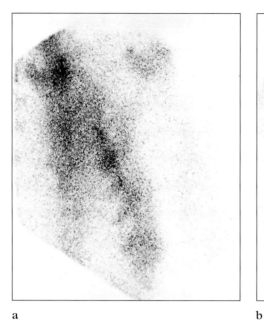
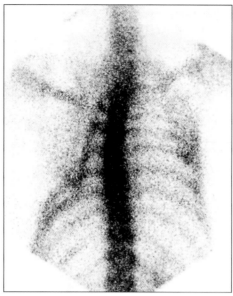
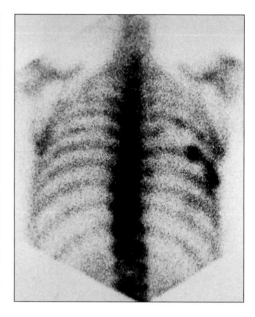

a   b

Figure 4.128

Ribs, healed thoracoplasty. (a) DS, chest, anterior, and (b) DS, chest, posterior. Typical scan appearances of previous thoracoplasty are seen in the left upper ribs.

Figure 4.129

Rib, resection, and healing fractures. DS, chest, posterior. Photon deficiency associated with the surgically absent right posterior sixth rib. Healing fractures associated with surgery involve the fifth and seventh ribs.

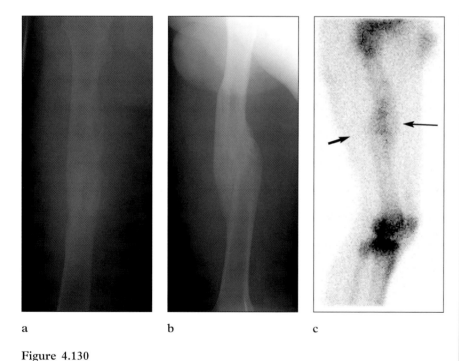
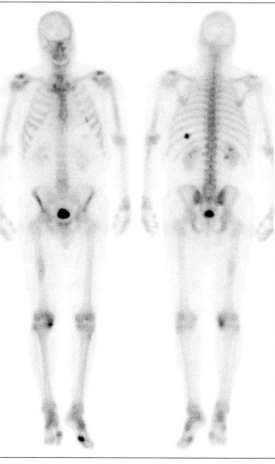

a   b   c

Figure 4.130

Femur, healed 40-year-old fracture. (a) X-ray, AP, and (b) X-ray, right lateral. Mid-shaft fracture with posterior offset of distal fragment healed with incorporation of bridging callus. (c) DS, femur, right lateral. The posterior offset of the distal fracture fragment can be appreciated (short arrow), as can the metabolic activity associated with the anterior bridging callous (thin arrow). (d) WB. Minimal increased tracer uptake in the right femoral diaphysis represents biomechanical stress changes secondary to altered alignment after prior fracture. Medial compartment degenerative changes in the right knee with more focal increased activity in the tibial subarticular surface. Incidental healing left posterior tenth rib fracture.

d

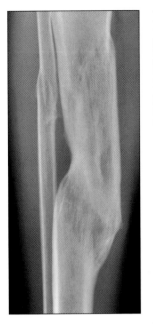

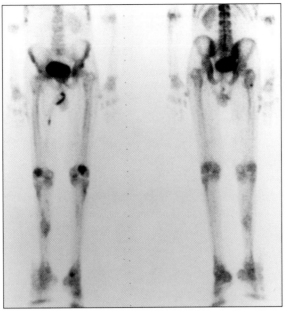

a　　　　　　b

Figure 4.131

Tibia. Healed fracture 27 years post-injury. (a) X-ray. Note the slight malalignment with development of stress trabecula and buttressing bone which has been well incorporated into the cortical structure. (b) WB. Slightly increased uptake, associated with minimal continued stress remodeling change. The patient was being staged for prostate cancer, which accounts for the abnormal uptake in the lumbar spine. (Reprinted with permission *Skeletal Nuclear Medicine*, p. 229, Figure 13–5.)

Abnormal healing

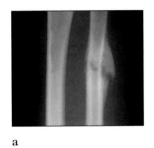

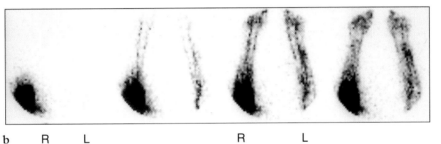

a　　　　　　b　R　L　　　　　　R　L

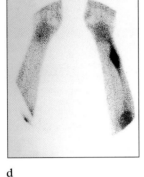

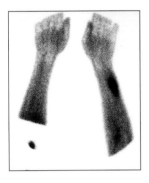

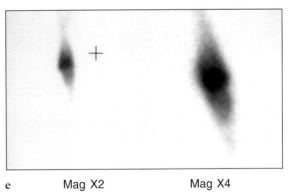

c　　　　　　d　　　　　　e　Mag X2　　　Mag X4

Figure 4.132

Ulna, atrophic nonunion. Six months post-trauma. (a) X-ray. The fracture line and the larger callus arising from the distal fragment. (b) RNA, palmar view. Activity associated with injection being made in right antecubital fossa is very intense. On the left side, mild focal increased perfusion to the area of the distal fragment. (c) BP, palmar. Moderate increased relative vascularity is larger than the fracture line. (d) DS, palmar. Intense fusiform-shaped increased tracer uptake. This would suggest a healing fracture. (e) DS, palmar, magnified view. The intense increased activity is associated only with the distal fragment.

Nonunion has been defined as that point in time after which spontaneous healing can no longer be expected to occur. Healing has stopped before bony continuity has been re-established. Clinically, differential considerations include slow union, delayed union, and nonunion. The pattern of a photon-deficient separation of activity between the edges or ends of bone has been termed atrophic nonunion. When there is only a single focus of increased activity encompassing both sides of a fracture site such that the fracture site itself cannot be identified, the term reactive nonunion has been utilized. Reactive nonunion has also been called hypertrophic nonunion, and is thought to be caused by continued motion at the fracture site. Usually, on a single radionuclide scan, reactive nonunion cannot be differentiated from delayed union. Nonunion can be caused by synovial, fibrous, or infected tissue interposed between fracture fragments. The differential diagnosis is also important because patients with delayed union often respond to more aggressive therapy resulting in eventual healing, whereas patients with atrophic nonunion will usually not heal with conservative treatment.

Figure 4.133

Hip, subcapital fracture, reactive nonunion, two years post-fracture and fixation. (a) X-ray, left hip, anterior. Three Knowles pins transfix the subcapital fracture. There is foreshortening of the femoral neck. There is sclerosis at the fracture site (arrow). (b) X-ray, right hip, AP. For comparison. Also note the osteophyte at the SL aspect of the acetabulum (arrow). (c) WB. Increased tracer uptake associated with the subcapital fracture on the left. (d) 3-D volumetric reprojection images, selected views from 0° to 50°. The normally metabolic femoral head could also be appreciated on these images. (e) SPECT, coronal images. The photon deficiency of the metallic Knowles pin could be seen (small arrow). The minimal increased tracer uptake associated with the right hip osteophyte could also be appreciated (thin arrow).

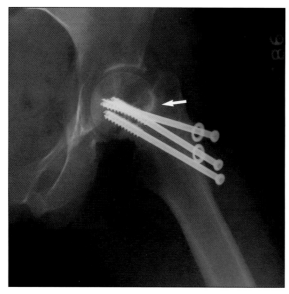

a

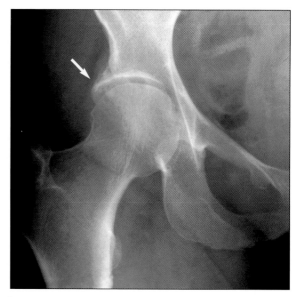

b

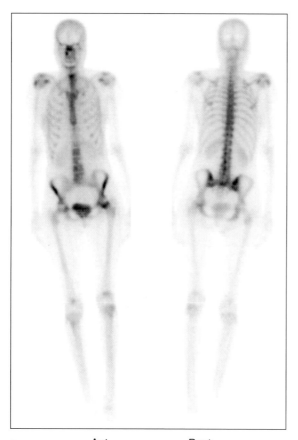

c   Ant   Post

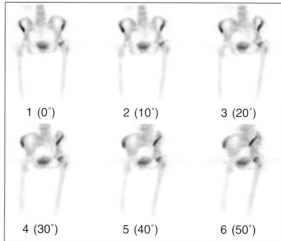

1 (0°)   2 (10°)   3 (20°)

4 (30°)   5 (40°)   6 (50°)

d

Teaching point

When the scintigraphic differential diagnosis is between reactive nonunion and delayed union, patient history and correlative imaging will be needed to supplement the bone scan. Even then a follow-up scan in several months might be necessary.

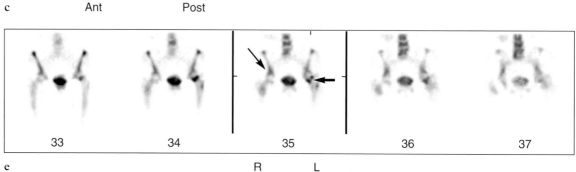

33   34   35   36   37

e   R   L

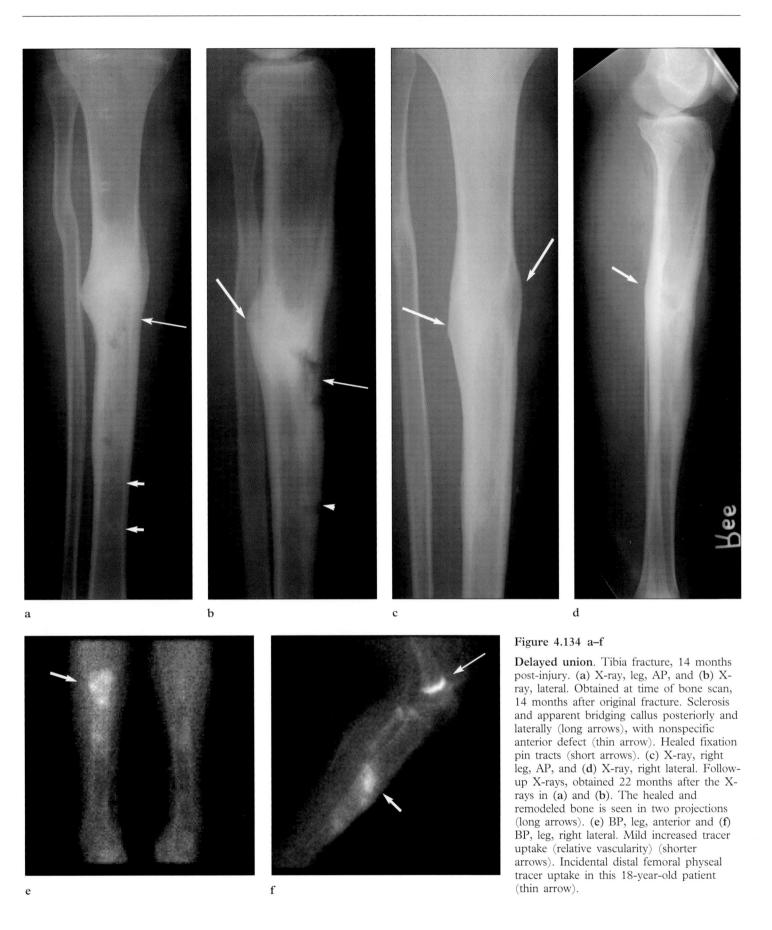

a

b

c

d

e

f

Figure 4.134 a–f

Delayed union. Tibia fracture, 14 months post-injury. (a) X-ray, leg, AP, and (b) X-ray, lateral. Obtained at time of bone scan, 14 months after original fracture. Sclerosis and apparent bridging callus posteriorly and laterally (long arrows), with nonspecific anterior defect (thin arrow). Healed fixation pin tracts (short arrows). (c) X-ray, right leg, AP, and (d) X-ray, right lateral. Follow-up X-rays, obtained 22 months after the X-rays in (a) and (b). The healed and remodeled bone is seen in two projections (long arrows). (e) BP, leg, anterior and (f) BP, leg, right lateral. Mild increased tracer uptake (relative vascularity) (shorter arrows). Incidental distal femoral physeal tracer uptake in this 18-year-old patient (thin arrow).

continued

Figure 4.134 g–i

(g) DS, right lateral. The detail of the moderate increased activity at the fracture site, most marked in the mid-portion, but extending posteriorly, is seen (short arrow). A nonspecific anterior defect (thin arrow). There is no significant increased uptake associated with the almost completely healed fibular fracture or of the round pin tracts. Minimal activity (arrowhead) in the mid-tibia corresponds to a larger fixation screw track seen on (b) (arrowhead). (h) 3-D volumetric reprojection images. Selected views from 120° to 170°. Anatomic location of increased tracer better appreciated on these images. (i) SPECT, coronal (bottom row) and sagittal (middle row) images also define the extent and orientation of abnormal tracer uptake. The coronal views (and the 3-D images in h) show minimal metabolic activity associated with radiographically completely healed, left tibial fractures. On this single radionuclide scan, the differential diagnosis between delayed union and reactive nonunion would not be possible without the correlative radiographs.

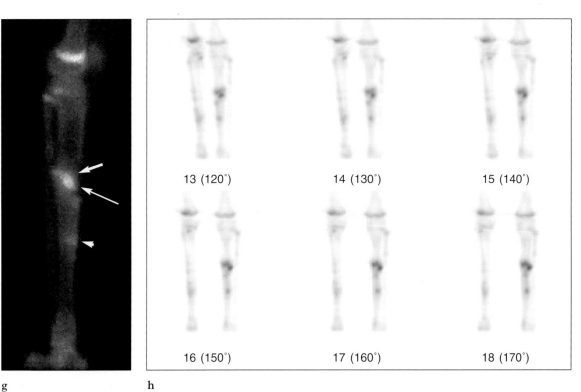

g   h

13 (120°)   14 (130°)   15 (140°)

16 (150°)   17 (160°)   18 (170°)

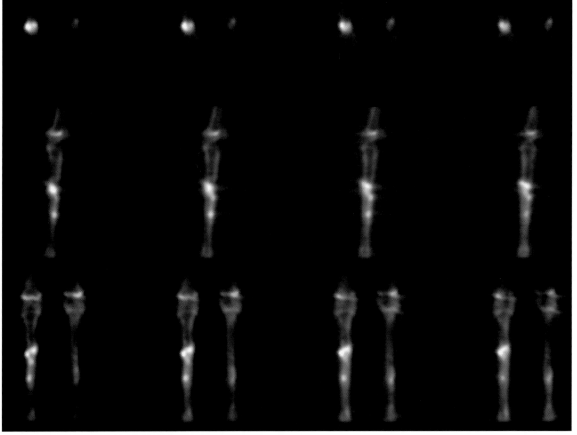

i

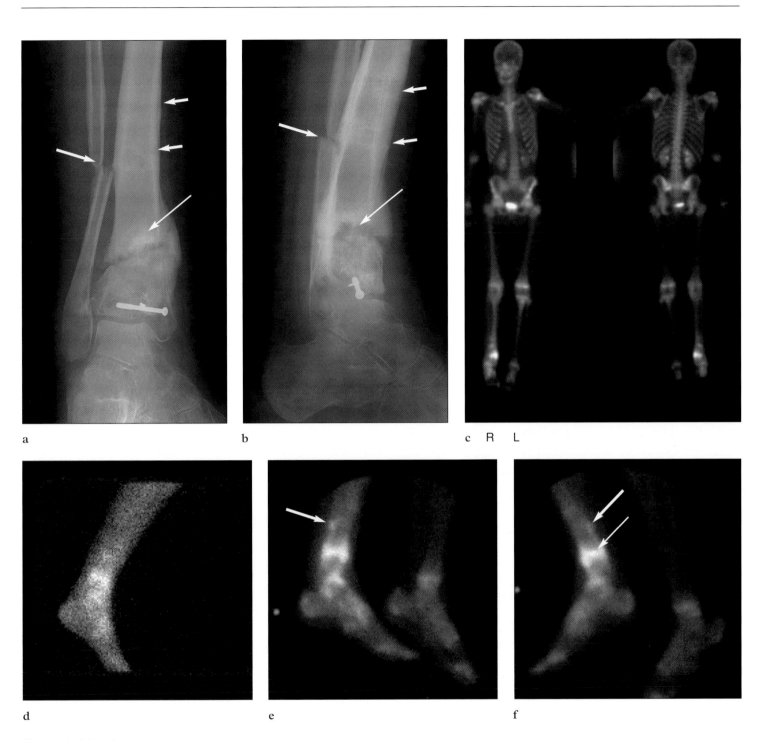

a   b   c R L

d   e   f

Figure 4.135 a–f

Tibia, nonunion, and chronic osteomyelitis. A 15-year-old gymnast approximately 2 years post-fracture, with drainage. (**a**) X-ray, lower leg and ankle, AP and (**b**) X-ray, lateral. Fracture seen in area of drainage (thin arrow). Screw fixation. Subtle lucencies at site of prior pin tracks (short arrows). Nonunited fibular fracture (long arrow). (**c**) WB. The relative intensity of the distal lesion can be appreciated. The mild asymmetry in activity between the right and left extremity was of uncertain significance. (**d**) BP, right lateral. Mild increased tracer uptake centered at the fracture site. (**e**) DS, lower leg and ankle, right lateral, and (**f**) DS, right medial. Increased activity at the fracture site. Although not well reproduced, there was slightly more focal increase in the mid-portion (thin arrow). Mild increased tracer at site of fixation pins (long arrows).

continued

Figure 4.135 g–j

(g) SPECT, triangulation display. The multiple foci of increased uptake at the fracture site can be best appreciated on the sagittal images (middle row) and the coronal images (bottom row). (h) Ga, WB. Observe the relative intensity of Ga uptake at the distal tibial fracture site compared with uptake in normal bone. (i) Ga, lower leg and ankle, anterior and (j) Ga, right lateral. The area of greatest Ga accumulation was in the middle half of the tibia at the superior side of the fracture site.

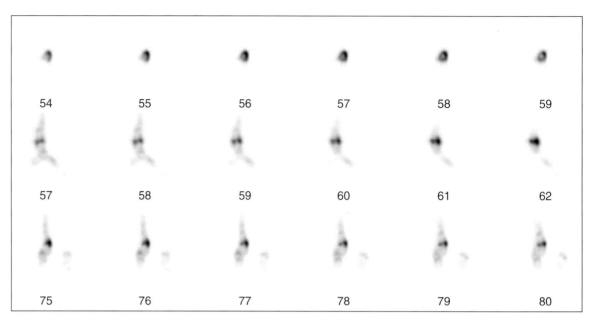

g

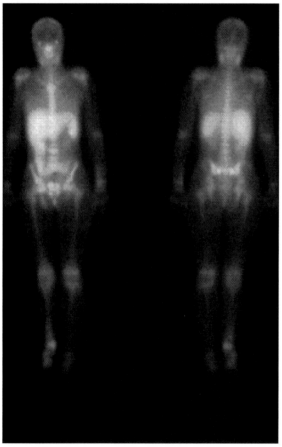

h

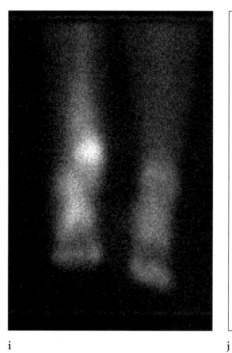

i

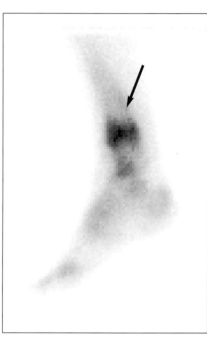

j

Teaching point

When the ratio of tracer uptake in abnormal bone to normal bone is greater for the bone agent, infection is less likely, and when the ratio is greater for gallium, infection is more likely. When ratios are similar, incongruence of gallium uptake in relation to areas of bone tracer uptake suggests infection.

Graft viability

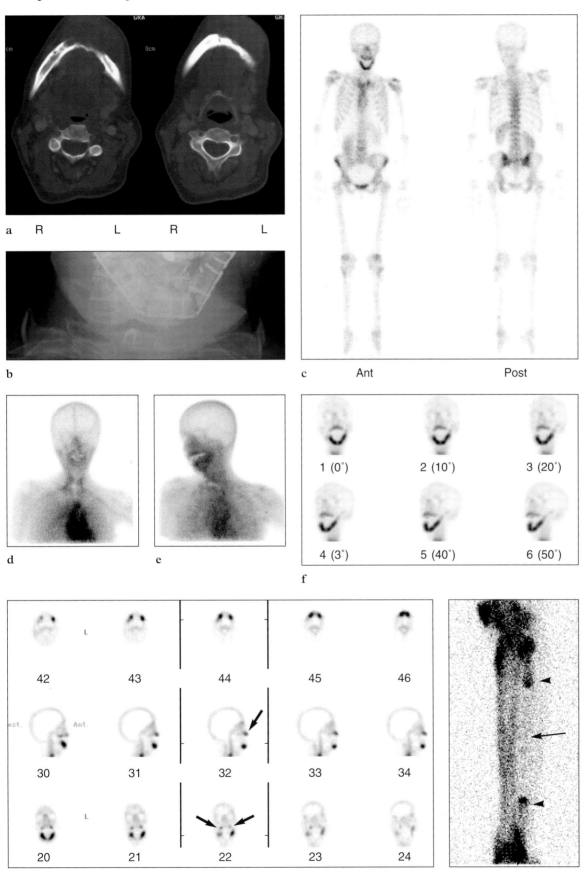

a   R   L   R   L

b

c   Ant   Post

d   e

1 (0°)   2 (10°)   3 (20°)

4 (3°)   5 (40°)   6 (50°)

f

42   43   44   45   46

30   31   32   33   34

20   21   22   23   24

g   h

Figure 4.136

Autogenic graft, normally vascularized and metabolizing. Fibula to mandible. Carcinoma, floor of mouth invading mandible. (**a**) CT. Pre-operative. The bone destruction is seen in the mid-line extending both left and right. (**b**) X-ray, mandible, AP. Post-operative with fixation bands and pins immobilizing the graft. (**c**) WB, 24-hour post injection. Patient returned for this image which was inadvertently not obtained at the time of the three-phase and SPECT imaging of the graft. No evidence for osseous metastasis. (**d**) BP, head and neck, anterior and (**e**) BP, left lateral. No evidence for photon deficiency on these tissue phase images. (**f**) 3-D volumetric reprojection images. The extent of mandibular uptake could be well appreciated. (**g**) SPECT triangulation display. The mandibular uptake is well defined. Symmetrical inferior maxillary uptake (arrows on coronal and sagittal views) was of uncertain significance. It was thought most likely to be related to dental disease. (**h**) DS, leg, lateral, 24 hours post-injection. The photon deficiency associated with the resected graft (thin arrow). Minimal activity at the borders of the resection (arrowheads) is normal healing.

Teaching point

Because of the relatively high target to background ratios obtained with technetium-labeled phosphorus bone scanning agents, images can be obtained up to 24 hours following injection. They are not of optimal quality, and require proportionately longer acquisition times with associated image degradation due to patient movement.

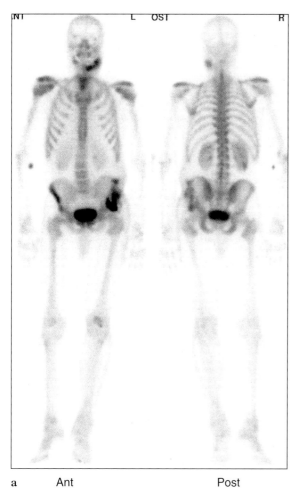

a   Ant   Post

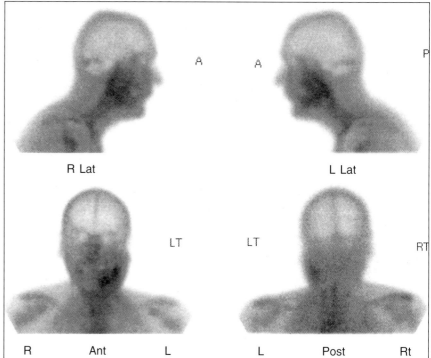

b

Figure 4.137

Autograft, normal vascularity and metabolism. Hip to mandible. (a) WB. Moderately increased tracer in the left mandible represents normally metabolic autograft. The activity involving the left ilium laterally represents healing at the donor site. (b) BP, head and neck, multiple views. The increased tracer uptake associated with the viable graft in the left mandible. There is some associated soft tissue uptake.

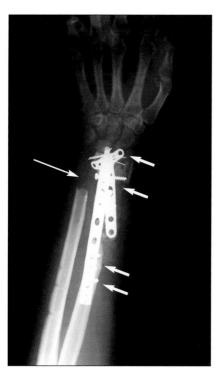

a

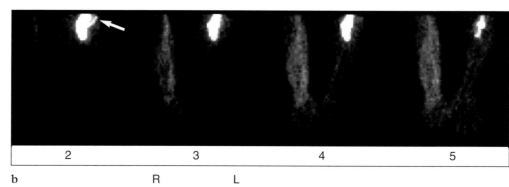

b   R   L

Figure 4.138 a and b

Autograft, nonviable. Vascularized fibula to radius. (a) X-ray, PA. Obtained several months prior to subsequent scan. The resected distal ulna (long arrow), the area of proximal side plate and screws (short arrows), the area of bone graft beneath the more distal compression plate (thin arrow), and the fixation of the distal plate on to the proximal carpal row (thick arrow). (b) RNA, arm, anterior. Five seconds per frame. The injection site in the left antecubital fossa shows some extravasation (short arrow). There is mild increased relative vascularity to the region of the right forearm.

continued

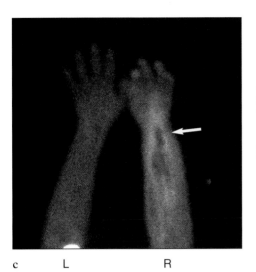
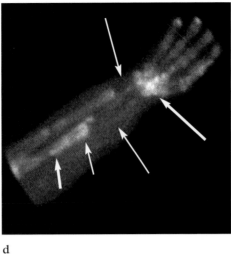

c   L   R   d

Figure 4.138 c and d

(c) BP, arm, anterior. Mild, diffuse, increased vascularity to the area of the right forearm and into the wrist. There is some photon deficiency (arrow) associated with de-vascularized graft and compression plate. **(d)** DS, arm, anterior. Photon deficiency of the surgically absent distal ulna (long arrow), minimal amounts of increased uptake associated with bone stress of the distal native radius underneath the compression plate and screws (short arrows), absent activity associated with the nonviable photon-deficient graft (thin arrow), and activity in the proximal carpal row (thick arrow) associated with the fixation of the distal compression plate.

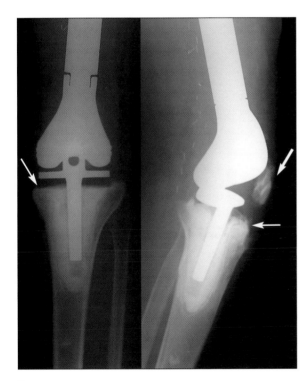
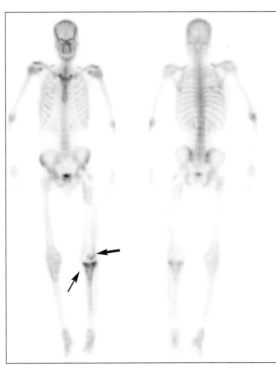

a   b

Figure 4.139 a and b

Allograft, viable. Proximal tibia. Osteosarcoma right femur. Limb salvage surgery. Scan 11 months after second prosthesis. **(a)** X-ray, anterior (left image) and right lateral (right image). The resected distal femur with metallic prosthesis. The tibial component with associated methyl methacrylate. Distal residual patella (thick arrow) and location of allograft bone (thin arrow) which is not well seen on this reproduction. **(b)** WB. The photon deficiency associated with the prosthesis in the left femur, which extends from hip to knee. Activity in the residual patella (thicker arrow) and surrounding the tibial component. Slightly more activity medially is at a site of allograft bone (thin arrow).

continued

Figure 4.139 c and d

(c) DS, femur and knee, left lateral. Activity at the patella (thicker arrow) and around the tibial component, with more focal uptake anteriorly (thinner arrow), which represents a site of allograft bone. (d) 3-D volumetric reprojection images, selected views from 0° to 50°. Lip of activity anteromedially where allograft bone has been placed (arrow). The degree of activity surrounding the tibial component in this case is postsurgical. On a single scan, this could not be easily differentiated from loosening or infection.

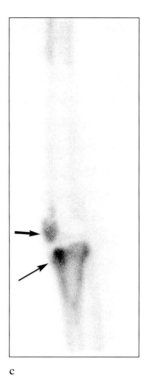

c

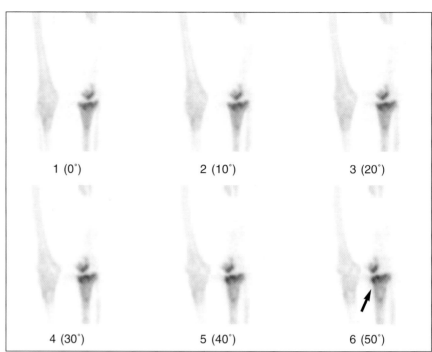

1 (0°)   2 (10°)   3 (20°)

4 (30°)   5 (40°)   6 (50°)

d

Figure 4.140

Dental implant to the mandible. WB, moderately intense, relatively well-defined, increased tracer uptake associated with the mandible extending from the mid-line. This uptake is nonspecific (compare it with Figures 4.136 and 4.137). Correlative history and correlative radiographs are required for differential diagnosis.

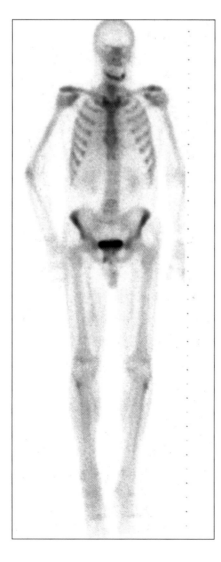

Figure 4.141 opposite

Below-knee amputation. PL inflammation without infection from prosthesis, postoperative HO and bilateral medial compartment osteoarthritis. (a) X-ray, knee, anterior and (b) X-ray, lateral. Two surgical screws are present within the tibial plateau. Bridging ossification between the tibial and fibular stumps (arrow). (c) Biplane RNA, leg, anterior and (d) posterior. Five (5) seconds per frame. The moderately intense, somewhat focal, lateral increased perfusion to the right knee at the level of the distal femur. (e) BP, leg, anterior, (f) posterior, and (g) right lateral. Focal, moderately intense, increased uptake laterally at the level of the distal femur (thicker arrow). Posterior location is confirmed on orthogonal lateral view. Popliteal vein activity seen on posterior view (thin arrow). (h) DS, leg, anterior, (i) posterior, and (j) right lateral. Moderate increased tracer uptake associated with the bridging HO (thin arrow); medial compartment osteoarthritis bilaterally; and on the lateral view some patellar femoral degenerative arthritis. The bone beneath the area of inflammation, manifested as increased tracer accumulation on the RNA and BP images, does not show any intense increased tracer, so that an underlying osteomyelitis could be excluded. The lateral view also demonstrates some minimal increased tracer at the tip of one of the proximal screws (arrow). This was thought to represent normal healing.

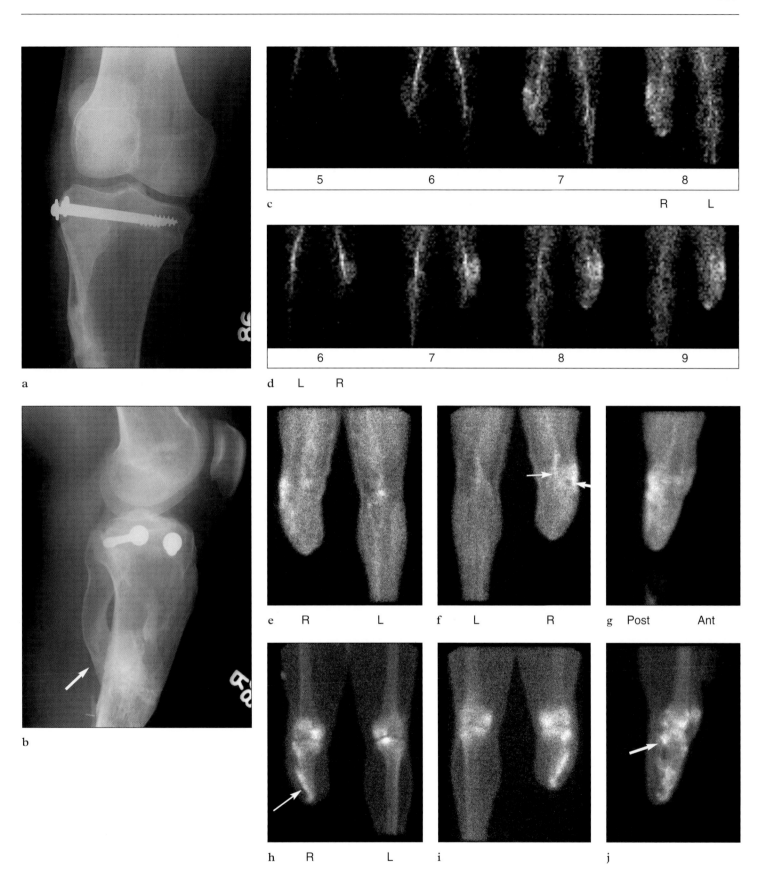

a

b

c 5 6 7 8

R L

d L R 6 7 8 9

e R L

f L R

g Post Ant

h R L

i

j

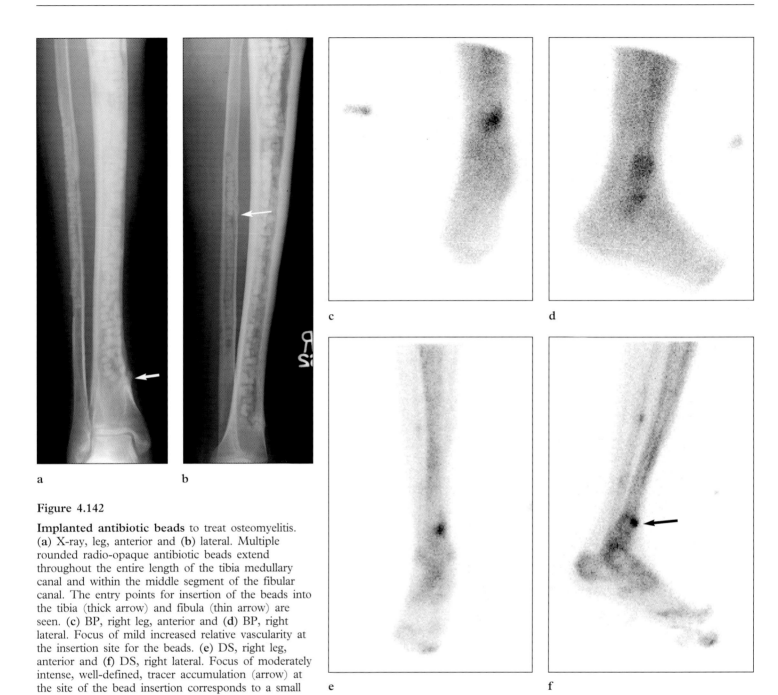

a   b

Figure 4.142

Implanted antibiotic beads to treat osteomyelitis.
(a) X-ray, leg, anterior and (b) lateral. Multiple
rounded radio-opaque antibiotic beads extend
throughout the entire length of the tibia medullary
canal and within the middle segment of the fibular
canal. The entry points for insertion of the beads into
the tibia (thick arrow) and fibula (thin arrow) are
seen. (c) BP, right leg, anterior and (d) BP, right
lateral. Focus of mild increased relative vascularity at
the insertion site for the beads. (e) DS, right leg,
anterior and (f) DS, right lateral. Focus of moderately
intense, well-defined, tracer accumulation (arrow) at
the site of the bead insertion corresponds to a small
amount of periosteal elevation at that point. This is
normal healing of a postsurgical defect.

c

d

e

f

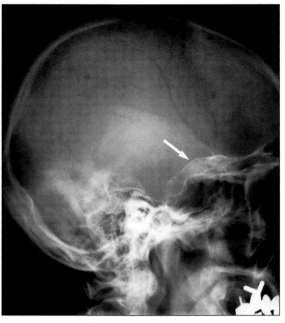

a

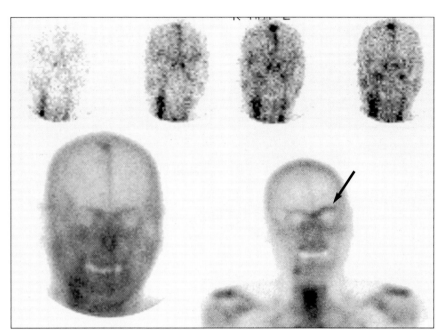

b

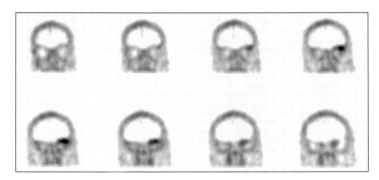

c

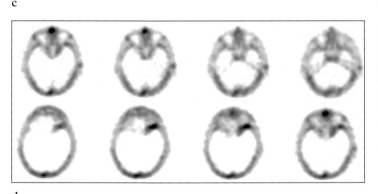

d

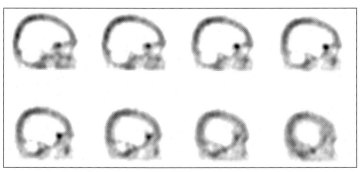

e

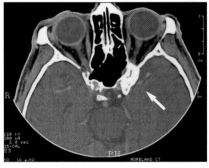

f

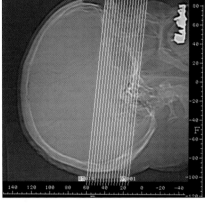

g

Figure 5.14

Fibrous dysplasia, left orbital bone. Double and impaired vision, left 4th nerve paresis. (a) X-ray. (b) Three-phase scan. RNA. No increased perfusion identified. BP, anterior. No increased vascularity. DS, anterior. Minimal increased uptake left superior orbit (arrow). (c) SPECT, coronal slice. (d) SPECT, transaxial. (e) SPECT, sagittal slice. (f) CT, transaxial slice. Note left orbital bone thickening (arrow). (g) CT, or localizer film. Lines demonstrate orientation of the study slices obtained. This study demonstrates the ability of multiplanar SPECT images to precisely localize the anatomic site of abnormal tracer uptake.

Correlative imaging comment

The plane or section for transaxial head CT is usually angled minus 10° from the horizontal canthomeatal line; thus the CT and SPECT images are not exactly comparable unless oblique angle reconstruction is utilized.

Giant cell tumors

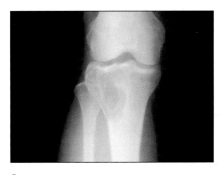

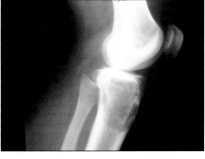

a

b

Figure 5.15

Giant cell tumor, proximal tibia. (a) X-ray, knee, AP and (b) Lateral. Lytic lesion without sclerotic margins involving proximal tibial metaphysis and epiphysis. (c) RNA and anterior BP demonstrate minimal increased tracer on BP image (arrow). (d) BP. Mild increased tracer uptake. (e) DS. Well defined, marked increased tracer uptake has same appearance as lytic lesion. (f) CT. Transaxial slice shows lytic lesion disrupting the cortex.

Giant cell tumors are locally aggressive lesions, which some authors categorize as malignant. Giant cell tumors involve epiphysis and metaphysis and almost always extend to the articular surface.

Teaching point

Some 75–90% of giant cell tumors are in long tubular bones especially around the knee, with the most common sites being the femur, tibia, radius, and humerus.

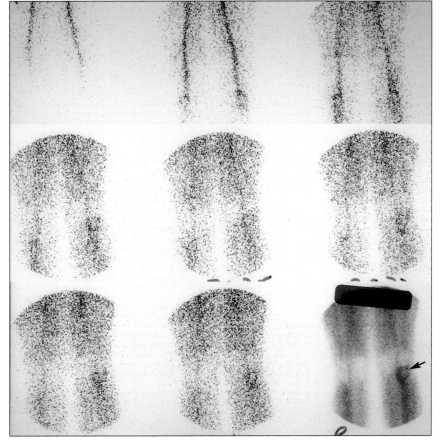

c

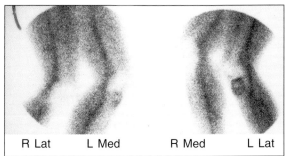

| R Lat | L Med | R Med | L Lat |

d

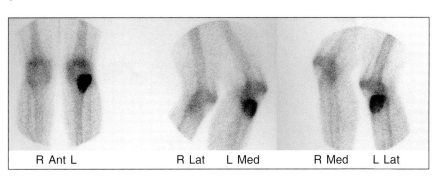

| R Ant L | R Lat | L Med | R Med | L Lat |

e

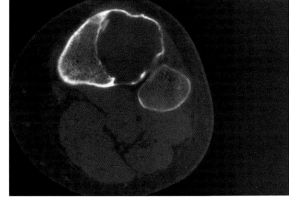

f

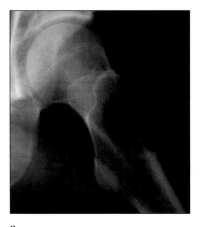
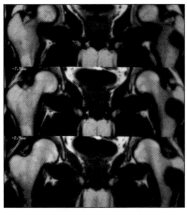
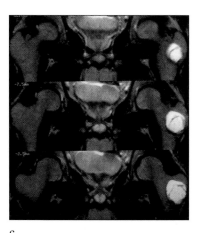

a   b   c

Figure 5.16

Giant cell tumor, hip.
(a) X-ray right hip. Lytic lesion. (b) MR T1 and (c) MR T2-weighted images show a well-defined lesion with low signal on T1 and bright signal on T2. (d) DS pelvis and hips. Well-defined focus of intense increased tracer uptake (arrow) corresponds to radiographic lesion.

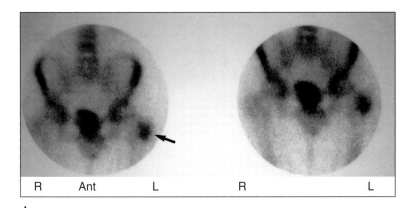

R   Ant   L   R   L

d

Giant cell tumors are most often found in epiphyseal or epiphyseal equivalent regions, and also in metaphyseal regions. This MR signal pattern is usually seen with malignant lesions, but is diagnostically nonspecific.

Teaching point

A lesion, which has intense abnormal increased tracer accumulation, is often overexposed on analog and digital display with standard settings.

SPECT imaging often allows precise localization of abnormal increased tracer uptake.

Figure 5.17

Giant cell tumor, femur. (a) WB. Scan is reatively overexposed, so that exact location of lesion is not optimally defined (arrow). (b) BP. Focus of mild increased uptake laterally in distal femoral (arrow) helps localize epicenter of lesion. (c) SPECT, transaxial. Slices through distal femoral localized the abnormal focus, which corresponded in this case to the lesion seen on a plain radiograph (not shown).

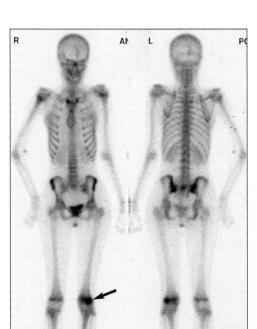

R Ant   L Post

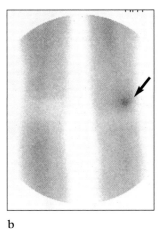

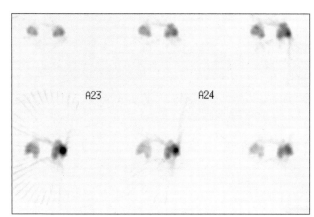

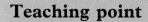

a   b   c

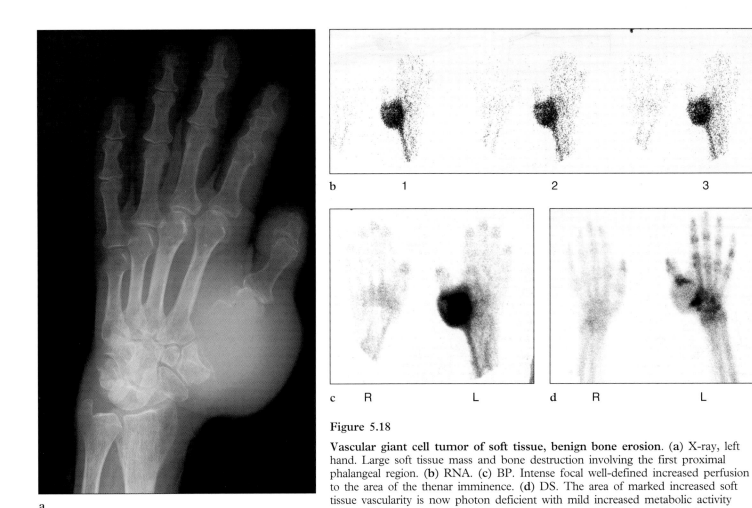

Figure 5.18

Vascular giant cell tumor of soft tissue, benign bone erosion. (a) X-ray, left hand. Large soft tissue mass and bone destruction involving the first proximal phalangeal region. (b) RNA. (c) BP. Intense focal well-defined increased perfusion to the area of the thenar imminence. (d) DS. The area of marked increased soft tissue vascularity is now photon deficient with mild increased metabolic activity associated with the benign bone erosion at the edges of the mass secondary to pressure of growing tumor mass.

Hemangioma

Figure 5.19 a–b

Hemangioma, L3. (a) Delay WB. The most minimal asymmetry in L3 vertebral body. (b) 3-D volumetric display (reprojection images), selected images. Accentuation of mild increased uptake in right side of L3 vertebral body (arrow).

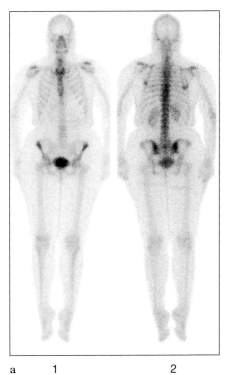

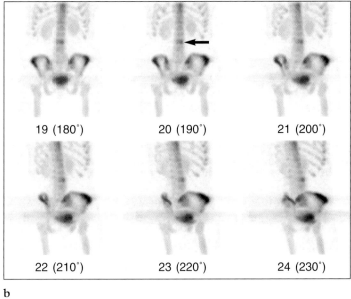

19 (180°)   20 (190°)   21 (200°)

22 (210°)   23 (220°)   24 (230°)

continued

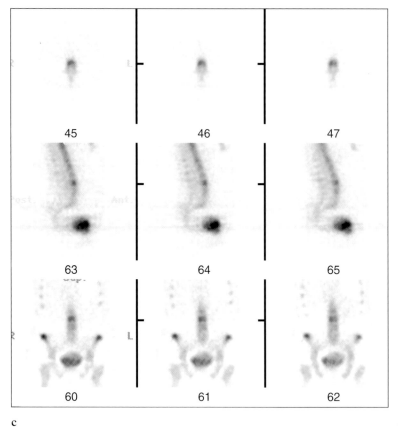

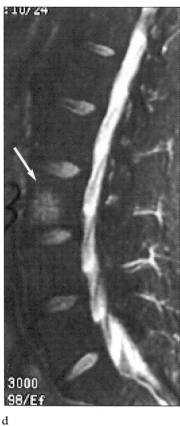

c

d

Figure 5.19 c–d

(c) SPECT images, triangulation display. Confirms location of L3 vertebral body activity. (d) MR T2-weighted, sagittal, image demonstrates subtle abnormal high signal (arrow).

Teaching point

The L2–L3 vertebral bodies are often more prominent on the anterior view, because normal lumbar lordosis places them closer to the camera's anterior head.

Teaching point

Hemangioma of the spine may appear photon deficient, normal, or show slightly increased tracer uptake.

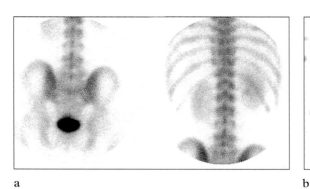

a

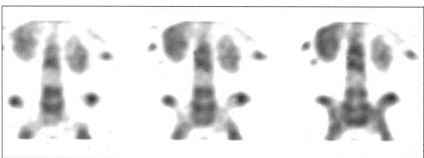

b

Figure 5.20 a–c

Hemangioma, L3. (a) DS, anterior and posterior. Decreased tracer involving L3 vertebra. (b) SPECT, coronal slice. (c) SPECT, sagittal slice. Photon deficiency confined to vertebral body is demonstrated.

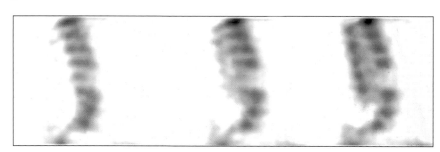

c

continued

Figure 5.20 d–e

(d) MR, T1 weighted.
(e) MR, T2 weighted.
Diffuse increased signal
on both sequences. More
subtle on T2.

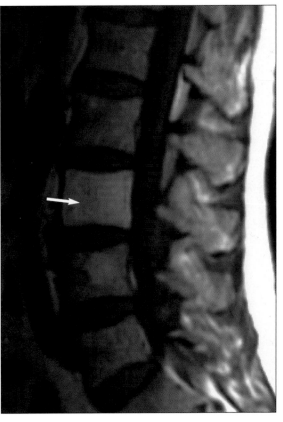

d

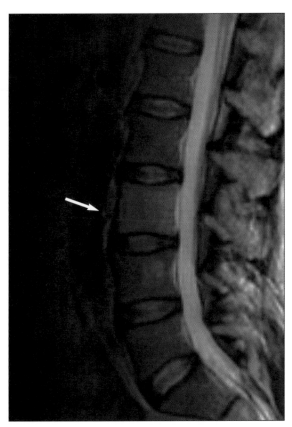

e

Intraosseous lipoma

Figure 5.21

**Intraosseous lipoma
and AC joint arthritis**.
(a) X-ray, left shoulder,
AP view. Lytic lesion
well marginated. (b) DS,
left shoulder. No
abnormal increased tracer
uptake associated with
lytic lesion. Pain
attributed to AC joint
arthritis. Asymmetric
increased uptake on left
side.

This benign lesion is not causing any reparative
bone response. The lytic appearing cavity is
most likely secondary to liquefaction.

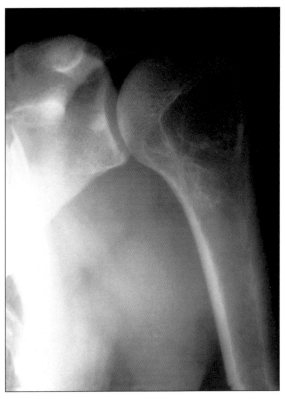

a

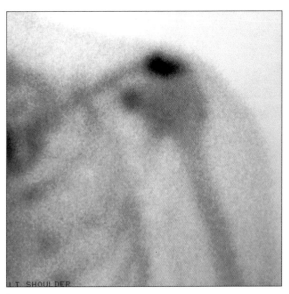

b

Meningioma

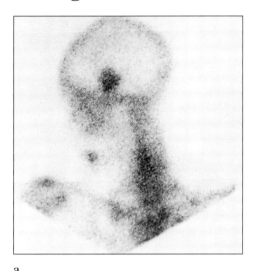 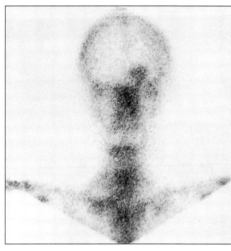

a

b

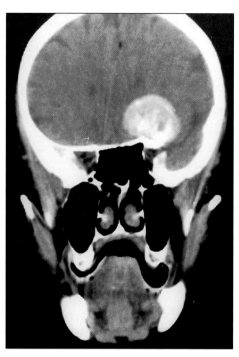

c

Figure 5.22

Meningioma. (a) DS, lateral view. Intense abnormal tracer uptake. (b) DS, anterior view. (c) CT, direct coronal.

Meningioma is a tumor of the meninges, which often incites a bone response. It is usually detected on RNBI as an incidental lesion when searching for metastatic bone disease.

Teaching point

Orthogonal views confirm intracerebral rather than calvarial location of abnormal tracer uptake.

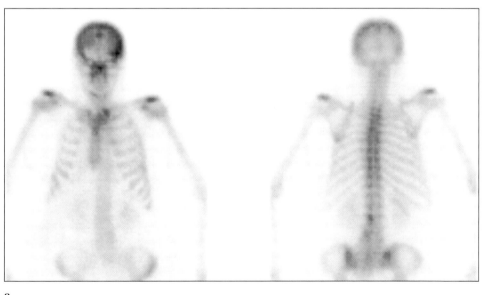 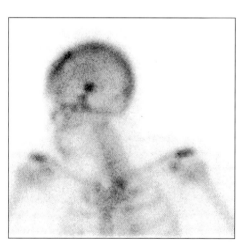

b

a

Figure 5.23 a–b

Meningioma, frontal bone. (a) WB. Moderately increased, poorly defined left frontal bone uptake. (b) DS, lateral view. Round focal area of intense increased tracer uptake.

continued

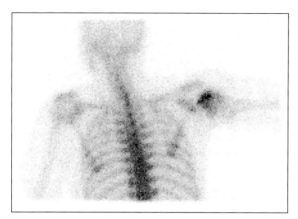

d

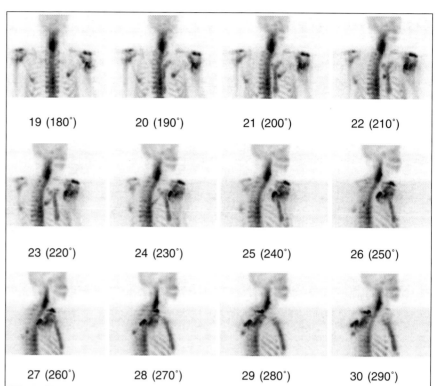

19 (180°)   20 (190°)   21 (200°)   22 (210°)

23 (220°)   24 (230°)   25 (240°)   26 (250°)

27 (260°)   28 (270°)   29 (280°)   30 (290°)

e

Figure 5.28 d–f

(d) DS, arm abducted. Better defines lesion. (e) 3-D. Selected images 180–290°. Posterior location and varying intensity of lesion uptake. (f) SPECT, triangulation display. Activity associated with metabolically active cap, especially well seen on sagittal sections (arrow).

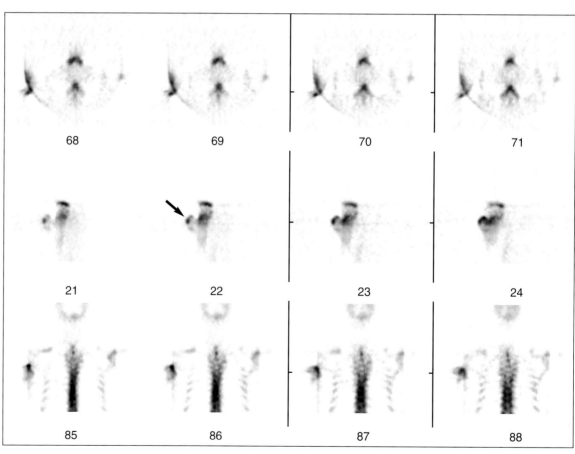

68   69   70   71

21   22   23   24

85   86   87   88

f

Exostoses

Pain associated with exostoses is usually secondary to mechanical irritation or impingement upon nerves or vessels.

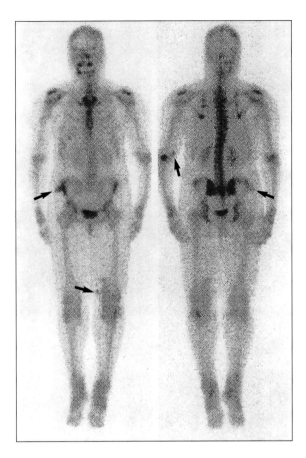

Figure 5.29

Multiple exostosis. WB. Multiple lesions of varying intensity, from mild to moderate, protrude away from the joint from long bones (arrows).

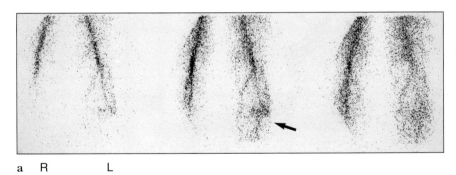

a   R   L

Figure 5.30

Multiple exostosis. (a) RNA, posterior projection. Occluded left popliteal artery. Analog 5 seconds per view images oriented to correspond to contrast angiogram. (b) Contrast angiogram. Selected frame demonstrates proximal tibia and fibula, osteochondroma viewed en face, and occlusion of popliteal artery.

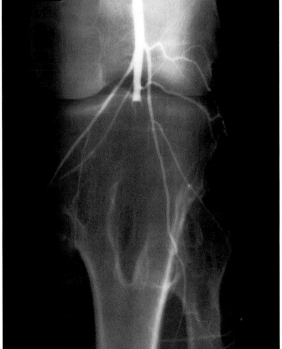

b

Osteoid osteoma

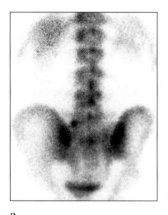

a

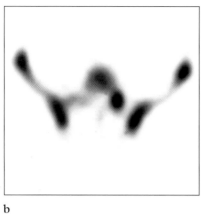

b

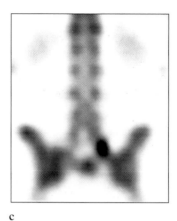

c

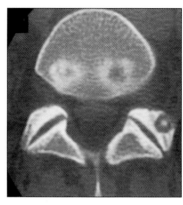

d

Figure 5.31

Osteoid osteoma, lumbar spine. 36-year-old with low back pain. Plain radiographs were normal. **(a)** DS, posterior view. Mild increased round focal uptake, left side L5. **(b)** SPECT, transaxial slice and **(c)** SPECT, coronal slice localize increased tracer to the region of the left L5–S1 facet joint. **(d)** CT, transaxial, demonstrates a well-defined lytic area with a central sclerosis (the nidus) in the superior facet of S1.

Teaching point

The rounded appearance of the increased tracer is not typical of activity associated with facet arthritis, which is more linearly oriented along the plane of the facet joint.

Figure 5.32 a–c

Osteoid osteoma, proximal phalanx. **(a)** X-ray, finger. Soft tissue swelling surrounding a slightly enlarged, elongated, second proximal phalanx, with chronic type cortical thickening, and distally, a tiny round area of lucency with a possible sclerotic center (arrow). **(b)** CT transaxial and **(c)** CT direct sagittal slice delineate the extent of reactive sclerosis, the lucent lesion, and the calcified center of the nidus (arrow).

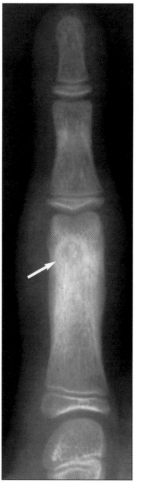

a

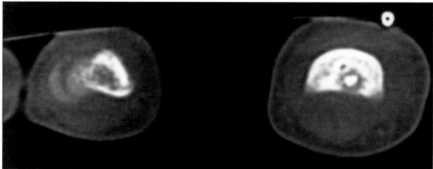

b

c

Correlative imaging comment

Radiographic evidence of phalangeal enlargement, which takes time to develop, is a sign that this lesion is chronic.

continued

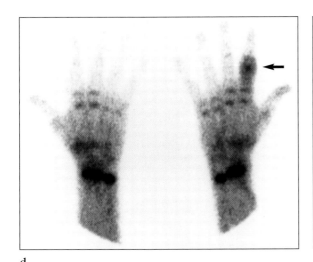

d

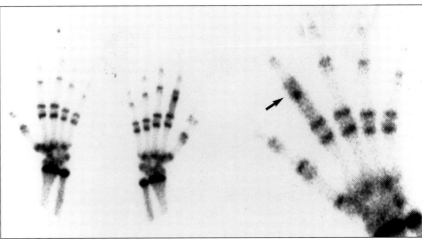

e

Teaching point

Most active osteoid osteoma lesions will demonstrate focal increased tracer on BP images, which is thought to represent the vascular tumor nidus.

Figure 5.32 d–e

(**d**) BP. Mildly increased activity about the proximal phalanx with a tiny round focus of more intense increased tracer corresponding to the area of central lucency (arrow). (**e**) DS. Mild diffusely increased tracer uptake involving all the proximal phalanges, and an intense round area of increased tracer corresponding to the radiographic lucency (arrow).

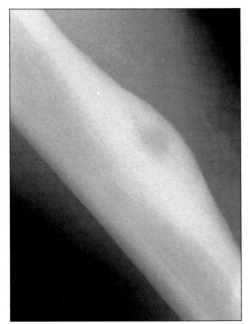

a

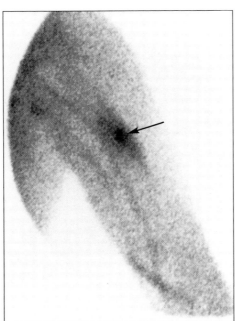

b

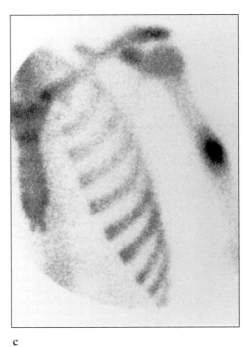

c

Figure 5.33

Osteoid osteoma, humerus. Insidious onset of pain in a young adult male. (**a**) X-ray, mid-humeral shaft. Longer lesion, cortical sclerosis with central lucency. (**b**) BP. Moderate hyperemia, with a central round focus of more intense tracer uptake (arrow). (**c**) DS, moderate tracer uptake, with central area of more focal intense uptake.

Osteomas are of uncertain etiology, and are thought to represent foci of periosteal new bone.

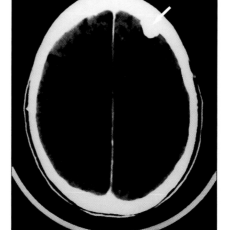
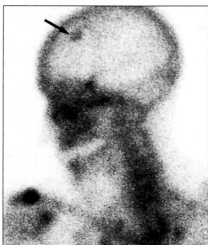

a   b

Figure 5.34

Osteoma, skull. (a) Small calcified lesion adjacent to inner table of left frontal bone (arrow). (b) DS, lateral view. Small, round focus of mild increased tracer accumulation (arrow).

Teaching point

Mature osteoma lesions, like mature bone islands, usually have only minimal increased metabolic activity on delayed images, which is used to confirm the diagnosis of a nonaggressive lesion.

Figure 5.35 a–b

Osteoid osteoma, knee. (a) BP, anterior view. Small round area of minimal increased uptake (relative vascularity) (arrow). (b) WB. Intense uptake, lateral condyle region. More focal on posterior view (arrow).

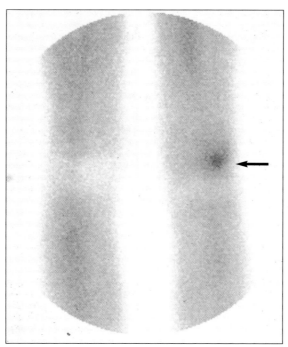
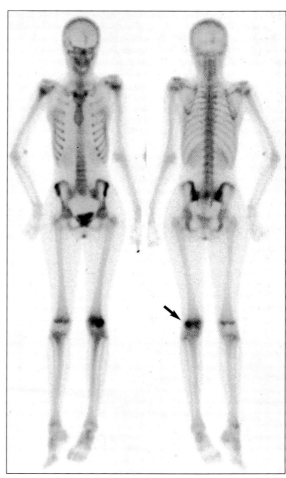

continued   a   b   L Ant   R Post

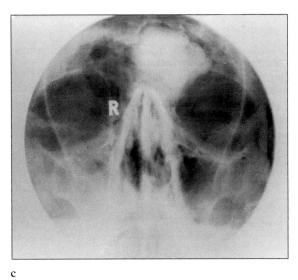

Figure 5.35 c–d

(c) SPECT, transaxial. Further localizes uptake. (d) X-ray knee, AP and lateral. Subtle increased bone density (arrows).

d   AP   Lat

Ivory osteoma

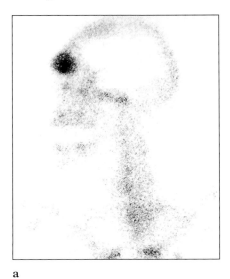

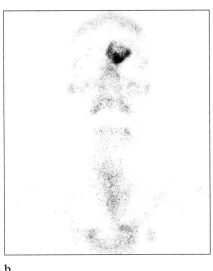

a   b   c

Figure 5.36

Ivory osteoma, skull. (a) DS, lateral and (b) DS, Water's view. Intense focus of increased uptake in left supraorbital area. (c) X-ray, Water's view. Demonstrates dense sclerosis.

Malignant bone tumors

RNBI cannot be used to provide a histologic diagnosis of primary malignant bone tumors. However, understanding of those histologic and growth characteristics considered by orthopedic surgeons, tumor surgeons, radiologists, pathologists, and oncologists during diagnosis, staging, and management of lesions allows the nuclear medicine physician to communicate effectively with these specialists. A simplified histologic classification of malignant bone tumors is found in Table 5.1. It is modeled from the teachings of Ed McCarthy.

Table 5.1 Histologic classification of malignant bone tumors*

- Osteoblastic
    Osteosarcoma, conventional and variants
- Cartilaginous
    Chondrosarcoma, variants
- Fibrous
    Malignant fibrous histiocytoma
    Fibrosarcoma
- Small round cell
    Ewing's/PNET
    Lymphoma/leukemia
    Myeloma
- Chordoma
- Adamantinoma

---

*Developed from text: *Pathology of Bone and Joint Disorders with Clinical and Radiographic Correlation.* McCarthy EF, Frassica FJ, 1998, WB Saunders, Philadelphia.

Chondrosarcoma

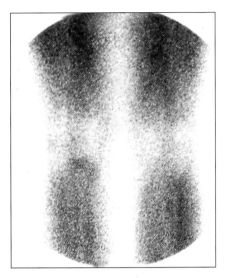

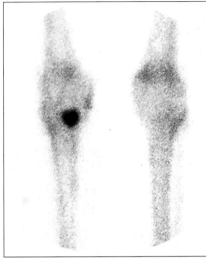

New pain in the area of an enchondromatous lesion, even if benign appearing radiographically, should be further investigated.

Teaching point

Unless totally absent, the degree of metabolic activity (tracer uptake) in an enchondromatous lesion in a mature adult cannot be used to exclude malignancy, although minimal increased activity does suggest a lower-grade lesion.

a   b

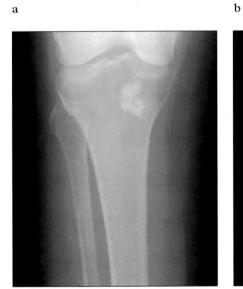

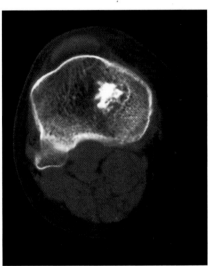

Figure 5.40

Low-grade chondrosarcoma in a 40-year-old female with knee pain and no history of trauma. (**a**) BP. Very minimal increase in tracer uptake (relative vascularity of the lesion). (**b**) DS. Intense increased tracer corresponds to X-ray bone lesion. (**c**) X-ray, knee. Moderately dense lesion with cartilaginous matrix is not radiographically aggressive. (**d**) CT. Lesion appears slightly more aggressive on CT.

c   d

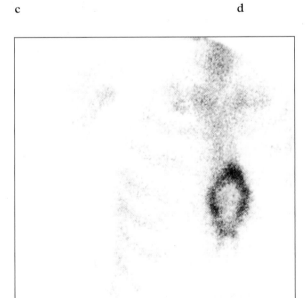

Figure 5.41

Low-grade chondrosarcoma. Elderly male presenting with a sternal mass. DS. Mild to moderate tracer uptake in the sternum, surrounding a more central area of relative photopenia.

Figure 5.42

Chondrosarcoma, right ilium. (a) X-ray, slight RAO. Irregular chondroid calcification projects almost stalk-like from upper ilium. (b) CT. The relationship of the tumor to the ilium. (c) RNA. No significant increased perfusion. (d) BP, anterior (left image) and posterior (right image). Very faint increased relative vascularity noted as asymmetry on anterior view. (e) DS, anterior. The stalk-like intense increased tracer with irregular borders laterally. (Image courtesy of F Frassica, Baltimore, MD.)

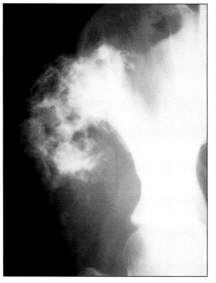

a

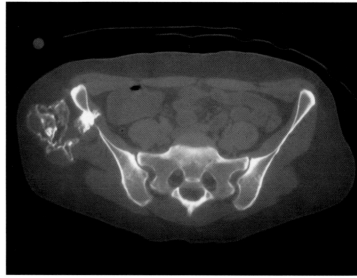

b

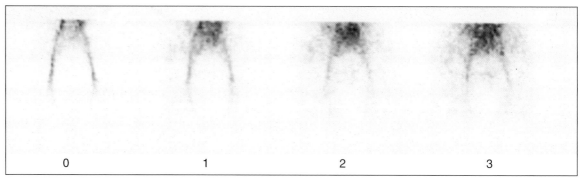

0   1   2   3

c

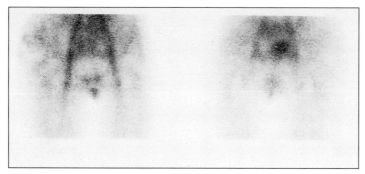

d   R Ant   L Post

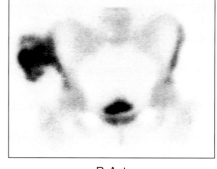

e   R Ant

Teaching point

Even without increased perfusion on RNA or intense increased relative vascularity on BP images, the irregularity of the uptake on the delayed images suggests a more aggressive lesion.

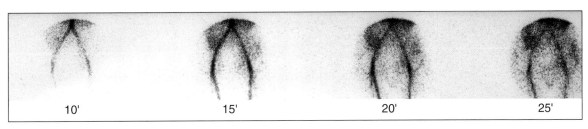

a

Figure 5.43

Chondrosarcoma, left ilium. (a) RNA, anterior, 5 seconds per view. Mild to moderate increased perfusion left ilium. Blood pool image not available. (b) WB. Irregular tracer accumulation projects laterally, medially, and inferiorly. The more posterior location is appreciated by the relative increased intensity of activity on the posterior compared with the anterior view.

Teaching point

Although SPECT is preferred, orthogonal views, which should be used frequently in bone imaging and can localize lesions in three dimensions, are often satisfactory.

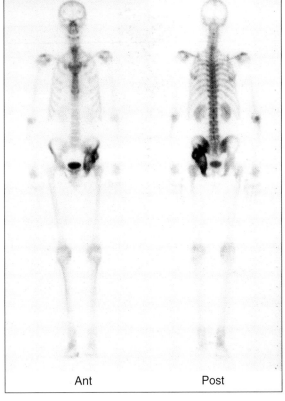

Ant   Post

b

Eosinophilic granuloma

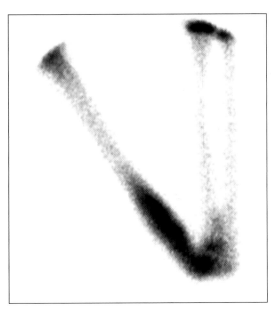

a

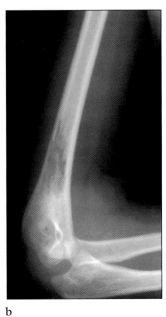

b

The term histiocytosis X, which had been used to describe three related disorders – eosinophilic granuloma of the bone, Hand–Schüller–Christian disease and Letterer–Siwe disease – is no longer utilized because the proliferating cells are not true histiocytes. The disorder is now called Langerhans' cell granulomatosis, which may be unifocal or multifocal. Localized lesions are known as eosinophilic granulomas.

Figure 5.44

Eosinophilic granuloma, right humerus. Ten-year-old boy with right arm pain. (a) DS. Intense abnormal uptake over a long area of the proximal most humerus. (b) X-ray. Permeative aggressive appearing lesion.

Fibrosarcoma

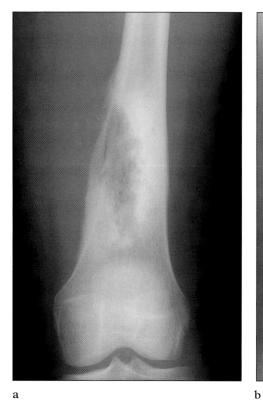

a

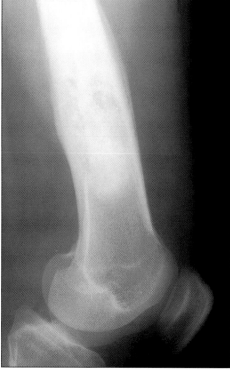

b

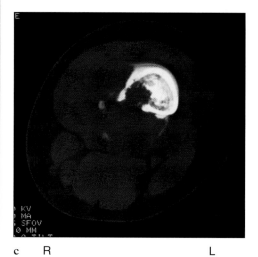

c R   L

Fibrosarcomas are not common. Many are now classified as malignant fibrous histiocytomas (MFH).

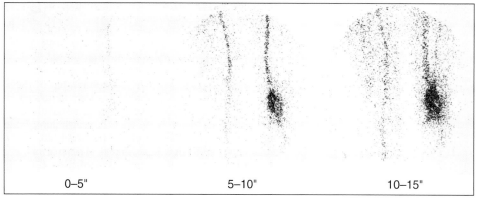

d R   L   R   L

0–5"   5–10"   10–15"

e

Figure 5.49 a–e

Fibrosarcoma. (a) X-ray, AP and (b) X-ray, lateral. A poorly defined lytic area with a permeative growth pattern. The cortical disruption and a soft tissue component are well appreciated on the AP view. (c) CT. The productive intramedullary component is illustrated, as is the cortical break. (d) MR, T2-weighted image, coronal. The soft tissue extent of the tumor is well seen on MR. (e) RNA, anterior, 5 seconds per view. Intense focal increased perfusion.

continued

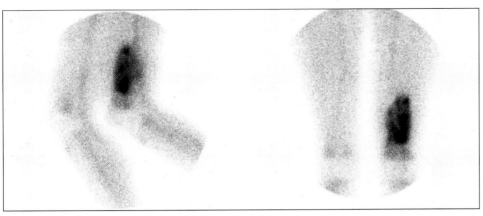

f   R Med   L Lat   R   L

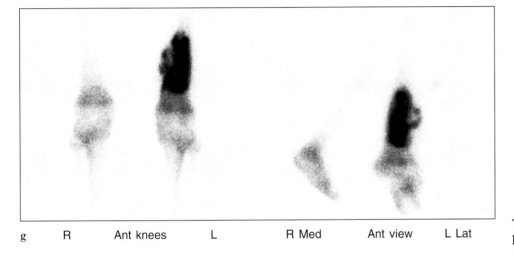

g   R   Ant knees   L   R Med   Ant view   L Lat

Figure 5.49 f–g

(f) BP, left lateral (left image) and anterior (right image) shows irregular distribution of the hypervascularity. (g) DS, anterior (left image) and left lateral (right image) shows the intense metabolic activity in comparison to adjacent bones. In this teenager the physeal activity is minimal.

The malignant proliferation of hemopoietic stem cells in leukemias takes place primarily in the bone marrow and the normal hemopoietic cells are replaced.

Leukemia

Figure 5.50

Leukemia, chronic lymphocytic. 68-year-old white female who presented with CLL and leukemia cutis. (a) Leukemia cutis over shoulders and neck. (b) WB. Diffuse abnormal bone uptake accentuated in the metaphyseal regions and in the spine.

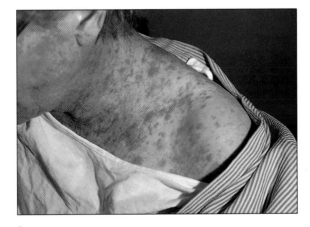

a

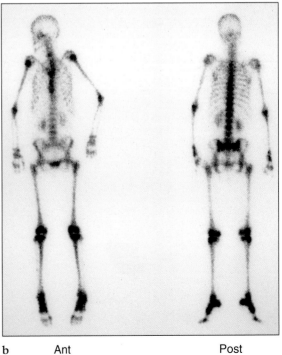

b   Ant   Post

Teaching point

The osseous lesions of acute leukemia are the result of replacement of the bone marrow by malignant cells. The exact etiology of increased deposition of tracer in these cases is uncertain, especially during the early stages when radiographs are normal or only diffuse osteopenia is present.

Figure 5.51

Leukemia, acute lymphocytic. Thirty-year-old patient who died 3 weeks after scan. WB. The epiphyseal uptake resembles that of a child.

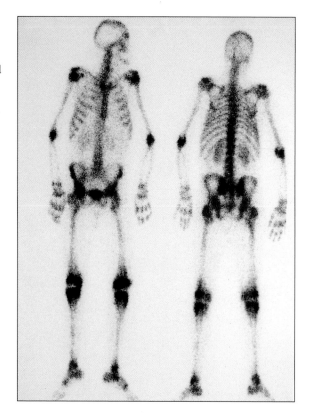

Lymphoma

Figure 5.52

Lymphoma, primary malignant lymphoma of bone. (a) DS, pelvis. Intense tracer uptake in lesser trochanter and adjacent intertrochanteric region. (b) Gallium-67, 48–72 hour image, pelvis. The lesion is gallium avid. (c) X-ray, pelvis, AP. Destructive lesion.

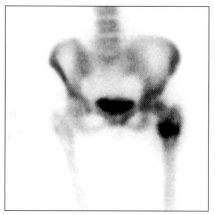

a

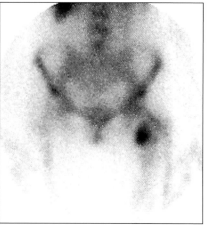

b

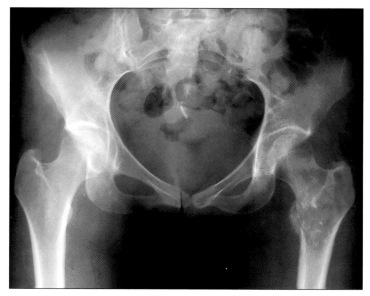

c

Malignant lymphoma that presents in bone without evidence of nodal or visceral disease is known as primary malignant lymphoma of bone. It has a more favorable prognosis than malignant lymphoma that secondarily involves bone marrow as a manifestation of disseminated disease.

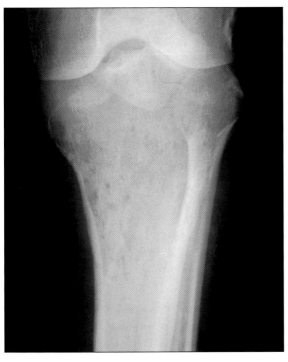

a

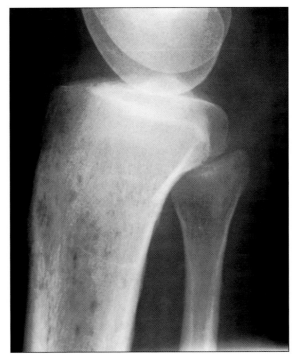

b

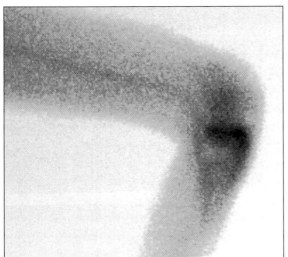

c

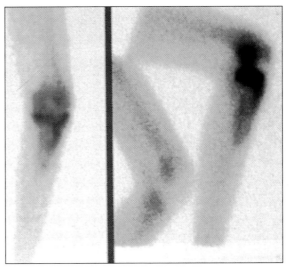

d

Figure 5.53

Lymphoma. (a) and (b) X-ray, AP and lateral. Permeative bone lesion. (c) BP. Lateral position only, because patient in such severe pain that she was imaged in bed in this position. (d) DS. Also only lateral view. Note activity most intense around periphery of lesion.

Lymphomas and leukemias are in the small round cell tumor group of lesions.

Teaching point

The location of greatest metabolic activity, as demonstrated on a bone scan, often represents the location of most active tumor growth and may guide the surgeon in the choice of biopsy site.

Figure 5.54

Lymphoma, Burkitt's.
(a) BP, anterior. Mild
increased relative
vascularity (increased
uptake) in proximal
humeri, and possibly the
ribs. (b) WB. Mild
homogeneous
symmetrical uptake in
proximal two-thirds of
both humeri and femurs.
Possibly rib uptake also.
(c) MR, T2-weighted
image, coronal. Diffuse
altered signal
characteristics of all the
visualized marrow except
the greater trochanter.

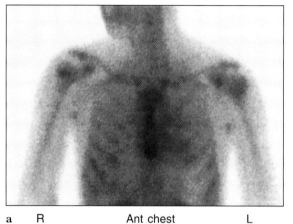

a   R   Ant chest   L

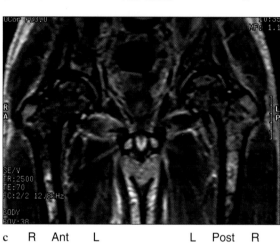

c   R   Ant   L   L   Post   R

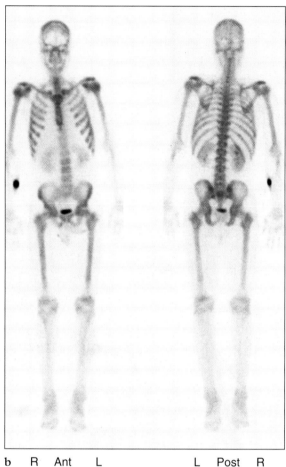

b   R   Ant   L   L   Post   R

Figure 5.55

**Lymphoma, malignant
small cell.** Seventy-nine-
year-old female. (a) WB.
Intense increased uptake,
entire right iliac wing,
lumbar spine, and
sternum. (b) CT. Mixed
sclerotic/lytic lesion right
iliac bone.

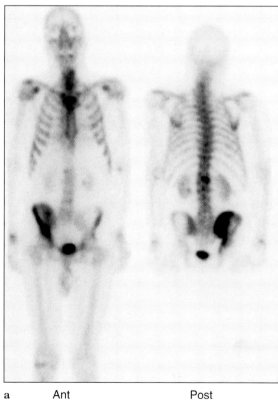

a   Ant   Post

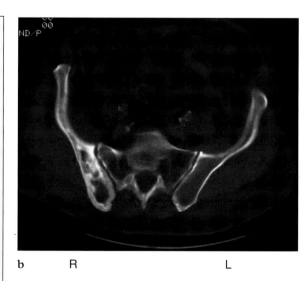

b   R   L

Any bone may be involved with malignant
lymphoma, with up to 30% of patients reported
with multiple osseous sites. The mandible, maxilla,
femur, pelvis, and spine are most common. Lesions
have varying amounts of intraosseous reactive
bone, which probably accounts for the variable
features on radionuclide bone imaging.

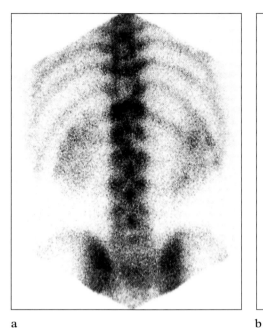

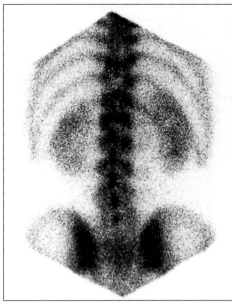

a

b

Figure 5.56

Lymphoma, T11 and paraspinal adenopathy. (**a**) DS, thoracic spine (TSP) and lumbar spine (LSP). Photon deficiency on the left at T11. Right kidney displaced laterally with axis rotated clockwise by adenopathy which does not take up bone tracer. (**b**) DS, 4 months later after radiotherapy. The photon-deficient lesion is less obvious and the kidney is now in normal position with a normal axis.

Teaching point

The position and orientation of the kidney, as well as the relative intensity, should be evaluated on all bone scans.

Malignant fibrous histiocytoma

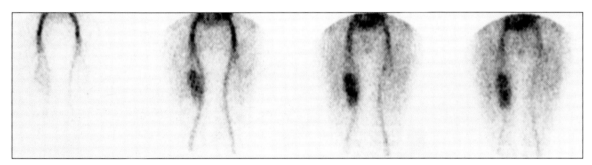

a

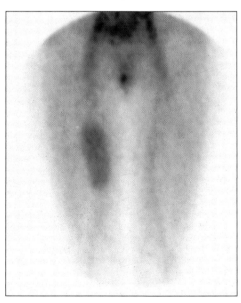

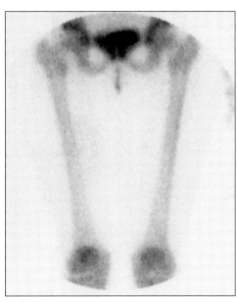

b

c

Teaching point

When there is no abnormal increased bone uptake associated with a soft tissue tumor, it is straightforward to exclude underlying bone involvement. When uptake on delayed images is only minimal, the differential between remodeling changes due to extrinsic pressure and those due to tumor destruction of bone is difficult. (Compare with Figure 5.18.)

Multiple myeloma

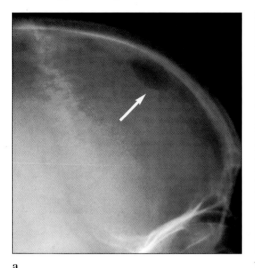

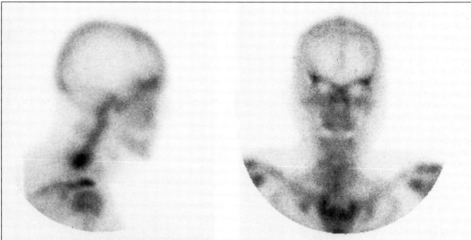

a

b

Figure 5.58

Multiple myeloma, normal scan. (a) X-ray, skull, lateral. Lytic lesions without any sclerotic margins in frontal bone (arrow). (b) DS, right lateral (left image) and anterior (right image). No abnormal uptake identified at site of lytic lesion.

Teaching point

The low sensitivity of bone imaging in detecting myeloma bone lesions is explained by the lack of new bone formation in this disease. In myeloma, bone resorption is in most cases uncoupled from new bone formation.

Osteosarcoma

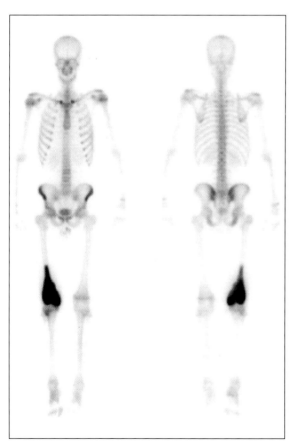

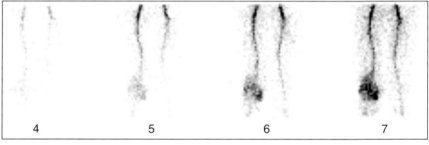

b

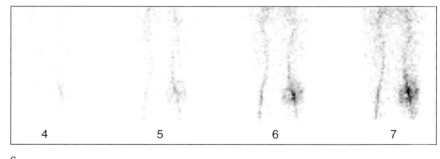

c

Figure 5.59 a–c

Osteosarcoma, conventional, distal right femur. (a) WB. Intense abnormal increased tracer in the distal third of the right femur. This is a monostotic lesion. (b) RNA, anterior and (c) RNA, posterior. Biplane RNA shows moderate focal increased perfusion to the distal femur.

a

continued

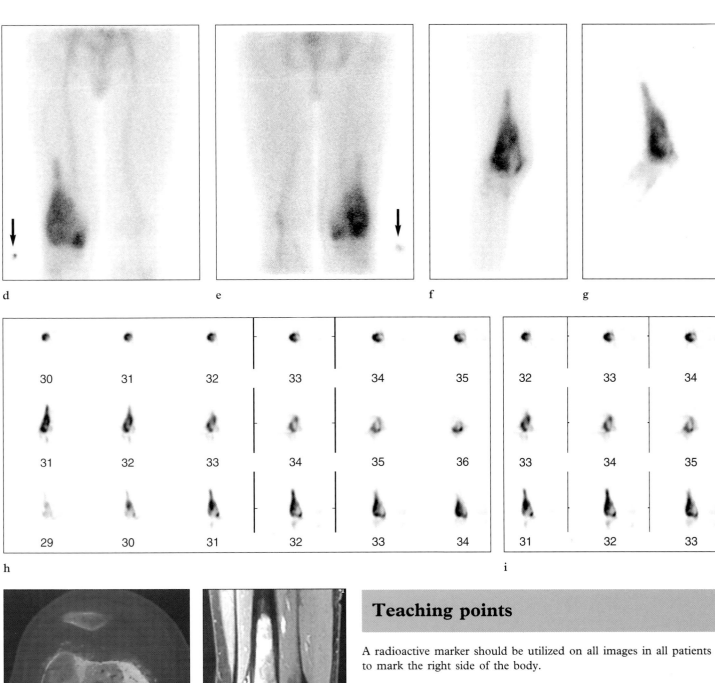

d   e   f   g

h   i

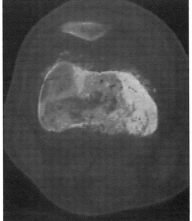 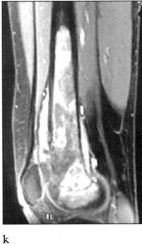

j   k

MR imaging with its ability to depict differences in soft tissue is excellent for determining the extent of intramedullary extension of tumors and the presence and characteristics of associated soft tissue extension. MR is now indispensable for preoperative therapeutic planning.

Teaching points

A radioactive marker should be utilized on all images in all patients to mark the right side of the body.

When viewing SPECT studies, the entire sequence in all reconstructed planes should be analyzed.

Figure 5.59 d–j

(d) BP, anterior and (e) BP, posterior. Intense somewhat irregularly distributed increased uptake (relative vascularity) throughout the lesion. Arrows point to the hot markers used on all images to indicate the right side of the patient's body. (f) BP, right lateral. Orthogonal view important for localization on BP as well as delayed images. (g) DS, right lateral. (h) SPECT, triangulation display. There is irregular distribution of metabolic activity throughout the lesion with localization of most intense areas. (i) SPECT, triangulation display, magnified views. Often larger views allow for better correlation with other imaging modalities. (j) CT, transaxial. Correlate with image (i). (k) MR, T1-weighted image. The intramedullary and soft tissue extent of the tumor are identified.

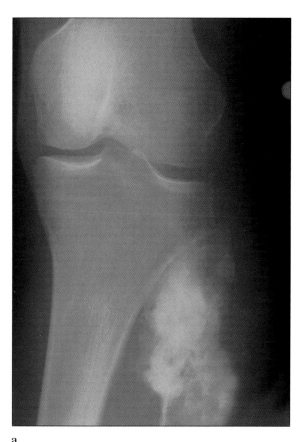

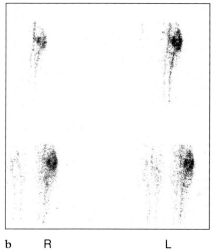

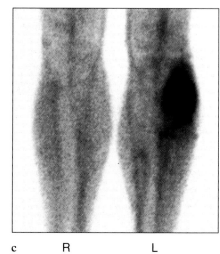

This is the most common type and the most common scintigraphic appearance of osteosarcoma.

a

b   R   L

c   R   L

Figure 5.60

Conventional osteosarcoma in 17-year-old. (a) X-ray AP. Proximal fibula lesion with typical tumor bone. (b) RNA, anterior. Moderate generalized increased perfusion to left knee region, more focal laterally. (c) BP. Moderate to marked increased tracer uptake (increased vascularity) proximal leg region. (d) WB. Intense abnormal increased tracer, proximal leg, with activity projecting off the expected outline of normal fibula. (e) DS, lateral. Well-defined, marked increased tracer uptake corresponds to lesion on radiograph.

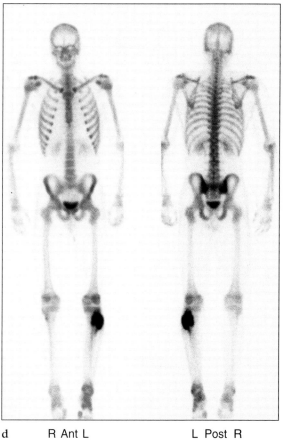

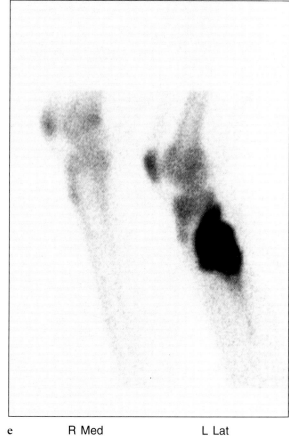

d   R Ant L   L Post R

e   R Med   L Lat

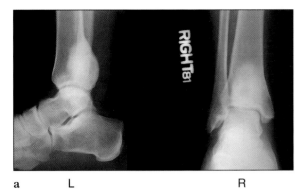

a   L   R

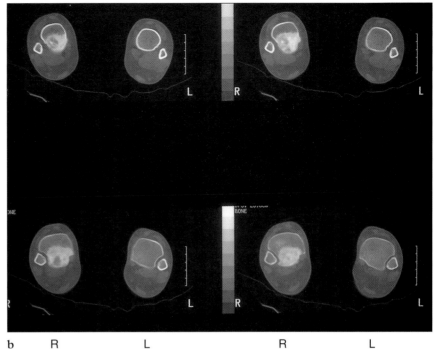

b   R   L   R   L

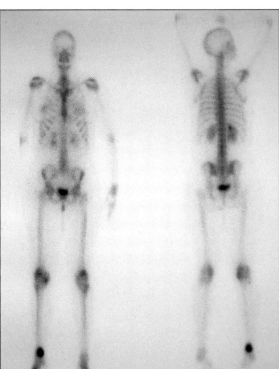

c   R Ant L   L Post R

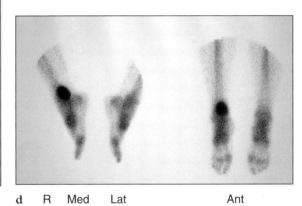

d   R   Med   Lat   Ant

Figure 5.61

Low-grade osteosarcoma, originally thought to be fibrous dysplasia. (**a**) X-ray, AP and lateral. Demonstrates intramedullary ossification. (**b**) CT, transaxial slices. Demonstrate intramedullary location of ossification. (**c**) WB. Intense abnormal tracer generally corresponds to radiographic lesion. (**d**) DS. Orthogonal views for better localization. Note the relative overexposure of this analog image.

This examination emphasizes again that RNBI depicts the metabolic activity associated with bone lesions, and that other anatomic imaging modalities, the clinical presentation, and often the tissue biopsy are all required for specific diagnosis.

Teaching point

RNBI is the most efficacious examination to evaluate the entire skeleton for determining whether a known lesion is monostotic or part of a polyostotic process.

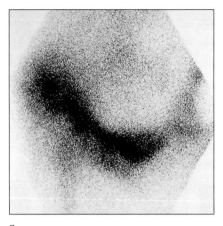

a

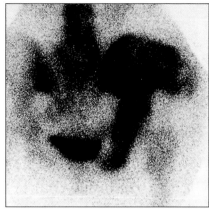

b

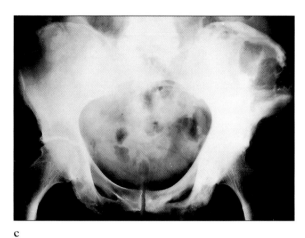

c

Figure 5.62

Osteosarcoma, left ilium, superimposed on Paget's disease. (a) DS, anterior, (b) DS, posterior and (c) X-ray of pelvis. The bone scan shows extensive abnormal tracer accumulation throughout the right hemipelvis, with gross disruption of the anatomic borders in the lateral portion of the iliac wing. Note that there is some tracer uptake in associated soft tissue. The X-ray shows evidence of gross destruction at the corresponding site, together with the changes of Paget's disease. The expanded destructed appearance laterally is caused by the sarcomatous change.

Teaching point

While sarcomatous change normally appears as increased activity on the bone scan, this is not always the case.

If sarcomatous change is suspected in a patient with known Paget's disease, radiographic investigation is required for evaluation because, as with fracture, increased uptake may not always be apparent when superimposed on an already tracer avid lesion.

Figure 5.63

Parosteal osteosarcoma. (a) Lateral X-ray. Productive lesion with tumor bone. (b) RNA. Moderate generalized increased perfusion to left distal femur, with more focal increase in distal medial aspect. (c) BP. Well-defined marked increased uptake (increased relative vascularity) primarily to anteromedial aspect of lower leg. (d) DS. Intense tracer uptake defines the metabolically active tumor.

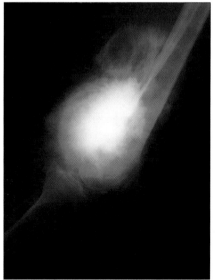

a

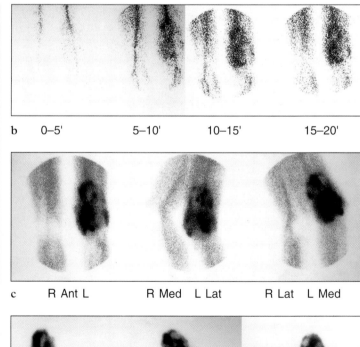

b 0–5'   5–10'   10–15'   15–20'

c R Ant L   R Med L Lat   R Lat L Med

On these spot views, taken for counts, the relative intensity of tumor uptake is such that, on the images, no demonstrable counts are contributed by normal bone.

d R Ant L   R Lat L Med   R Med L Lat

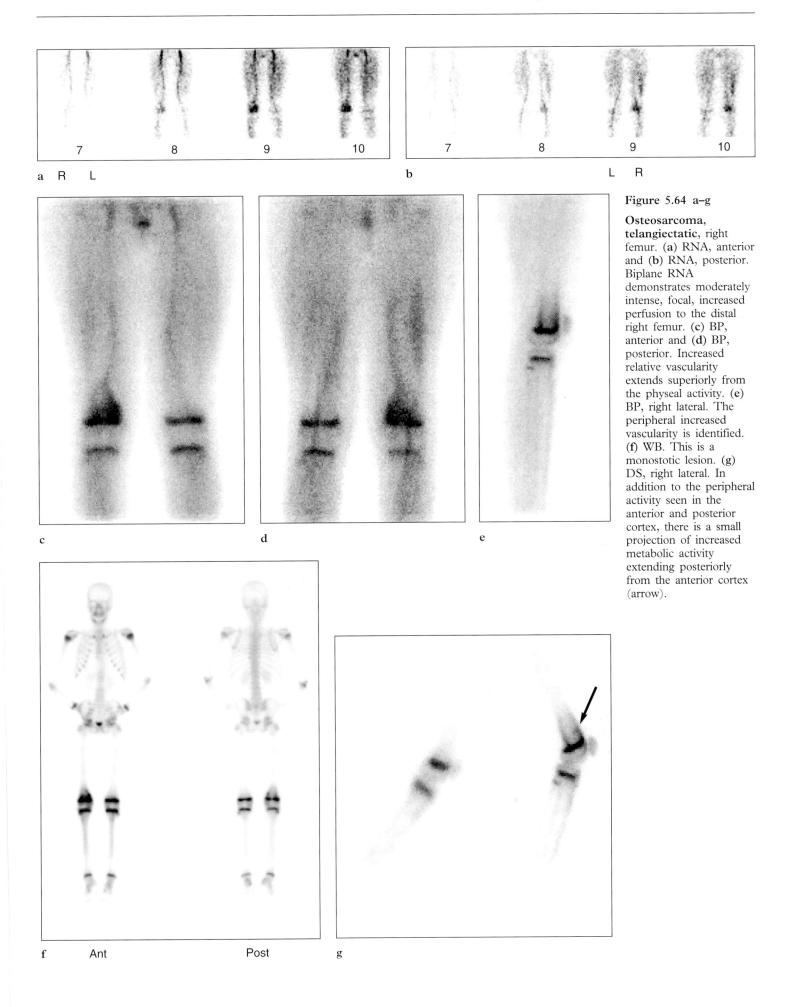

a   R   L

b   L   R

c

d

e

Figure 5.64 a–g

Osteosarcoma, telangiectatic, right femur. (a) RNA, anterior and (b) RNA, posterior. Biplane RNA demonstrates moderately intense, focal, increased perfusion to the distal right femur. (c) BP, anterior and (d) BP, posterior. Increased relative vascularity extends superiorly from the physeal activity. (e) BP, right lateral. The peripheral increased vascularity is identified. (f) WB. This is a monostotic lesion. (g) DS, right lateral. In addition to the peripheral activity seen in the anterior and posterior cortex, there is a small projection of increased metabolic activity extending posteriorly from the anterior cortex (arrow).

f   Ant   Post

g

Blood-borne metastasis

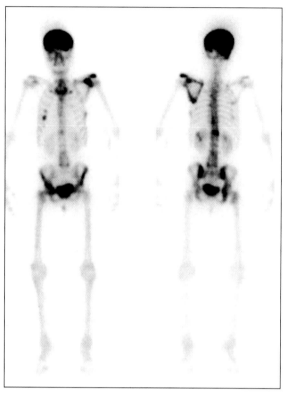

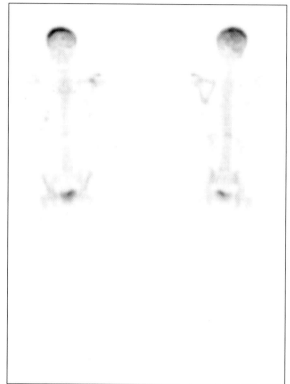

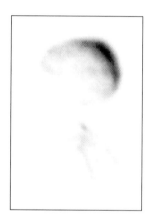

a

b

c

Figure 6.1

Breast cancer. (a) WB. Scaled so that normal ribs look 'normal'. With this scaling setting all the bone lesions are identified. The skull activity is so intense that Paget's disease could be suspected. (b) WB. Scaled to hottest count per pixel. The skull activity seems less geographic. Other bone lesions, however, are not identified. (c) DS, skull, left lateral. Irregular skull activity in orthogonal view. Radiographs confirmed multiple lytic lesions most compatible with metastatic disease.

Teaching point

Although many geographic lesions and lesions involving the entire bone can suggest Paget's disease, that diagnosis should not be made without careful correlative imaging and consideration of the patient's presenting signs, symptoms, and history.

Figure 6.2 (*images on facing page*)

Lung cancer, orbital and temporal bone metastasis. (a) WB. Both the right temporal and right orbital lesions are very subtle. (b) DS, right lateral. Abnormal foci, although still subtle, are better seen (arrows). (c) SPECT, triangulation display. Right temporal lesion. Abnormal uptake is at the junction of the squamosal and petrous portions of the temporal bone (as more precisely localized on MR image (f)). (d) SPECT, triangulation display. Coronal section through right medial superior orbital lesion (arrows). The value of viewing the entire series of images in all planes is emphasized by this study. (e) SPECT, triangulation display, enlarged images from (d). (f) MR. Anatomic imaging confirms a lesion corresponding to the abnormal increased tracer on bone scan, transaxial images on (c).

continued

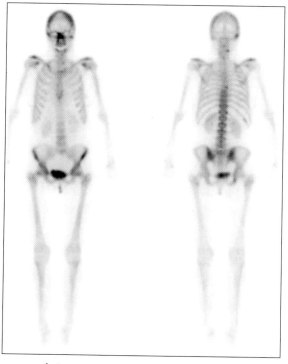

a   Ant   Post

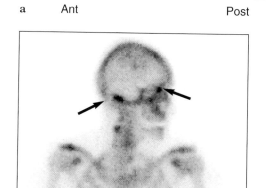

b

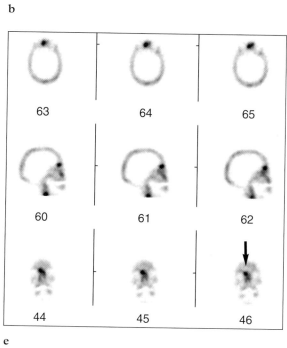

e

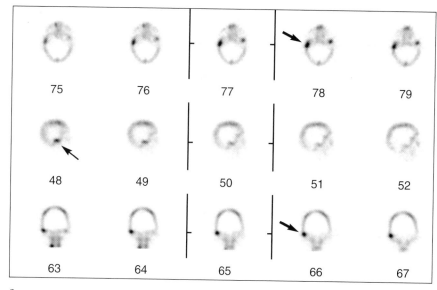

c

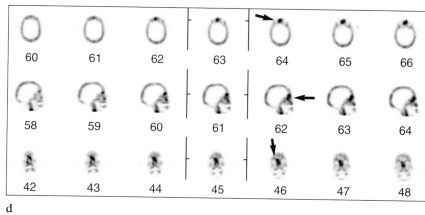

d

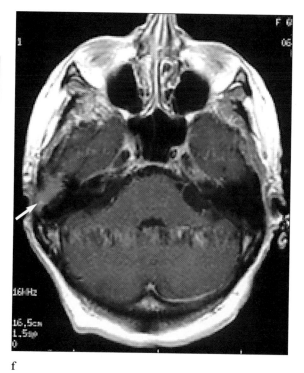

f

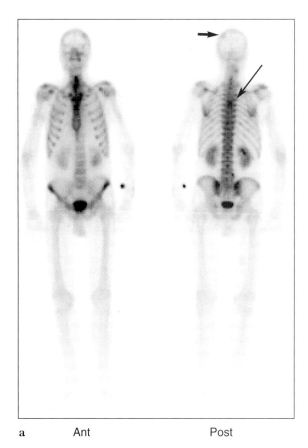

a   Ant   Post

Figure 6.3

Lung cancer, thoracic spine and parenchymal brain metastasis. (a) WB. Focal activity right side of head projects from inner table (straight arrow). Poorly defined thoracic spine uptake appreciated on posterior view (long thin arrow). (b) DS, left lateral, head. Orthogonal view localizes uptake to posterior parietal region. (c) 3-D. Selected images from 10° to 60°. In addition to the head activity, anterior cervical spine and anterior body thoracic spine activity are identified. (d) SPECT, triangulation display. Coronal sections through skull lesion. Transaxial view (especially numbers 19 and 20) (arrow) demonstrates the uptake separate from the bone. On correlative MR imaging this was thought to represent necrosis within a brain metastasis. (e) SPECT, triangulation display. Coronal image through upper thoracic lesion. Transaxial view demonstrates abnormal uptake confined to the body.

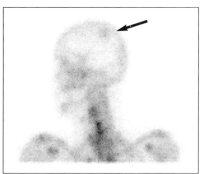

b

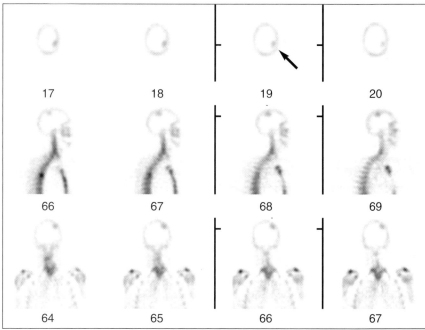

d

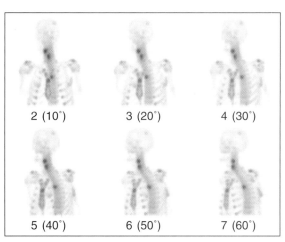

c

e

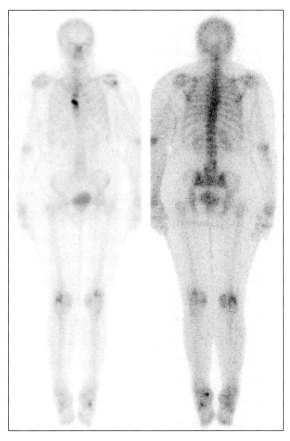

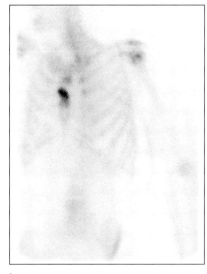

b

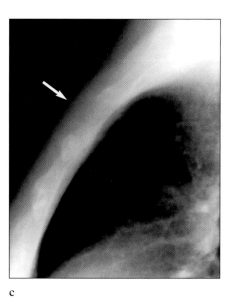

c

Figure 6.4

Breast cancer, sternal metastasis. (a) WB. Intense, obliquely oriented activity in midsternum is not typical of the horizontal activity at the angle of Louis, which is often a normal variant. (b) DS, chest LAO. This semi-orthogonal view demonstrates the lesion. (c) X-ray, lateral sternum. Focus of bone destruction with minimal associated soft tissue mass identified (arrow).

a

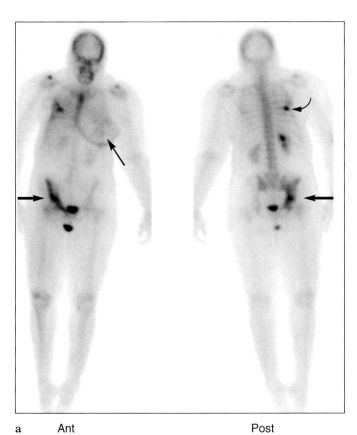

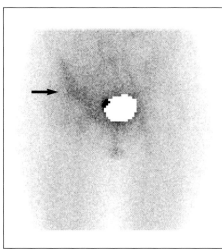

b　　　　Ant

a　　Ant　　　　Post

Figure 6.5 a–b

Breast cancer metastasis to pelvis and rib. Status post left breast reconstruction. (a) WB, 6/98. More focal acetabular activity (straight arrow on anterior and posterior view) is slightly more superior and medial than typical location for activity associated with biomechanical stress degenerative joint disease (DJD), and also extends into the ilium. Rib versus scapular activity dilemma on posterior view (curved arrow). Solved in (c). Skin-fold activity surrounds subtle photon deficiency of recent muscle flap breast reconstruction procedure (thin arrow on anterior view). (b) BP, anterior. Mild relative increased vascularity of right ilium and acetabulum.

continued

Figure 6.5 c–f

(c) DS, arms elevated. Focal uptake localized to rib. (d) X-ray, pelvis, 6/98. Large irregular partially lytic lesion (arrows) corresponds to region of abnormal tracer. (e) WB, 11/96. Earlier study demonstrates more subtle uptake which, however, should still raise the suspicion of metastatic disease. (f) X-ray, pelvis, 1/95. Focal sclerosis (arrow) corresponds to abnormal uptake.

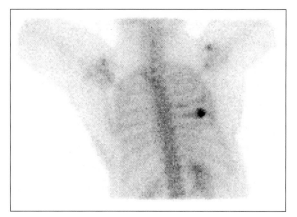

c

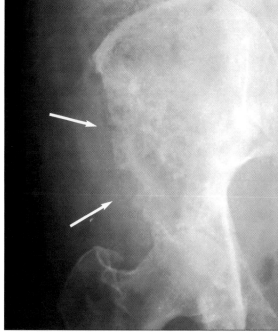

d

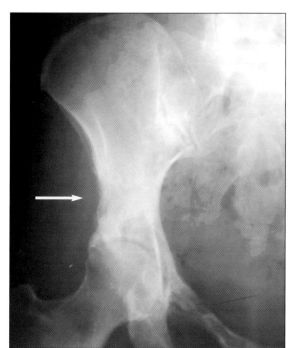

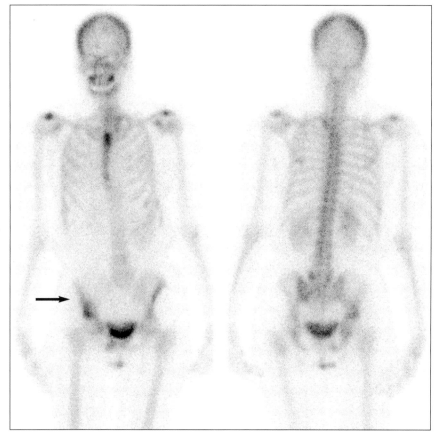

e   Ant   Post f

Teaching point

High-resolution planar images permit detailed anatomic localization and description of abnormal uptake, which can aid in differential diagnosis. Shape, orientation, extent, and severity can be determined.

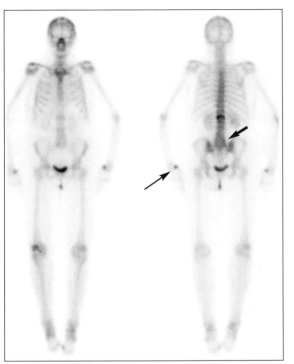

a

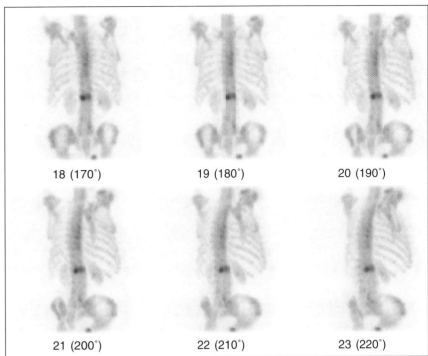

18 (170°)   19 (180°)   20 (190°)

21 (200°)   22 (210°)   23 (220°)

b

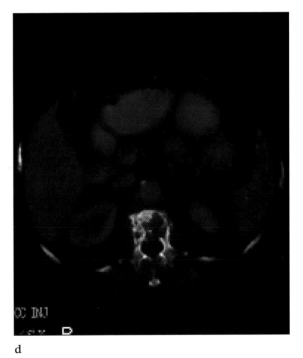

73   74   75   76

63   64   65   66

74   75   76   77

c

d

Figure 6.6

Breast cancer, lumbar spine. (a) WB. Asymmetric activity involving L1 vertebral body does not have the linear, superior endplate appearance of a fracture nor does it have the clear lateral location often associated with degenerative change, and hence it needs further evaluation. Minimally intense, laterally located activity at the L5/S1 level (straight arrow) is more typical of degenerative change. Focal activity in the region of the first carpometacarpal joint (thin arrow) represents the common basal joint arthritis. (b) 3-D volume-reconstructed image. Selected views from data set, which are usually viewed in movie mode, are valuable for detecting and localizing abnormal foci of uptake. (c) SPECT, triangulation display. SPECT localizes abnormal activity to the body, and on the left side possible extension into the pedicle (arrow). (d) CT, bone window. Lytic and blastic components of vertebral body lesion.

Figure 6.9

Breast cancer, photon-deficient 'cold' metastasis. (a) SPECT, coronal and (b) SPECT, transaxial, demonstrate photon deficiency. These images are processed with a filter to give a smoother image.

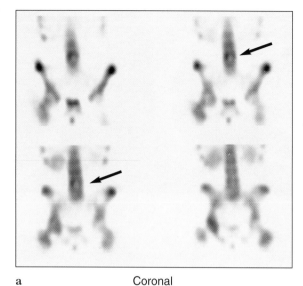

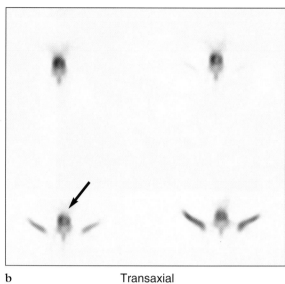

a   Coronal

b   Transaxial

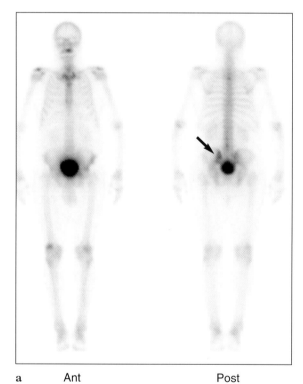

a   Ant   Post

Figure 6.10

Prostate cancer, left ilium. (a) WB. Subtle asymmetry in left SI region seen on posterior view (arrow); anterior sacrum and medial ilium obscured by full bladder. Patient could not void and refused catheterization. (b) SPECT, triangulation display, (c) SPECT, transaxial and (d) SPECT, coronal. The coronal sections begin at the level of posterior bladder and move posteriorly. Transaxial sections begin upper ilium, above bladder and move caudally. Abnormal tracer in ilium (arrows) and posteriorly. Note: Excellent lesion delineation (straight arrows) since the bladder-filling artifact and reconstruction-related bladder intensity scaling problems (curved arrows) are not in these planes of section.

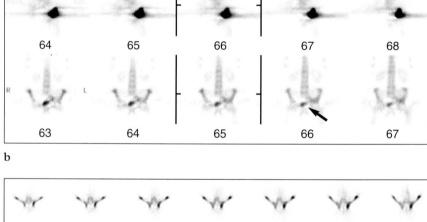

b

c

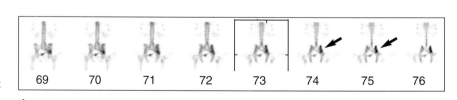

d

Teaching point

Review of SPECT images should be done on a computer monitor. Display manipulations such as window and leveling are usually required. Often lesions are satisfactorily seen on only one of two planes of section because of bladder-filling or reconstruction hotspot artifacts.

Figure 6.11 a–d

Prostate cancer, sacral lesion. (a) WB. L5/S1 region activity bilaterally could easily be mistaken for facet arthritis. **(b)** 3-D. Selected images from 180° to 230°. Note the more rounded configuration and inferior extent of the left-sided focus of increased tracer accumulation (arrow). **(c)** SPECT, triangulation display. Especially on coronal images the inferior extent of the left-sided focus of uptake is appreciated (arrow). **(d)** SPECT, triangulation display. Magnified images from **(c)**.

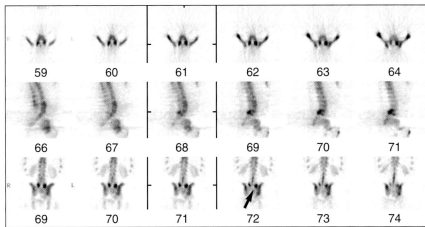

c

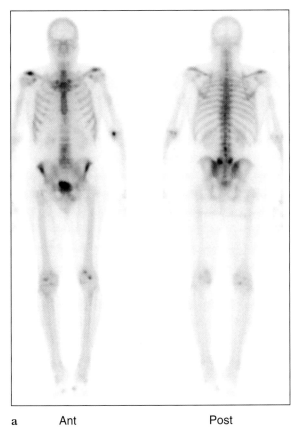

a   Ant   Post

19 (180°)   20 (190°)   21 (200°)

22 (210°)   23 (220°)   24 (230°)

b   d   *continued*

Figure 6.11 e–g

(e) SPECT, oblique angle reconstruction, triangulation display. The inferior extent of the left-sided uptake is appreciated on the transaxial images which are en face views (arrow). (f) SPECT, oblique angle reconstruction triangulation display. Magnified views of images from (e). (g) MR. Transaxial image, T2 weighted, abnormal signal (arrow).

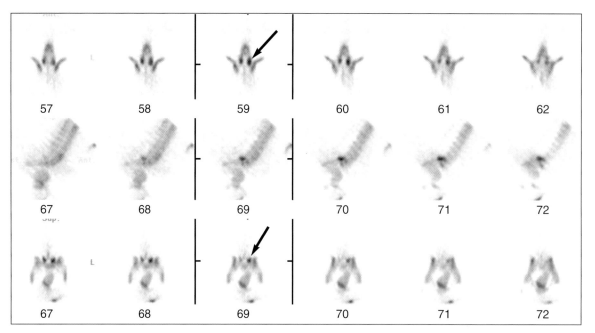

e

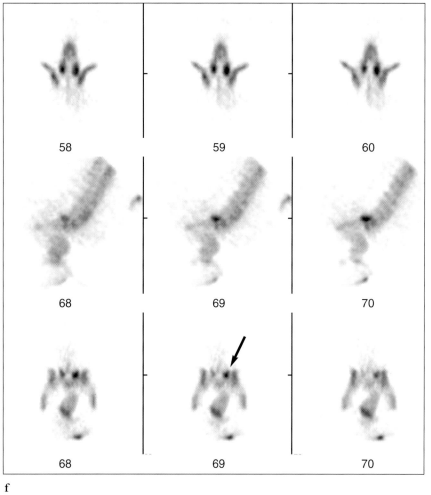

f

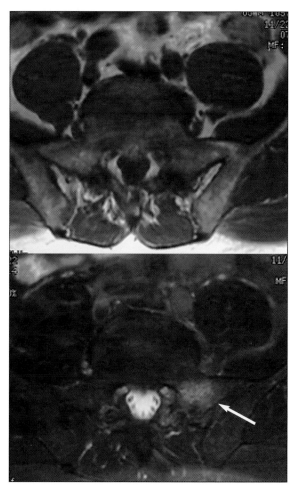

g

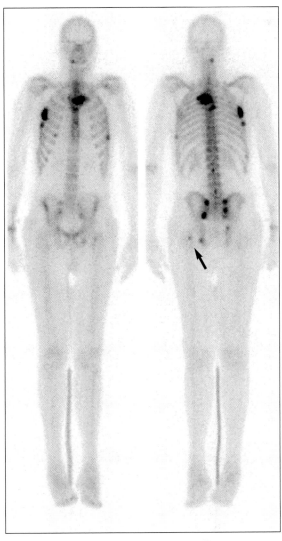

a   Ant   Post

Teaching point

Lesions in weight-bearing areas, which weaken the bone and increase the probability of fracture, are called 'critical lesions'. The referring physician should be contacted prior to the patient leaving the Nuclear Medicine Department.

Figure 6.12

Prostate cancer. (a) WB. Four rounded foci of uptake in SI joint region are unusually symmetric for metastatic disease. Femoral neck activity in weight-bearing area is so-called 'critical' lesion (arrow). (b) DS, RPO view. Oblique view demonstrates elongated rib lesion typical for metastasis. This contrasts with the focal round lesions usually associated with healing rib fractures. (c) SPECT, triangulation display. The sacral location of the round pelvic foci is identified. Compare the transaxial view with the CT scan in (d). (d) CT, soft tissue window. Unfortunately bone windows were not obtained. Image reproduced to illustrate relationship of sacrum to ilium at this level of section.

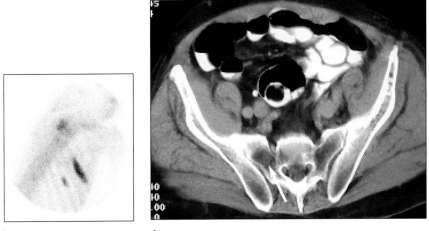

b   d

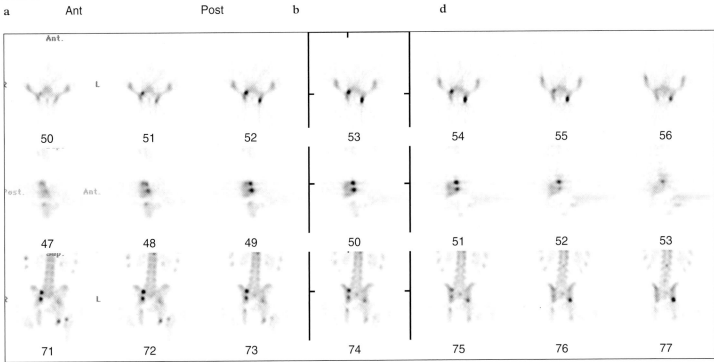

c

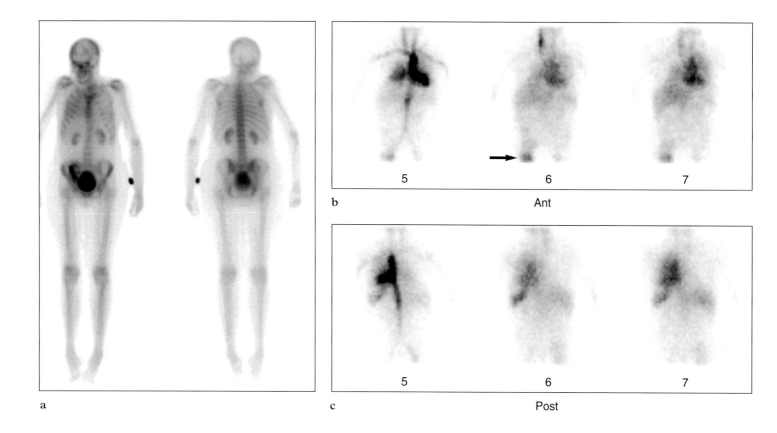

b   Ant

c   Post

a

Figure 6.13 above

Breast cancer, status post renal transplant. (a) WB. Activity in calyces in transplant kidney in right pelvis should not be mistaken for a metastasis. Often the native kidneys are left in place, and can still show minimal function as in this patient. Biplane radionuclide angiography was performed because of low back pain. On the anterior RNA (b) the perfusion to the transplant kidney is noted at the bottom of the field of view (arrow). On the posterior RNA (c) there is no significant perfusion to the minimally functioning native kidneys.

Figure 6.14

Neuroblastoma, pelvis and femurs. Incidental sutural activity in skull. Eight-year-old female. WB. Subtle activity in distal right femurs (arrow), just above the more intense normal linear uptake of the distal femoral physes, illustrates that in these pediatric tumors uptake can be very subtle and the imager needs a strong index of suspicion. Similarly, asymmetry in the SI joint regions, particularly well appreciated on the posterior view, deserves further evaluation. In this case the entire pelvis was involved with tumor. Incidental round foci of very minimally intense uptake in the skull are seen. These usually represent normal variants.

Teaching point

Small, round, and generally minimally intense foci of uptake in the skull, usually in the frontal or immediately adjacent parietal or temporal bone, are usually normal variants even in patients with malignancy. When the intensity of uptake or size gives the experienced imager pause for concern, correlative plain X-ray or CT images can be performed. They are usually normal, although an occasional osteoma or bone island may be present. Similarly in children small foci can be seen in association with sutures.

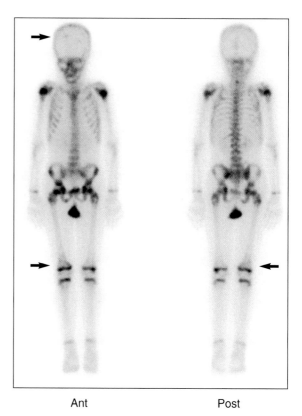

Ant   Post

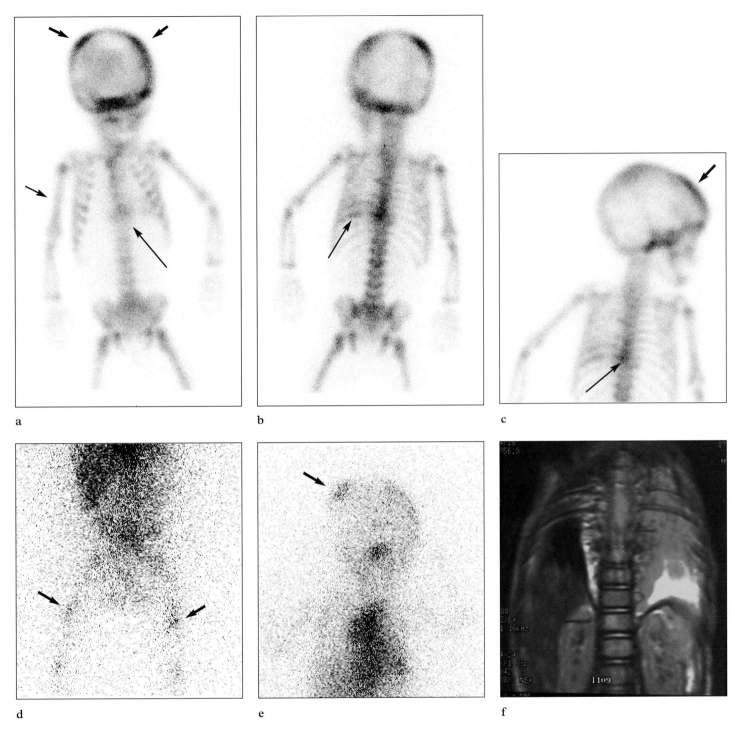

Figure 6.15

Neuroblastoma. Nine-month-old. (**a and b**) DS, anterior and posterior. Abnormal foci, skull (arrow) are more obvious than the subtle abnormalities in the humeri. Also subtle increase involving the left femur. There was some minimal uptake in the patient's primary tumor in the left chest appreciated on both the anterior and posterior views (long thin arrow). Compare with (**f**). (**c**) DS, right lateral skull with posterior chest. Orthogonal view demonstrates skull lesion (arrow). T9 activity (thin arrow) also noted. (**d**) MIBG tumor imaging. Twenty-four hour anterior. Femoral foci of activity identified (arrow). (**e**) MIBG. Anterior chest with right lateral skull. Skull lesion identified (arrow). (**f**) MR, coronal T2 image. Bright signal associated with tumor.

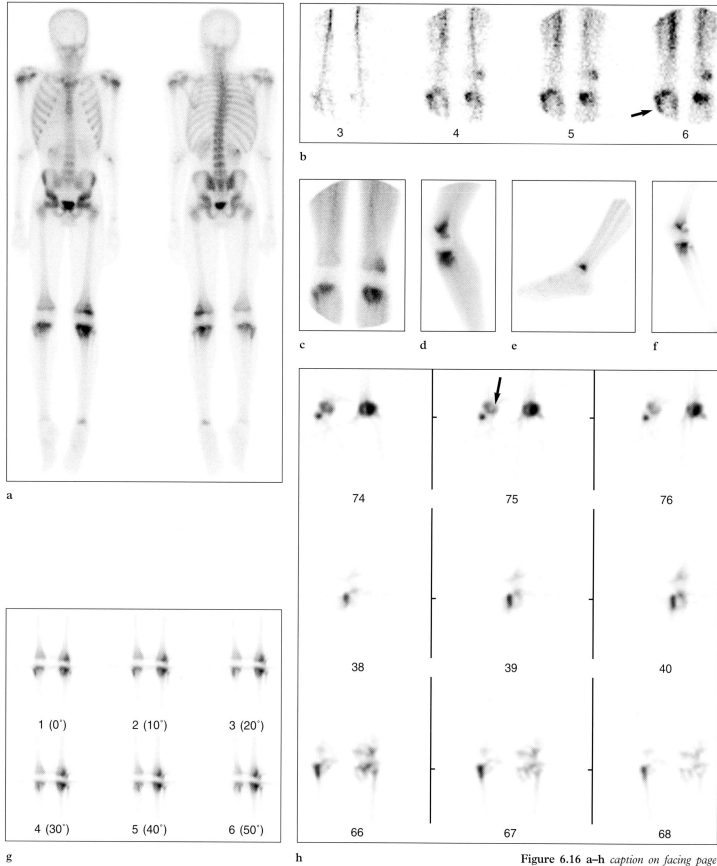

a

b

c d e f

g

1 (0°)   2 (10°)   3 (20°)

4 (30°)   5 (40°)   6 (50°)

3   4   5   6

74   75   76

38   39   40

66   67   68

h

Figure 6.16 a–h *caption on facing page*

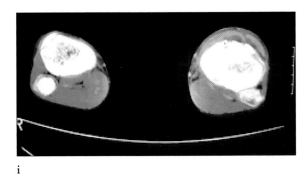

i

Variable histologic expression of tumor metastasis in the same patient makes radiographic detection of metastasis more difficult, and demands careful evaluation of all areas of abnormal tracer uptake seen on the bone scan.

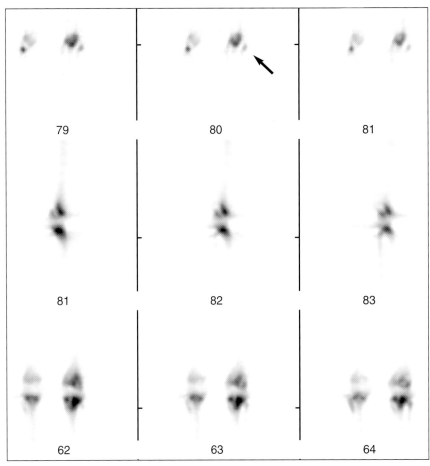

j

Figure 6.16

Malignant thymoma, 15-year-old male. (a) WB. Varying intensity of abnormal uptake in distal left femur, proximal left tibia, proximal right fibula, and distal left tibia represents different expressions of the same tumor. (b) RNA, anterior view, 5 seconds per frame. Focal area of increased perfusion seen in the distal left femur, proximal left tibia more medial than lateral, and in the proximal right fibula (arrow). (c) BP, anterior. Abnormal increased vascularity confirmed. (d) BP, left lateral. Orthogonal blood pool image helps confirm location of abnormal increased relative vascularity. (e) DS, left ankle, lateral triangular focus of increased tracer localized to distal tibia. (f) DS, left knee lateral. Varying intensity represents varying degrees of metabolic activity within the tumor. (g) 3-D, selected images from 0° to 50°. Shown in movie mode, these images highlighted the abnormal tracer in the proximal right fibula. (h) SPECT, triangulation display. Coronal images through proximal fibulas. The transaxial images demonstrate the relationship of the posterolateral fibula to the more anteromedial tibia (arrow). On the left the abnormal metabolic activity in the tibia is laterally located. (i) CT, bone windows. Level corresponding to the transaxial image in (h) demonstrates the relationship of the fibula to the tibia. (j) SPECT, triangulation display. Coronal image through the level of the tibial lesions. At this level the fibula on the left is better delineated from the tibia (arrow). (k) X-ray, right knee, anterior. Subtle proximal fibula changes seen medially consists of subtle cortical erosion and periosteal new bone formation. (l) X-ray, left knee, AP. Note the mixed radiologic appearance of the tumor with a lytic component in the lateral distal left femoral metaphysis and the proximal tibial metastasis both laterally and medially. (m) X-ray, left ankle, lateral. The subtle sclerotic triangular lesion just above the articular surface corresponds to the abnormal bone scan activity (arrow).

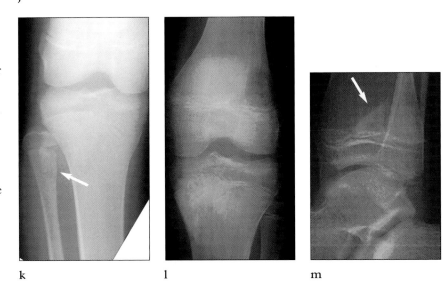

k   l   m

Teaching point

The anatomic location of abnormal increased perfusion (tracer accumulation) on the RNA can often be better localized by viewing the higher count BP image which is taken immediately, without moving the patient. Orthogonal BP images should also be obtained when abnormal tracer accumulation is identified.

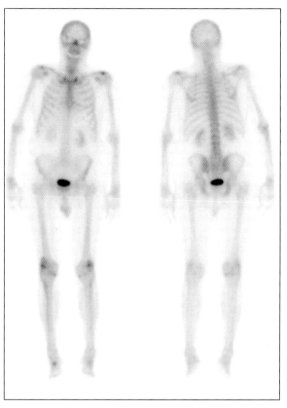

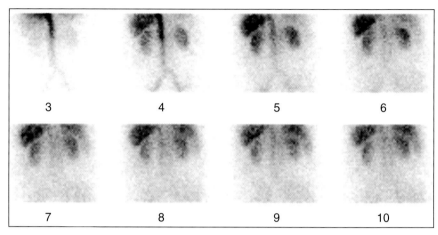

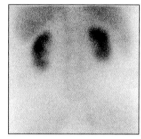

b

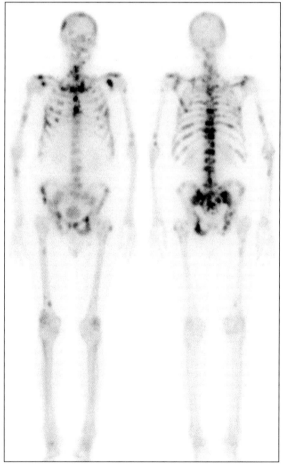

a

c

Figure 6.17

Prostate cancer, rapidly progressive disease. (a) WB, (b) RNA, posterior, and (c) BP, posterior. At time of staging. Normal examination. (d) WB, (e) RNA, and (f) BP. Nine months later. The WB (d) demonstrates intense diffuse multifocal uptake primarily in axial but also in appendicular skeleton. The RNA (e) demonstrates early increased perfusion to the spine and pelvis. Although subtle this is confirmed on the BP (f) images. Compare (e) and (f) with (b) and (c).

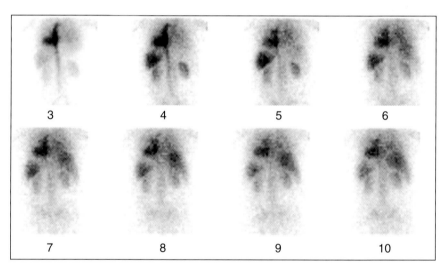

e

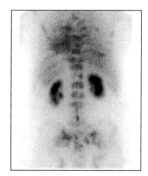

d   Ant   Post

f

Teaching point

Increased activity on BP or tissue phase images, when associated with passive diffusion of tracer because of soft tissue inflammation or infection, is usually diffuse. This contrasts with the more focal early bone uptake secondary to both increased blood flow and 'early fixation' of tracer in metastatic disease, which is illustrated in Figure 6.17 (f).

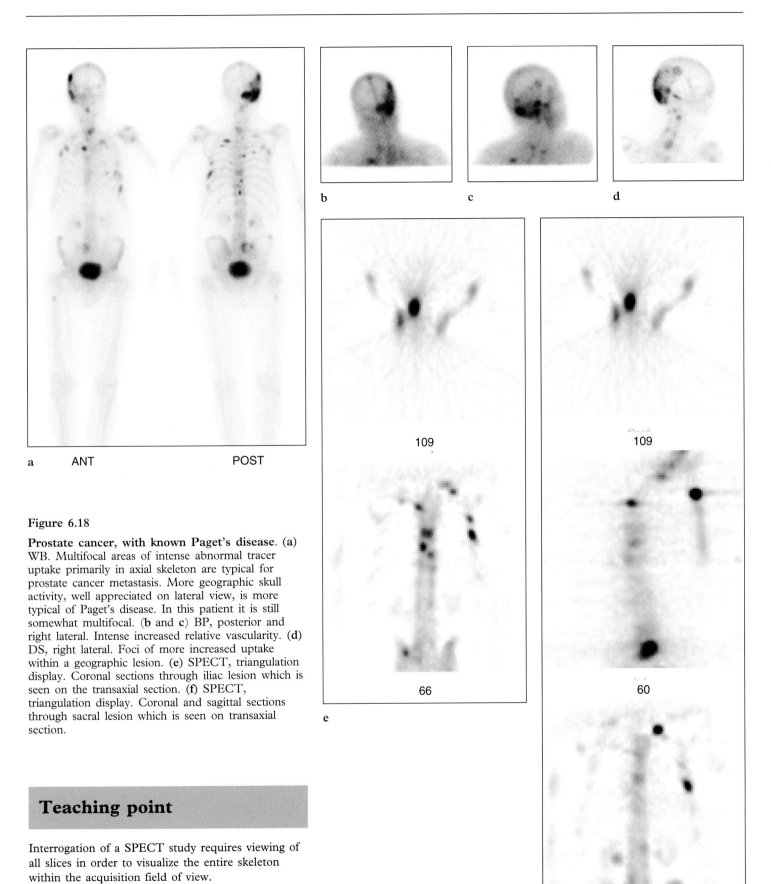

a   ANT   POST

b   c   d

109   109

66   60

e

61

f

Figure 6.18

Prostate cancer, with known Paget's disease. (a) WB. Multifocal areas of intense abnormal tracer uptake primarily in axial skeleton are typical for prostate cancer metastasis. More geographic skull activity, well appreciated on lateral view, is more typical of Paget's disease. In this patient it is still somewhat multifocal. (b and c) BP, posterior and right lateral. Intense increased relative vascularity. (d) DS, right lateral. Foci of more increased uptake within a geographic lesion. (e) SPECT, triangulation display. Coronal sections through iliac lesion which is seen on the transaxial section. (f) SPECT, triangulation display. Coronal and sagittal sections through sacral lesion which is seen on transaxial section.

Teaching point

Interrogation of a SPECT study requires viewing of all slices in order to visualize the entire skeleton within the acquisition field of view.

Figure 6.19

Hodgkin's lymphoma.
Radiographically these
widespread lesions were
almost purely lytic. Note
subtle femoral shaft
activity (arrow). Renal
uptake is compatible with
the nonspecific renal
uptake associated with
chemotherapy.

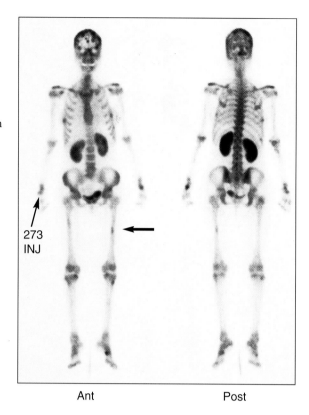

Ant   Post

Figure 6.20 a–b

**Prostate cancer,
vascular pelvic bone
metastasis.** (a) WB,
9/95. 'Super scan' of
diffuse metastatic disease.
Note absent visualization
of renal activity. For
comparison with (b)–(d).
(b) WB, 7/97. More
typical multifocal areas of
abnormal tracer. Note
the almost geographic
pattern of right ilial
uptake. This could be
confused with Paget's
disease.

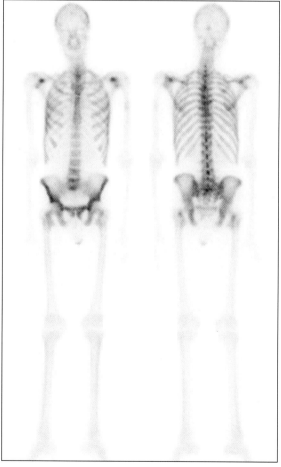

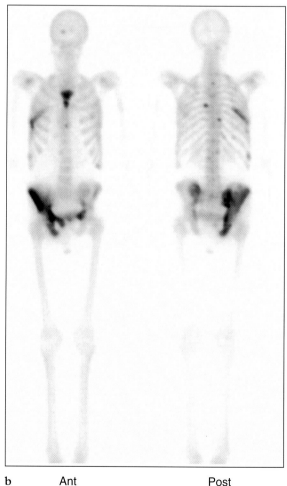

continued

a   Ant   Post

b   Ant   Post

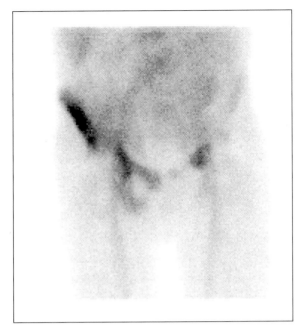

c

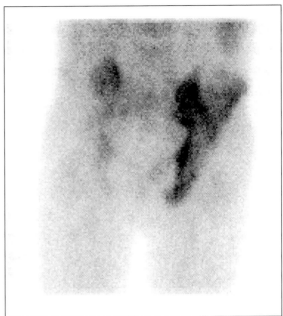

d

Figure 6.20 c–d

(c) BP, anterior. When a three-phase scan is performed because of focal pain, areas of rapid bone turnover will have intense early tracer uptake, which represents passive diffusion of tracer because of increased relative vascularity, as well as early fixation of tracer. (d) BP, posterior.

'Super scan' may be defined as a bone scan where there is increased and relatively uniform tracer uptake throughout the skeleton, with high contrast between bone and soft tissues. Renal activity, when images are displayed with standard scaling or film intensity settings, is usually not visualized because of increased relative bone uptake and decreased renal excretion. In addition high uptake of tracer by the skeleton leaves less available for excretion via the urinary tract, and bladder activity may not be seen. Although originally described in association with malignancy, the super scan has been reported in a variety of other situations, primarily hyperparathyroidism.

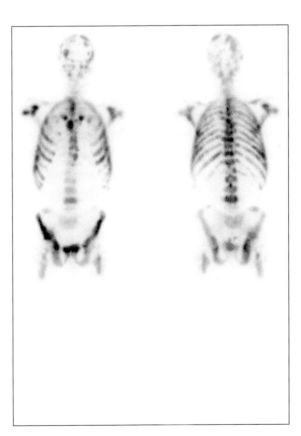

Figure 6.21

Prostate cancer, pseudo super scan. WB. Very intense abnormal tracer throughout the axial skeleton and proximal appendicular skeleton. With standard acquisition parameters, the overwhelming amount of tracer in the visualized areas results in apparent absent extremities. Renal activity is also not visualized. Because of the multifocal uptake, this scan would not be confused with a normal study.

Figure 6.22

Lung cancer with axial and appendicular metastasis. (a) WB. Moderately intense foci of tracer uptake in spine; contrast with mild uptake in left humerus (arrow). (b) DS. Image in orthogonal plane confirms abnormal humeral focus. (c) 3-D, volumetric reprojection. Selected images from 180° to 230°. (d) SPECT, triangulation display. Transaxial image through the T9 vertebra. Increased activity confined to vertebral body. (e) SPECT, triangulation display. Transaxial image through the T12 pedicle. Increased activity involves left pedicle. Coronal and sagittal planes detect more abnormal foci than seen on planar WB.

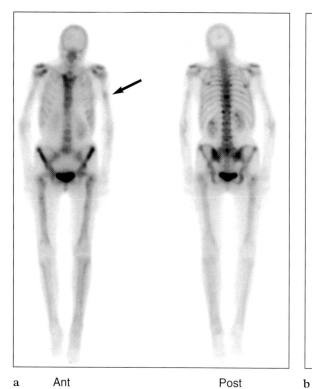

a   Ant   Post

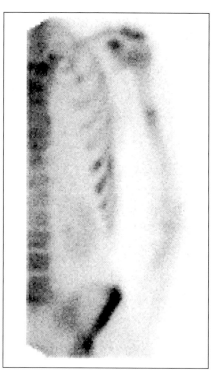

b

19 (180°)   20 (190°)   21 (200°)

22 (210°)   23 (220°)   24 (230°)

c

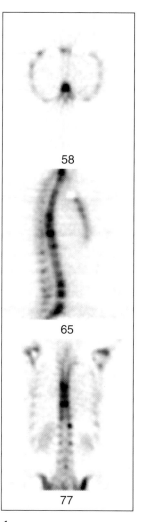

58   65   77

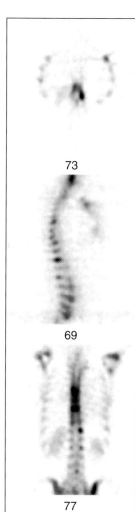

73   69   77

d   e

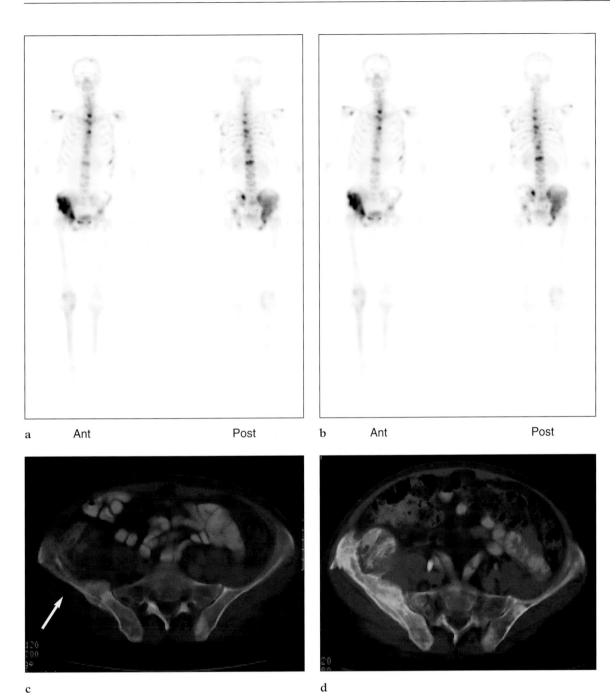

a   Ant   Post   b   Ant   Post

c   d

Figure 6.23

Prostate cancer, flare phenomenon. (a) WB, at time of initial staging. Multiple foci of intense abnormal tracer accumulation typical for widespread osseous metastasis. **(b)** WB, 3 months later following course of Lupron therapy. Some subtle increase in intensity of lesions previously present. **(c)** CT, at time of staging. Combined lytic and productive lesion right ilium. **(d)** Three months later at same time as **(b)**. Progressive sclerosis associated with ilial lesions. Healing of treated lytic bone lesions often occurs with sclerosis, which can appear on bone images as foci of increased tracer.

Teaching point

The flare phenomenon represents the tracer accumulation in areas of metastatic foci during the first 3–5 months following therapeutic intervention, which can represent healing with new bone formation rather than progressive metastasis. When the original radiographic lesions are lytic, healing is often associated with sclerosis, compared with the lysis of progressive metastasis.

Extraosseous metastasis

Nonosseous accumulation of bone-seeking radio-pharmaceuticals is covered more fully in Chapter 10. In this section, uptake of tracer in association with metastatic tumor will be illustrated. The mechanisms are probably similar to those operating in all cases of nonosseous accumulation.

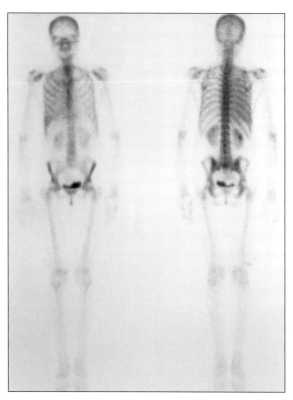

a

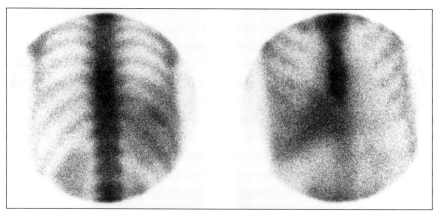

b

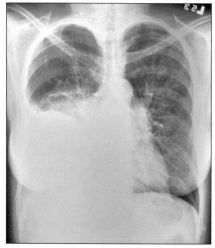

c

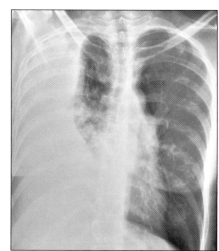

d

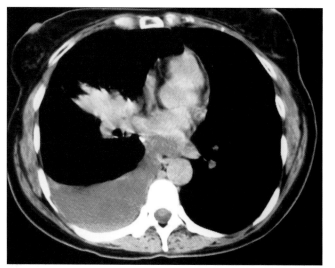

e

Figure 6.24

Pleural effusion, malignant, from breast cancer.
(a) WB. Diffuse increased activity involving right chest better seen on posterior view. Scan obtained with patient supine. **(b)** DS, chest, patient erect. Note layering of tracer within malignant effusion. Perhaps best appreciated on anterior view (right image). **(c)** X-ray, AP, **(d)** right decubitus chest X-rays. Layering of pleural fluid identified. **(e)** CT. Taken with patient supine. The posterior layering of the fluid is well seen.

Teaching point

Uptake in pleural effusions or ascitic fluid should be considered malignant until proven otherwise. The exact etiology of such accumulation is uncertain. Some authors have suggested altered tracer handling dynamics secondary to an expansion of interstitial fluid compartment, with slower washout of tracer. Scintigraphic confirmation of location in free-flowing fluid can be obtained by imaging the patient in positions designed to view the gravitational movement of fluid (upright, decubitus).

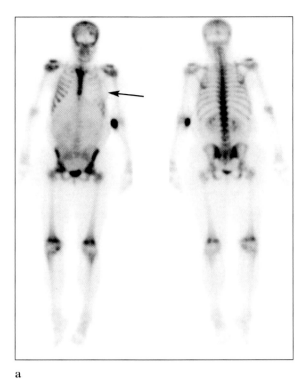

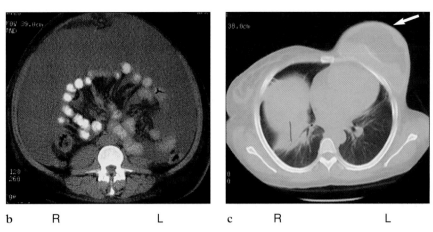

a

Figure 6.25

Ascites, malignant, from breast cancer. (a) WB. Mild to moderate intense diffuse uptake throughout a protuberant abdomen and pelvis. Round focal uptake in the left skull was not confirmed as a metastasis. Asymmetric appearance of the chest with decreased visualization of left anterior ribs secondary to breast prosthesis (arrow) attenuating photons. (b) CT, abdomen. Homogeneous diffuse fluid density of ascites throughout the abdomen, with opacified bowel loops floating in the center. (c) CT, chest. Soft tissue density of left breast prosthesis visualized (arrow).

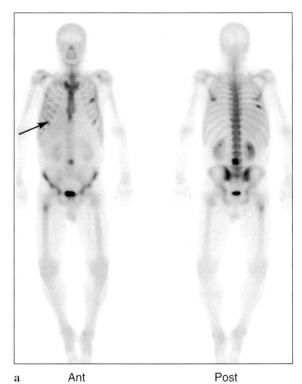

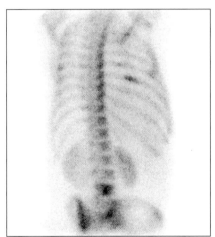

a   Ant   Post

b   c

Figure 6.26

Liver, diffuse uptake from lung cancer. (a) WB. Diffuse uptake in area of right upper abdomen corresponds to the region of the liver (arrow). Also noted were osseous metastasis involving fourth left anterior rib, seventh right posterior rib, L4 vertebra, and right proximal femur. (b) DS, RPO and (c) DS, LPO demonstrate the described bone lesions in orthogonal planes. (d) CT scan demonstrated multiple focal abnormalities which were simply not resolved on the nuclear medicine scan..

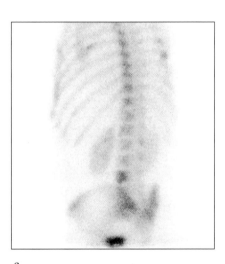

d   R   L

Figure 6.27

Liver, focal from mucinous cystadenoma carcinoma of the colon. WB. Intense focal uptake involving large area in right upper quadrant which is separate from kidney.

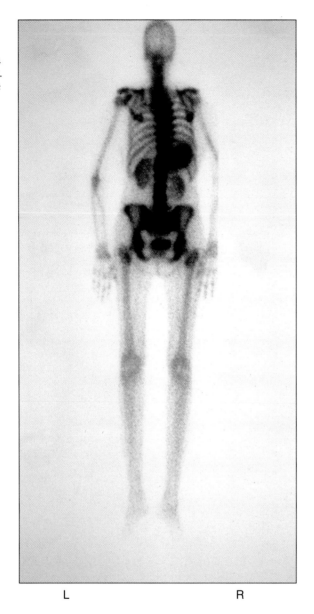

L   R

Figure 6.28

Lung, pleural and parenchymal from osteogenic sarcoma.
(a) Massive abnormal tracer accumulation such that with normal scaling techniques no rib activity is visualized. (b) In this patient massive abnormal tracer accumulation throughout the parenchyma and pleura.

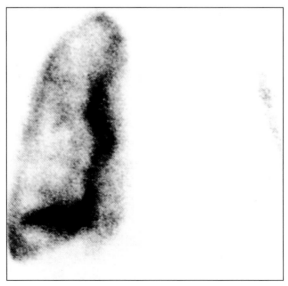

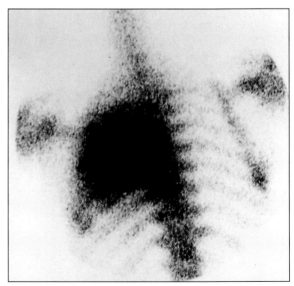

a   b

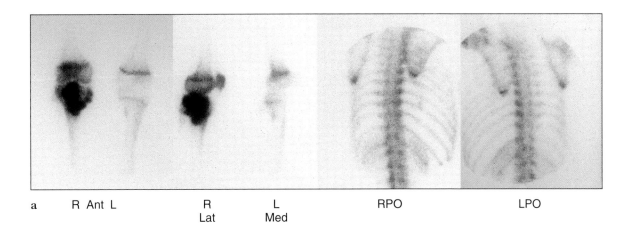

a   R Ant L   R   L   RPO   LPO
                      Lat   Med

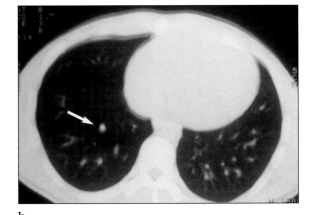

b

Figure 6.29

Lung, focal from osteogenic sarcoma. Thirteen-year-old male. (**a**) DS, knees anterior and right lateral, and CH, RPO and LPO. Intense abnormal tracer typical of osteogenic sarcoma. No other foci of abnormal uptake on planar images. (**b**) CT, chest. Dense, small, round lesion, mid-posterior portion of right lung (arrow). (**c**) SPECT, transaxial. Intense focus of tracer accumulation right posterior lung corresponds to lesion seen on CT (arrow). (**d**) SPECT, coronal sections. Intense focus of tracer seen on posterior sections (arrow).

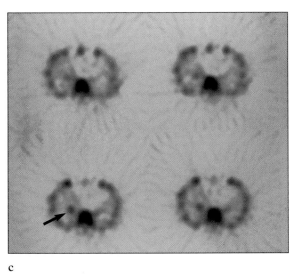

c

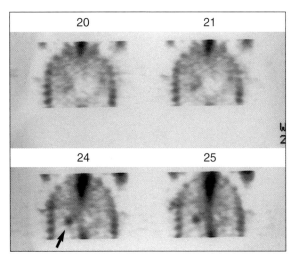

d

Teaching point

Calcified granulomas do not have abnormal increased tracer accumulation on bone scan.

Direct extension of tumor

Primary parenchymal lesions such as the Pancoast tumor in the apex, and pleural tumors such as mesothelioma or pleural based metasta-sis may all grow and directly extend into bone. The findings are generally similar to metastasis that primarily seeds the bone.

Figure 6.30

Chest wall invasion, pleural mesothelioma. (a) DS, chest, RPO. Multiple rib lesions, many of which are in a linear pattern. However, most show extension along the rib, involving longer segments than typically occur with simple fractures. (b) CT scan, chest. Diffuse pleural thickening with associated bone erosions (arrow).

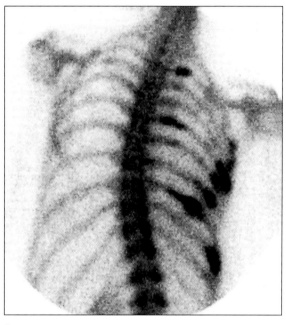

a

b

Teaching point

A linear pattern of clustered focal rib lesions 1–2 cm or less in length is characteristic of fractures, while lesions involving longer segments of rib are suspicious for malignancy.

Figure 6.31

Sacral invasion, colon cancer. Posterior (left image) and 'tail on detector' view (right image). Unusual pattern of uptake appreciated on posterior view is not uncommon with direct extension.

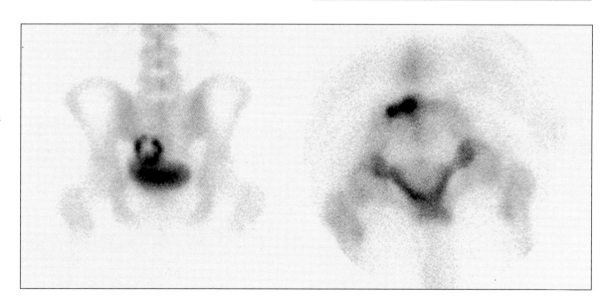

Teaching point

The special 'tail on detector', squat shot, or caudal upshoot view allows localization to the sacrum.

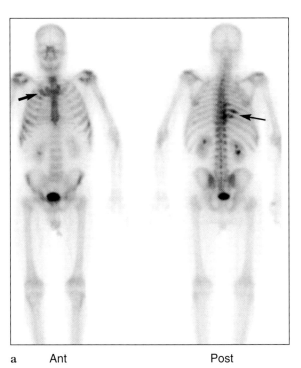

a   Ant   Post

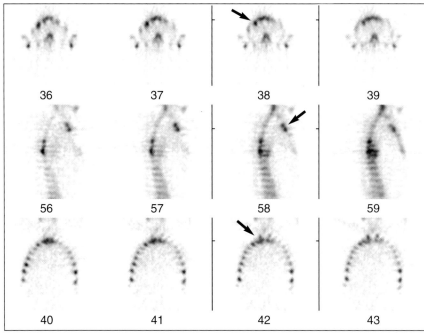

c

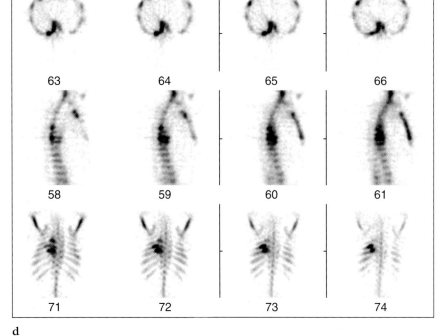

d

b

Figure 6.32

Rib erosion, lung cancer. (a) WB. Adjacent rib uptake, right apex on anterior view (arrow) and seventh, eighth, and ninth posterior ribs and posterior costovertebral junction region (thin arrows on posterior view) are not typical for fractures. (b) 3-D. Additional rib lesions from blood-borne metastasis which were not seen on planar imaging are identified. (c) SPECT, triangulation display. Images through anterior right apical lesions. Although the asymmetry on all three views is noted (arrows), rib lesions are always difficult to see on sectional imaging. Oblique angle reconstructions are sometimes helpful (see Figure 5.48). (d) SPECT, triangulation display. Views through posterior lesions. Because these lesions are larger they are easier to identify. Note that sagittal section passes through midline sternum. (e) CT. Section through anterior right apical lesion. Rib destruction identified (arrow). Lateral to the rib lesion is an additional pleural based mass. Please correlate with (c). (f) CT. Section through posterior lesion shows mass and rib destruction (arrow). Please correlate with (d).

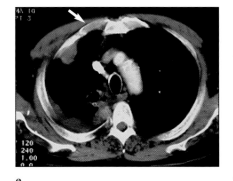

e

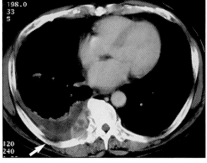

f

Figure 6.33

Muscle extension, from adenocarcinoma of the lung with multiple pulmonary nodules. WB. Asymmetric soft tissue along left lateral chest and abdominal wall (arrow) represents uptake in muscle. This is another example of non-osseous accumulation of tracer.

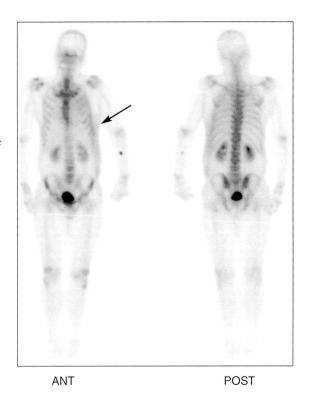

ANT   POST

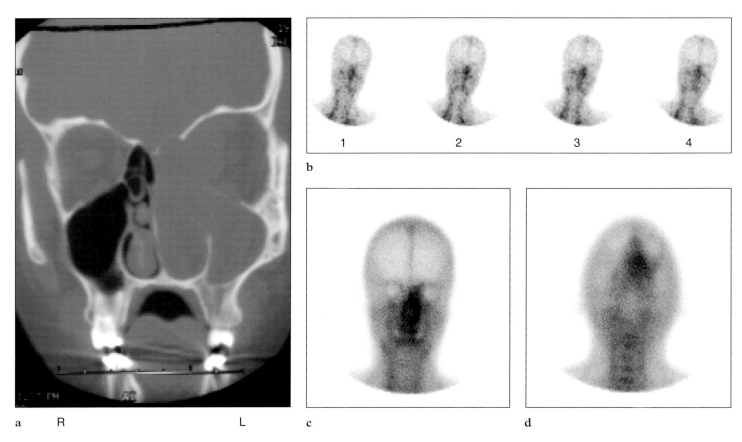

a   R   L   c   d

Figure 6.34 a–d

Rhabdomyosarcoma presenting as a nasal mass, with extension into the left orbit, maxillary and ethmoid sinuses, and through the cribiform plate. Nineteen-year-old female. **(a)** CT, direct coronal, bone windows, Homogeneous mass density with expansion of the left maxillary sinus and extension into the orbit. The black air of the right maxillary sinus can be used for comparison. **(b)** RNA. **(c)** BP, anterior and **(d)** BP, exaggerated Water's view. Mild increased vascularity to the left face.

continued

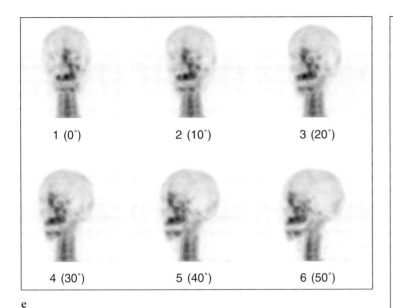

1 (0°)   2 (10°)   3 (20°)

4 (30°)   5 (40°)   6 (50°)

e

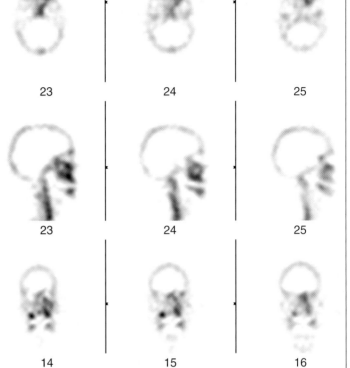

23   24   25

23   24   25

14   15   16

f

Figure 6.34 e and f

(e) SPECT, 3-D reprojection images. The extent of the abnormal tumor uptake into the sinuses and orbit was well seen with these images. (f) SPECT, triangulation display. The coronal image (bottom row) can be directly compared with the coronal CT (a).

Pathologic fractures

A pathologic fracture is a subset of an insufficiency fracture. In this specific group the bone is abnormal because of tumor infiltration. Although some patients with pathologic fractures of large weight-bearing bones present with a diagnosis of fracture, more often since these fractures occur with minimal or unrecognized trauma, the patients present with pain of unknown etiology.

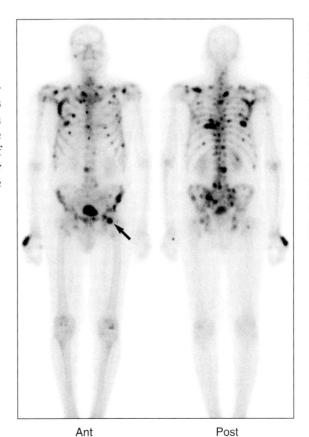

Ant   Post

Figure 6.35

Prostate cancer, critical lesion, right femoral neck. WB. Typical appearance for widespread osseous metastasis. The focal uptake in the left femoral neck is a so-called 'critical lesion' (arrow). When recognized, treatment with local radiation therapy is often undertaken in order to prevent a pathologic fracture.

Figure 6.36

Small cell cancer of the lung. (a) WB, linear scaling to hottest count per pixel. Spiral nature of abnormal uptake extending from superolateral to inferomedial and then inferolateral is identified. Best seen on anterior view. (b) WB, scaling with window and leveling so that 'normal ribs look normal'. Especially on anterior view, detail of fracture is obscured by uptake associated with tumor.

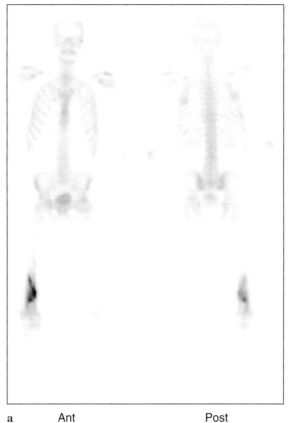

a   Ant   Post

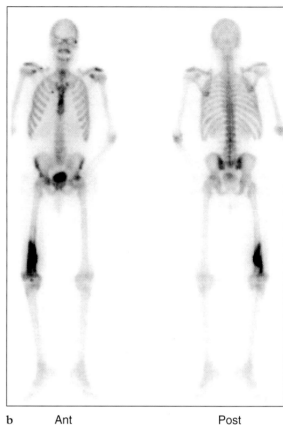

b   Ant   Post

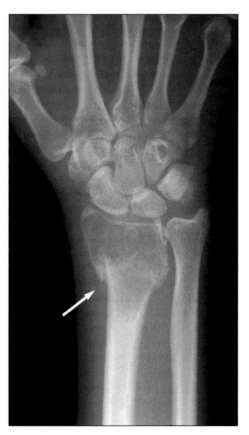

a

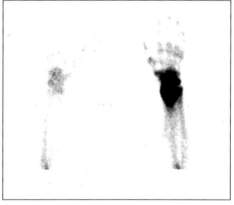

b

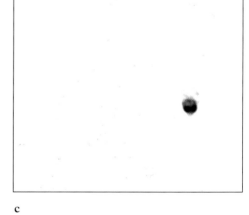

c

Figure 6.37

Giant cell tumor, distal radius. (a) Lytic lesion extends to end of bone. Fracture identified (arrow). (b) DS, palmar view. Intense uptake involves not only the fracture line and the remainder of the distal radius, but there is a so-called 'recruitment' phenomenon involving some of the carpal bones. (c) DS, palmar view, background subtracted image. The detail of the fracture line is seen, but there is still extended activity surrounding the lytic focus.

Teaching point

A pathologic fracture should be suspected if the size of the fracture is out of proportion to the reported traumatic event or when the scintigraphic intensity is more extended than expected, or if background subtracted views fail to demonstrate a more linear focus of greatest uptake corresponding to the fracture line.

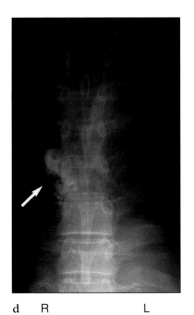

d R   L

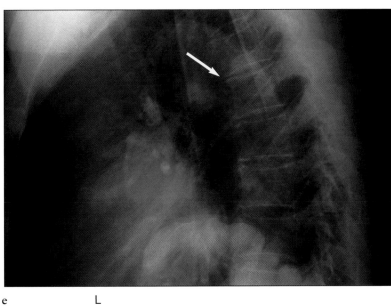

e   L

Figure 7.7 d–e

(d) X-ray, thoracic spine, anterior and (e) X-ray, thoracic spine, lateral. The area of abnormal tracer uptake is obscured on the anterior view by calcified hilar lymph nodes (arrow). On the lateral view the changes in the vertebrae anteriorly are very minimal anatomically.

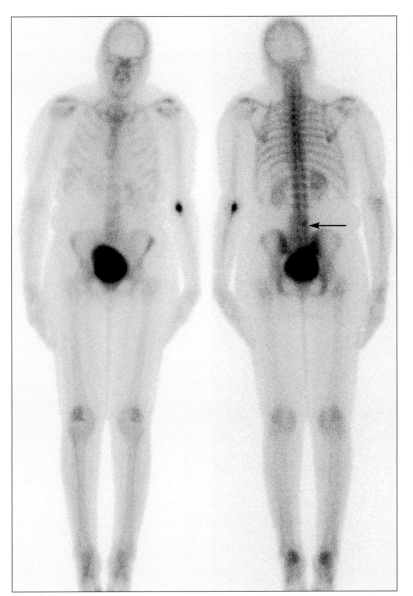

a

Figure 7.8 a

Lumbar spine, facet arthritis. (a) WB. Patient with severe pain could not void, which accounts for the full bladder. There may be faint uptake of tracer on the right posteriorly at L5/S1 area (thin arrow), but this was not certain.

continued

Figure 7.8 b–c

(b) 3-D volumetric reprojection images (selected views from 140° to 190°). The focal increased tracer can be localized to the facet region (arrow). Note the lack of bladder-filling artifact, since this bladder had a relatively constant volume during data acquisition. (c) SPECT, triangulation display. Focal round moderately intense increased tracer localized to facet region. Note the space (arrow) between the vertebral body activity and the abnormal facet uptake.

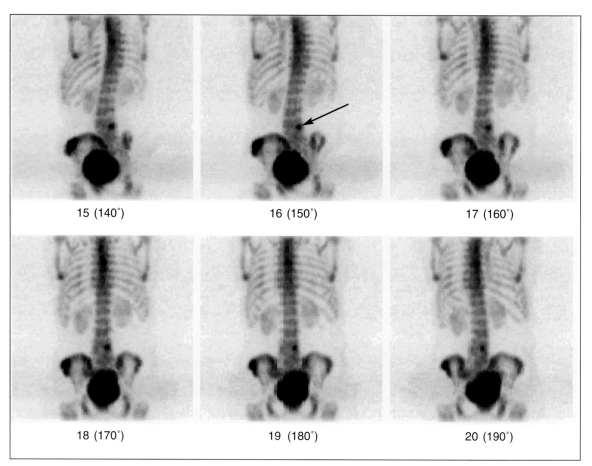

15 (140°) 16 (150°) 17 (160°)

18 (170°) 19 (180°) 20 (190°)

b

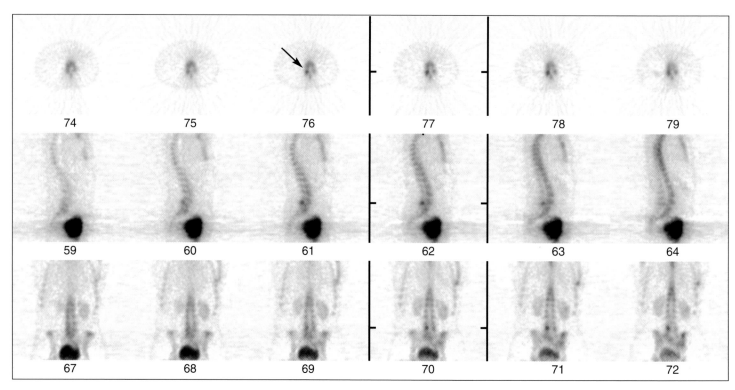

74 75 76 77 78 79

59 60 61 62 63 64

67 68 69 70 71 72

c

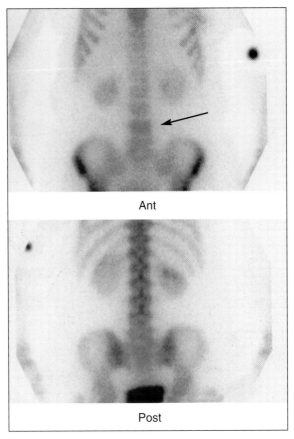

Ant

Post

a

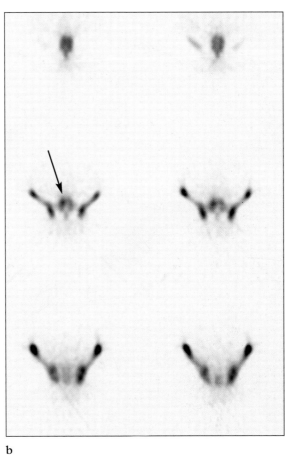

b

Figure 7.9

Lumbar spine, vertebral body osteoarthritis. (a) DS, lumbosacral spine, anterior (upper image) and posterior (lower image). Normal uptake. The accentuation of the L4 vertebral body (arrow) on the anterior view is a normal variation, because that vertebra is closer to the camera because of normal lumbar lordosis. (b) SPECT, representative transaxial, and (c) SPECT, representative sagittal. The anterior location of the abnormal tracer is well seen on both views (arrows).

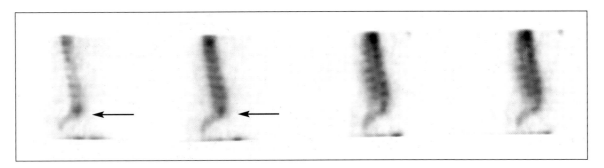

c

Teaching point

The projection of activity anterior to the expected outline of the vertebral body is more typical of degenerative osteophyte than a focal metastasis. Isolated vertebral body lesions do require correlative imaging for complete differential diagnosis.

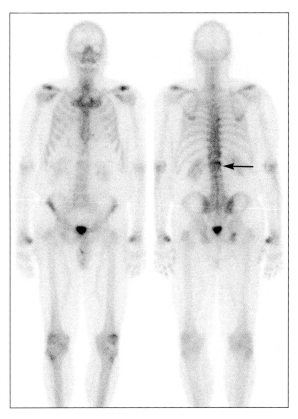

a

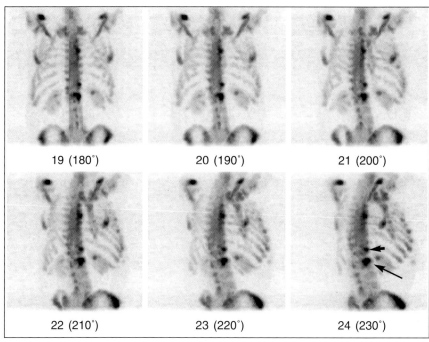

b

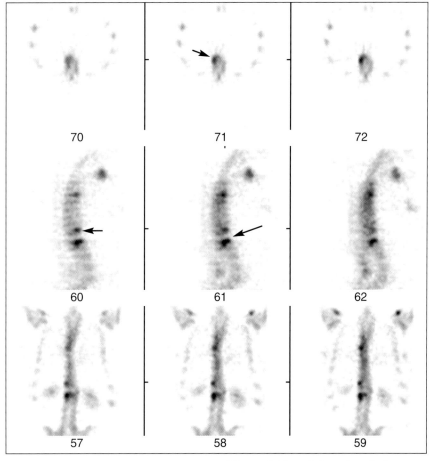

c

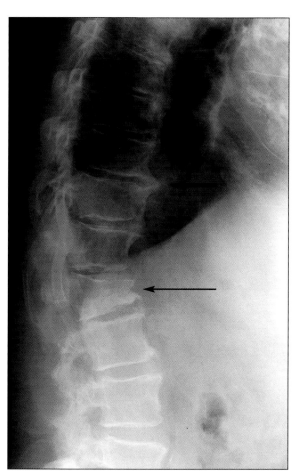

d

Figure 7.10 a–d *Legend on facing page.*   *continued*

Figure 7.10 (*images on facing page*)

Thoracic spine, anterior vertebral body osteophytes and lumbosacral spine, anterior wedge compression fracture. (a) WB. Abnormal increased uptake, more on the right side at approximately L1 (thin arrow) is of uncertain location. (b) 3-D volumetric reprojection images, selected views from 180° to 230°. The unusual shape of the L1 vertebral body activity on planar images and on anterior and posterior projection views has a wedge shape on the steeper oblique images (thin arrow). The anterior osteophyte activity in the lower thoracic spine (short arrow) is also appreciated. (c) SPECT, triangulation display. Transaxial view through the thoracic osteophyte. The anterolateral location of activity in relation to the vertebral body can be appreciated (short arrows). Relative photon deficiency of the T12 vertebral region (thin arrow) is partly due to reconstruction artifact. (d) X-ray, thoracolumbar spine, lateral. Anterior wedge compression (thin arrow) and anterior osteophyte (thick arrow).

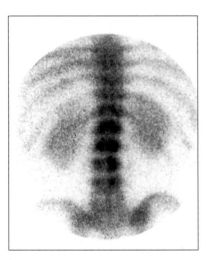

a

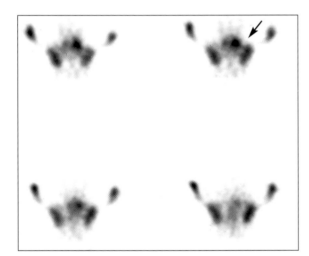

b

Figure 7.11

Lumbar spine, Schmorl's node. (a) SPECT. Bony reaction at anterior left side of vertebral body at site of Schmorl's node (arrow). (b) DS, lumbar spine, posterior. Normal. (c) CT, transaxial and sagittal reformatted. The sclerotic bony reaction at the node (arrow).

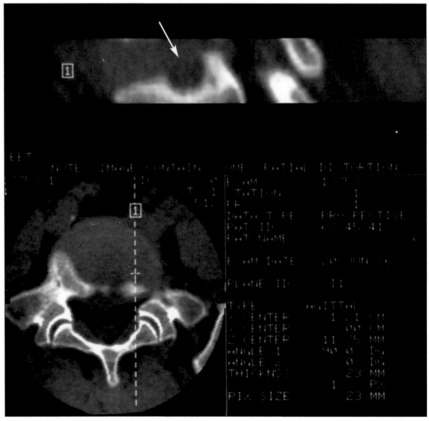

c

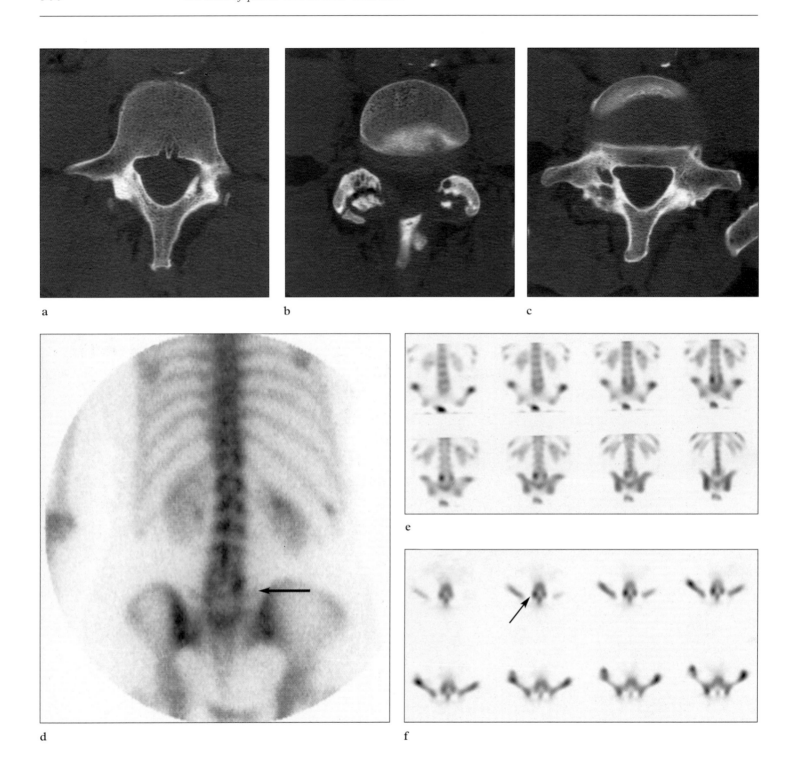

Figure 7.12

Lumbar spine, articular facet osteoarthritis right L4–L5. (a)
CT, level of the L4 pedicles; (b) CT, at level of L4–L5 articular
facets; and (c) CT, at level of L5 pedicles. Dysmorphic pars
interarticularis with sclerotic changes (arrow). Sclerosis, osteophyte
formation, and subchondral cysts involving facets. (d) DS, posterior
thoracolumbar spine. Minimal activity in the area of the L4–L5
facet region on the right (arrow). (e) SPECT, coronal and (f)
SPECT, transaxial. Six-millimeter thick slices demonstrate the focus
of increased tracer accumulation localized to the right-sided L4–L5
articular facet region (arrows). Heavy (smoothed) filter.

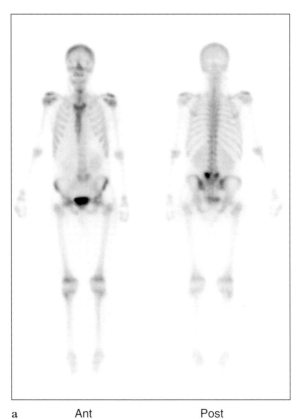

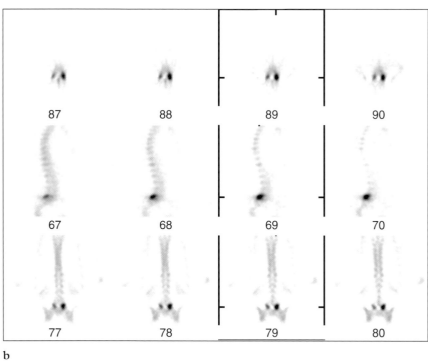

a   Ant   Post

b

Figure 7.13

Degenerative arthritis, pars interarticularis. Lumbosacral spine. Transitional vertebral S1, bilateral pars interarticularis defects L5, grade 1 spondylolisthesis L5 on S1. (**a**) WB. Abnormal increased tracer uptake is asymmetric with more activity on the left than on the right. (**b**) SPECT, triangulation display. Sagittal images through the left-sided pars region.

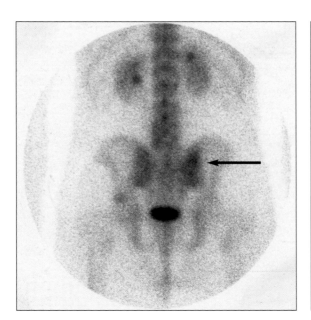

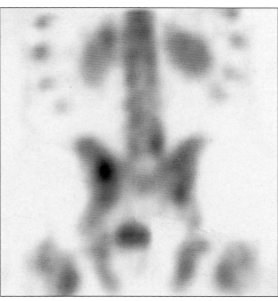

a   b

Figure 7.14

Sacroiliac joint, osteoarthritis. (**a**) DS, lumbosacral spine and pelvis, posterior. Faint subtle increase in tracer uptake in superior portion of right SI joint (arrow). Minimal asymmetry in the lateral elements at L5 and S1, and some mild increase in the superolateral portion of the left acetabulum. (**b**) SPECT, coronal, selected image. The increased uptake in the right SI joint is now more easily seen. There is some uptake in the left-sided L5/S1 articular facets.

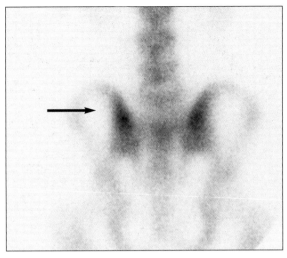

a

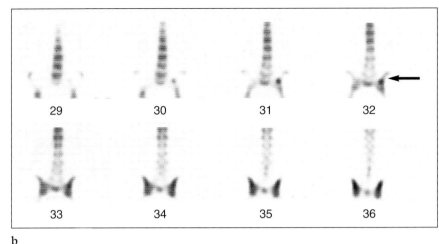

b

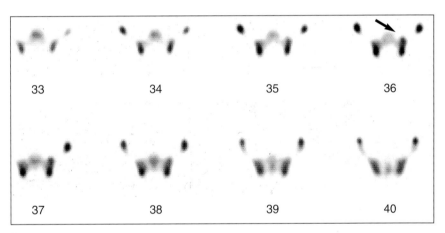

c

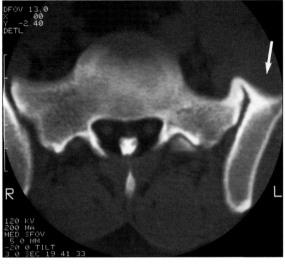

d

Figure 7.15

Sacroiliac joint, osteoarthritis. (a) DS, lumbosacral spine, posterior. In retrospect, there may be some very subtle relative increased tracer accumulation in the upper part of the left SI joint, compared with the right (arrow). (b) SPECT, coronal and (c) SPECT, transaxial. The location of moderate increased tracer uptake in the upper ligamentous portion of the left SI joint (arrows). (d) CT, for comparison. Joint narrowing, subchondral sclerosis, and osteophyte formation (arrow).

Figure 7.16

Shoulder, acromioclavicular joint osteoarthritis, following ACJ separation one month prior to image. DS, chest, anterior. The intense abnormal uptake at the right AC joint more on the clavicular side.

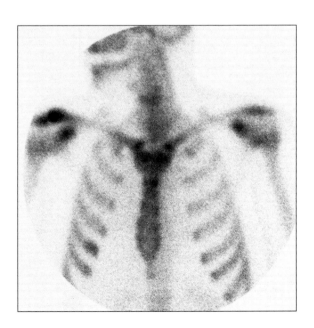

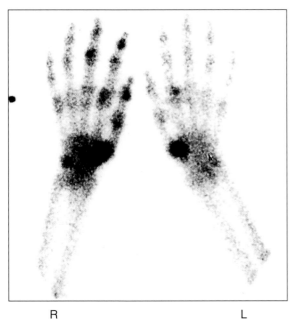

R   L

Figure 7.17

Hand and wrist, osteoarthritis. Multiple focal areas of increased tracer uptake are present in the inter-phalangeal joints, particularly involving the distal joints. The first carpo-metacarpal joints (basal joints) are also typically involved (contrast with more symmetrical uptake in rheumatoid arthritis seen in Figure 7.30).

R   L

Figure 7.18

Hand, scaphoid–trapezium osteoarthritis. DS, palmar view. Moderately intense activity at the right scaphoid–trapezium joint. Mild activity at the lunate carpal and at the third distal interphalangeal joint.

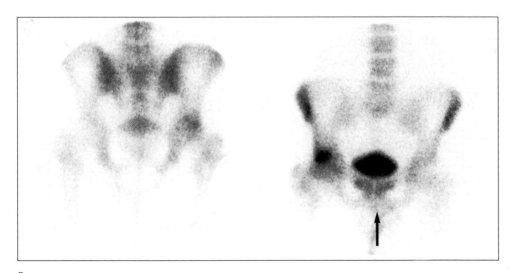

a

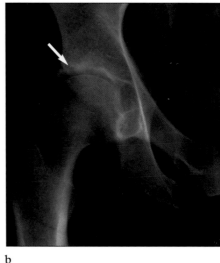

b

Figure 7.19

Right hip, osteoarthritis. Forty-three-year-old male. RNA and BP normal. **(a)** DS, pelvis and hips. Posterior (left image) and anterior (right image). Intense increased tracer at the superolateral portion of the right acetabulum. Note the normal photon deficiency associated with cartilage at the pubic symphyses (arrow). **(b)** X-ray, right hip, AP. The subchondral sclerosis, joint narrowing, and osteophyte formation (arrow) are classic findings for osteoarthritis.

Teaching point

Every focus of relative increased tracer uptake on delayed images represents an area of increased bone turnover and implies a response to an insult. Most of these foci are of mild intensity and in the hand and feet are usually encountered almost incidentally. In these cases, they usually represent a nonspecific stress remodeling response and are of no clinical significance. When these correlate to a possible site for symptoms, or the intensity is slightly more intense, then careful clinical examination and often correlative radiographs are warranted.

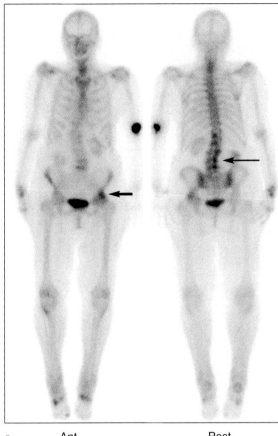

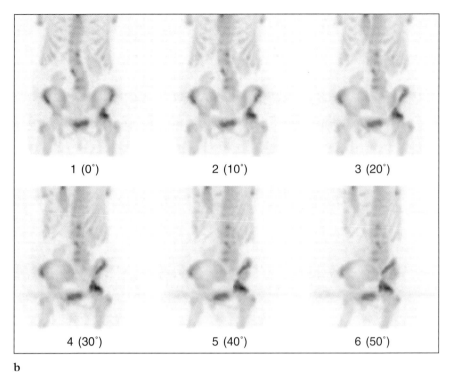

a   Ant   Post

b

Figure 7.20

Left hip, osteoarthritis with degenerative cyst formation. (a) WB. The mild activity associated with the superolateral acetabulum (arrow) is better seen on anterior than posterior view. Degenerative changes with stress response on the concave side of a lumbar levoscoliosis (thin arrow). (b) 3-D volumetric reprojection images. Selected views from 0° to 50°. Uptake in lower lumbar spine represents degenerative changes associated with scoliosis. The round focal superolateral acetabular increased tracer uptake is well seen. (c) SPECT, triangulation display. The intense increased tracer uptake extends slightly more superiorly than the immediate subarticular surface (arrows). (d) X-ray, left hip, AP. Very marked joint narrowing to the point of obliteration, osteophyte (longer arrow), and the radiolucency (shorter arrow) associated with the degenerative cyst.

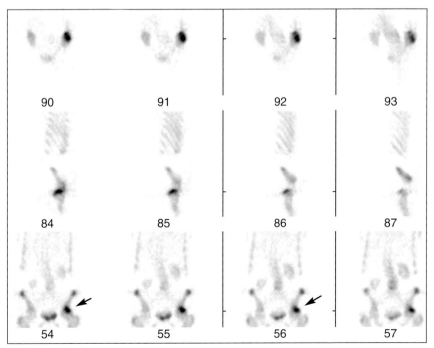

c

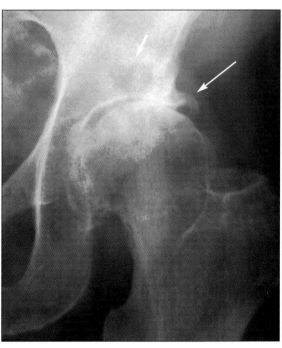

d

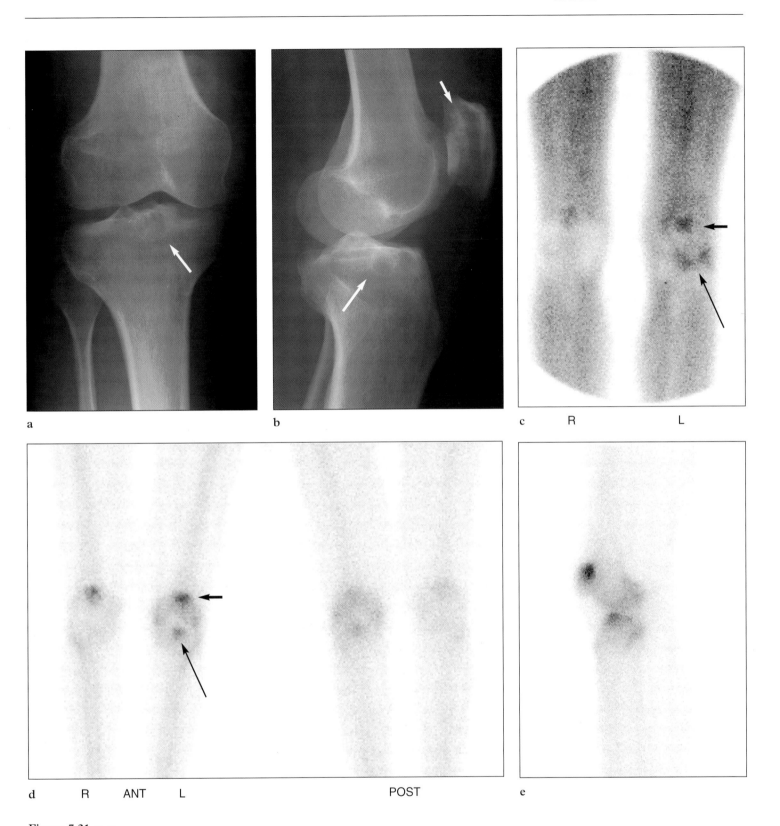

Figure 7.21 a–e

Knee, osteoarthritis, patellar femoral and central femoral tibial. Mild inflammatory component. **(a)** X-ray, left knee, AP and **(b)** X-ray, left lateral. Subchondral cyst formation, proximal tibia (long arrow). Posterior patellar subchondral sclerosis and cyst formation (short arrow). **(c)** BP, knees, anterior. Mild increased tracer uptake (increased relative vascularity) at patellar femoral (short arrow) and central femoral tibial (long arrow). There is also some mild patellar femoral increased uptake on the right side. **(d)** DS, knee, anterior (left image) and posterior (right image). Mild to moderate focal increased tracer at the patellar femoral regions bilaterally more intense on the left (short arrow) than on the right. Mild central femoral tibial uptake (long arrow). **(e)** DS, knee, left lateral. Moderate superior patellar femoral uptake. On this relatively true lateral view it is difficult to separate the patella from the sub-adjacent femur. There is also mild proximal tibial uptake.

continued

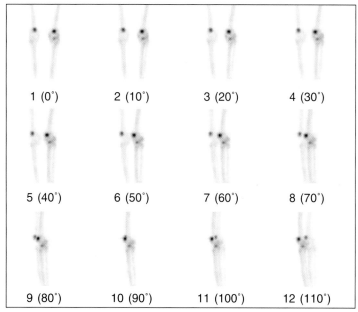

1 (0˚)   2 (10˚)   3 (20˚)   4 (30˚)

5 (40˚)   6 (50˚)   7 (60˚)   8 (70˚)

9 (80˚)   10 (90˚)   11 (100˚)   12 (110˚)

f

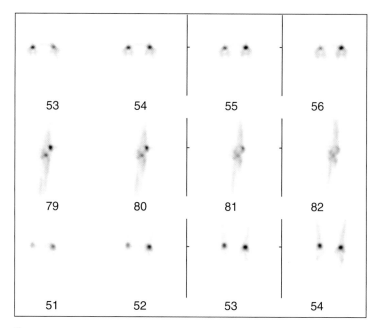

53   54   55   56

79   80   81   82

51   52   53   54

g

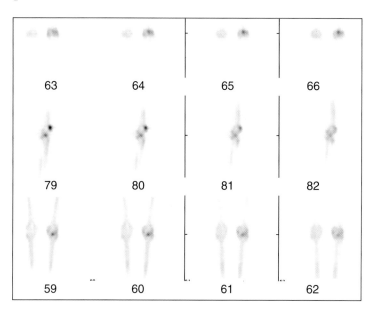

63   64   65   66

79   80   81   82

59   60   61   62

h

Figure 7.21 f–h

(f) 3-D volumetric reprojection, selected views from 0° to 110°. (g) SPECT, triangulation display. Transaxial images through patellar femoral uptake. (h) SPECT, triangulation display. Transaxial images through proximal tibial activity. All help localize the abnormal tracer uptake.

Figure 7.22

Knee, bilateral medial compartment osteoarthritis. (a) X-ray, knees, AP. Medial joint narrowing. (b) DS, knee, anterior. Increased tracer in the medial compartments bilaterally, more marked on the tibial surfaces. There is also some patellar femoral activity. (c) DS, right lateral/left medial and right medial/left lateral.

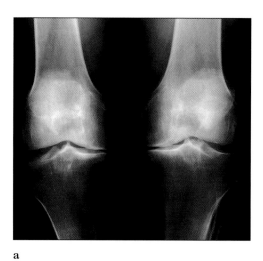

a

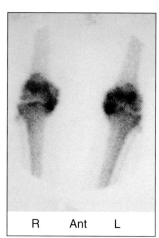

R   Ant   L

b

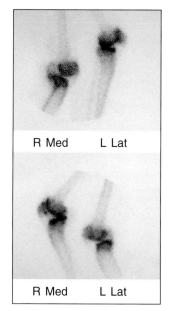

R Med   L Lat

R Med   L Lat

c

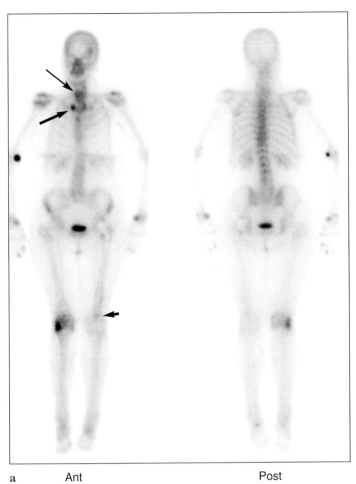

a   Ant   Post

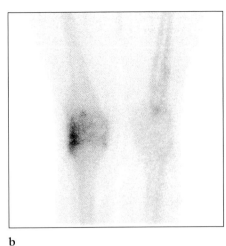

b

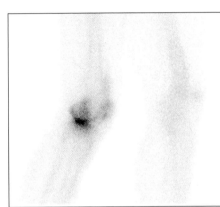

c

Figure 7.23

Knee, lateral compartment osteoarthritis. Patient status – post left total hip arthroplasty. (**a**) WB. A right genu valgus deformity is present with lateral compartment increased tracer uptake. Abnormal stress may be secondary to the left total hip arthroplasty. Normal hip prosthesis. No abnormal increased tracer at the tip of the femoral component (short arrow). Incidentally noted is mild uptake in tracheal cartilage (long thin arrow) and asymmetry in uptake at the sternoclavicular joints (long thicker arrow). (**b**) DS, knee, anterior and (**c**) DS, knee, right lateral. The lateral compartment osteoarthritis is more posterior than anterior.

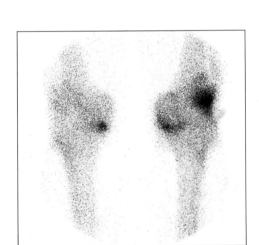

a

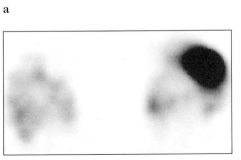

b

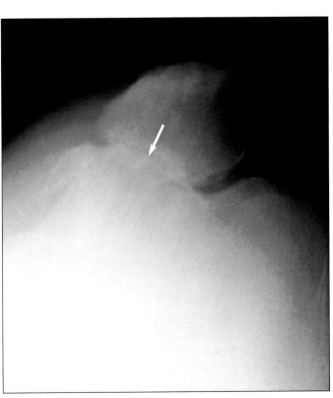

c

Figure 7.24

Knee, lateral patellar facet osteoarthritis. (**a**) DS, knee, anterior. Intense activity over the lateral aspect of left patella and milder activity in the medial compartment of both knees. (**b**) SPECT, transaxial, selected view through patella. Intense abnormal uptake extends far laterally. (**c**) X-ray, patella, sunrise view. Lateral joint narrowing and subchondral sclerosis (arrow).

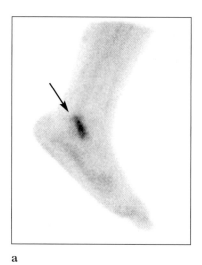
a

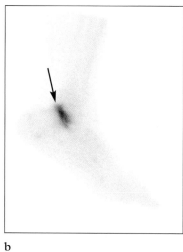
b

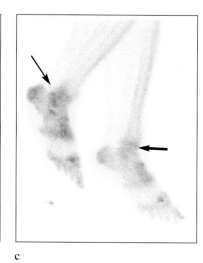
c

Figure 7.25

Subtalar joint. Osteoarthritis, with a mild inflammatory component. (a) BP, ankle, right lateral. The oblique moderate increased tracer uptake reflects increased relative vascularity. **(b)** DS, ankle, right lateral. Intense increased tracer uptake in the posterior subtalar joint. **(c)** DS, ankle and foot, right lateral/left medial. Another patient. Posterior subtalar activity on the right (thin arrow); the tibiotalar joint is defined on the opposite side (thick arrow). There is also some moderate activity at the first MTP joint bilaterally.

Miscellaneous joint disorders

Gout

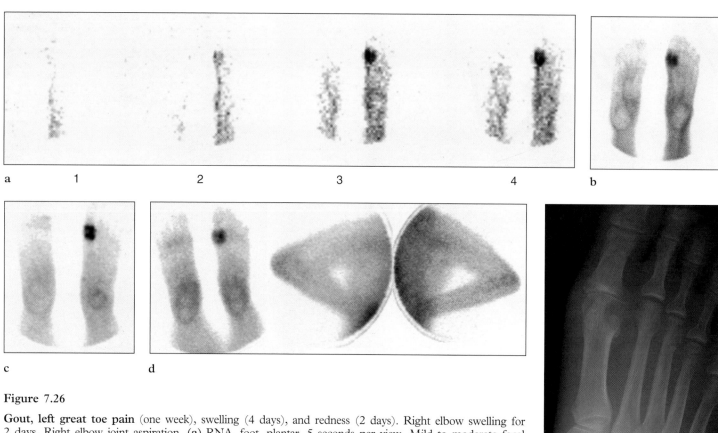

a   1   2   3   4   b

c   d   e

Figure 7.26

Gout, left great toe pain (one week), swelling (4 days), and redness (2 days). Right elbow swelling for 2 days. Right elbow joint aspiration. **(a)** RNA, foot, plantar, 5 seconds per view. Mild to moderate focal increased perfusion to first MTP joint region. **(b)** BP, foot, plantar. **(c)** DS, plantar. Focal increased tracer uptake, head of first metatarsal and base of proximal phalanx. This is the 'washed out' pattern of delayed activity, in which normal bone detail is not defined. **(d)** Gallium-67, foot, plantar (left image) and elbows (right image). Focal increased tracer in the right first MTP joint, but no significant uptake in the symptomatic right elbow when compared with the left. **(e)** X-ray, left foot, AP. The typical X-ray appearance of gout with well-defined erosion at the head of the first metatarsal.

Neuropathic joint

Denervation, either directly to a joint region, or leading to proprioceptive changes, can result in joint destruction with fragmentation, erosion, and osteophyte formation. Some authors characterize the result of neuropathic joint disease as a form of osteoarthritis. Diabetes mellitus is the most common underlying etiology. Syringomyelia, tabes dorsalis, alcoholism, amyloidosis, and other demyelinating diseases are also related.

Amyloid

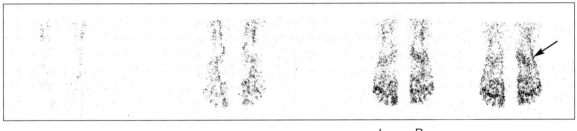

a   L   R

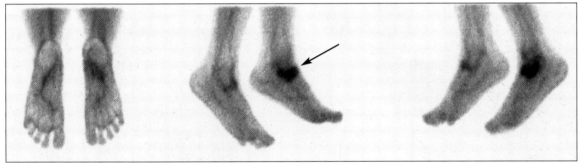

b   L   Plantar   R   L Med   R Lat   L Lat   R Med

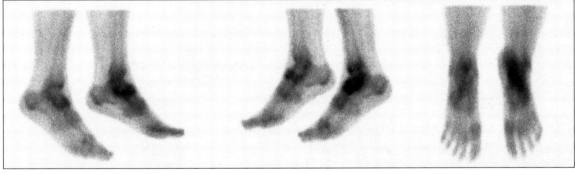

c   L Med   R Lat   L Lat   R Med   L   R

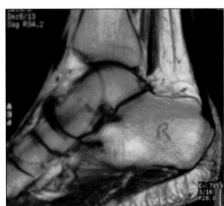

d

Figure 7.27

Amyloid arthritis involving right talonavicular, navicular cuneiform, and anterior subtalar joints. Thirty-nine-year-old male, 5 years of renal dialysis. Presents with pain and swelling in the right ankle of one week's duration. History prior AVN of hips. (a) RNA, plantar, 5 seconds per view. Although, in retrospect, there is subtle asymmetry with slight increased perfusion to the right mid-foot (arrow), this is an essentially normal RNA. (b) BP, plantar (left image), left medial/right lateral (mid-image), and left lateral/right medial (right image). Moderate increased tracer uptake (arrow) predominantly at the talonavicular joint region. (c) DS, ankle, left medial/right lateral (left image), left lateral/right medial (middle image) and plantar (right image). The areas of increased tracer in the symptomatic right ankle, predominantly at the talonavicular and posterior subtalar joints. There is incidental activity at the calcaneal cuboid, and at the tibiotalar joint. There is also activity in the asymptomatic left side. (d) MR, T1-weighted, ankle, sagittal. There is abnormal soft tissue of low signal intensity thought to be compatible with synovial thickening within the subtalar and talonavicular joints, which is more prominent on the right.

Diabetes

Figure 7.28

Diabetic neuropathy.
(a) DS, foot, plantar.
Mild asymmetric
increased uptake left hind
and mid-foot, and first
metatarsal. (b) DS, ankle
and foot, left lateral.
Abnormal mid-foot
uptake (arrow) extends
inferiorly below expected
outline of bottom foot.
(c) DS, foot, right lateral.
Similar inferior abnormal
uptake secondary to
subluxation.

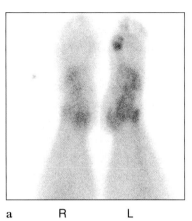
a   R   L

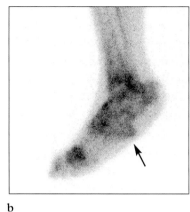
b

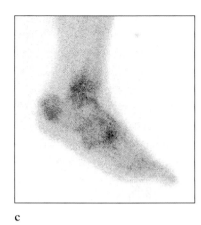
c

Pigmented villonodular synovitis

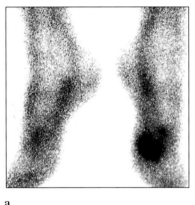
a

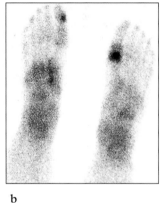
b

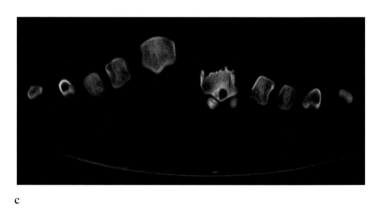
c

Figure 7.29

Pigmented villonodular synovitis. Forty-four-year-old male, one-year painful enlargement of left great toe. (a) BP, ankle and foot, anterior slightly oblique. Moderately intense, poorly marginated, but relatively focal increased tracer uptake in the region of the first MTP joint. (b) DS, foot, plantar. Moderate intense activity associated with the head of the first metatarsal. (c) CT bone windows, through metatarsals. Soft tissue fullness only suggested on these windows. Bony erosions and cyst formation are nonspecific. Biopsy proved diagnosis.

Rheumatoid arthritis

Figure 7.30

Rheumatoid arthritis.
DS, hands, palmar.
Increased uptake of
tracer in both wrists with
more focally increased
uptake in many small
joints of the hand. Ulnar
deviation is present.

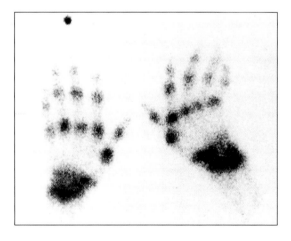

Teaching point

Joint uptake on RNBI is nonspecific. The diagnosis of rheumatoid arthritis can often be suggested when the presentation is symmetric and involves typical locations. These include PIP/MCP joints in the hands, MTP joints in the foot, the carpus and tarsus, the hips, the knees, and the cervical spine.

Seronegative spondyloarthropathies

The seronegative spondyloarthropathies are a family of disorders in which the HLA-B27 antigen can be demonstrated. Syndromes include ankylosing spondylitis, psoriatic arthritis, reactive arthritis, and many cases of sacroiliitis. Most of the lesions are associated with tendon or ligament insertions.

Ankylosing spondylitis

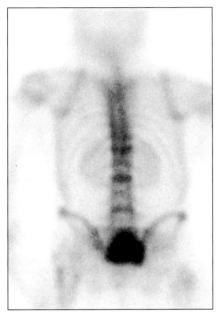

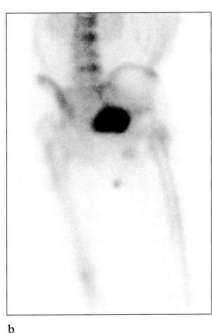

a   b

Figure 7.31

Ankylosing spondylitis. (a) DS, thoracolumbar spine, posterior. Abnormal increased tracer accumulation in calcified ligaments as well as uptake in areas of osseous fusion create the 'bamboo' spine appearance. (b) DS, lumbar spine and pelvis, slight RPO. Demonstrates the peripheral uptake associated with the calcified ligaments.

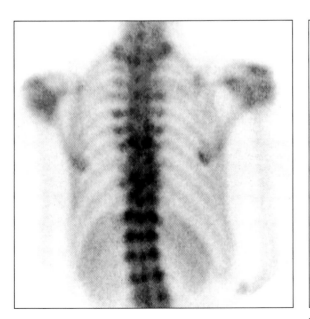

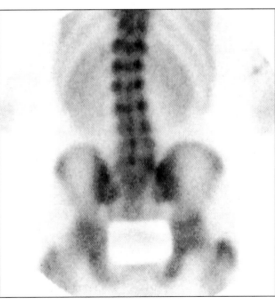

a   b

Figure 7.32 a–b

Ankylosing spondylitis. (a) DS, cervicothoracic spine, posterior and (b) DS, thoracolumbar spine, posterior. Increased tracer more prominent in the facet regions than in Figure 7.31.

continued

Figure 7.32 c–d

(c) SPECT, transaxial and (d) SPECT, coronal. Very symmetric abnormal increased uptake appreciated.

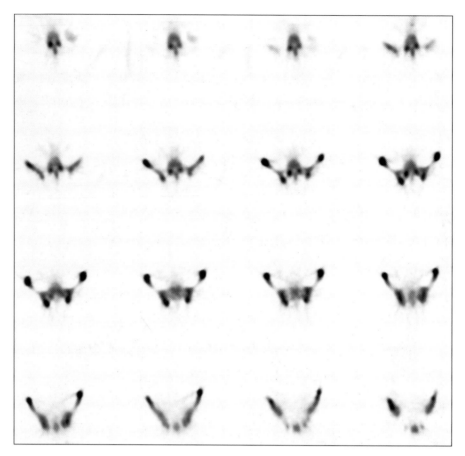

c

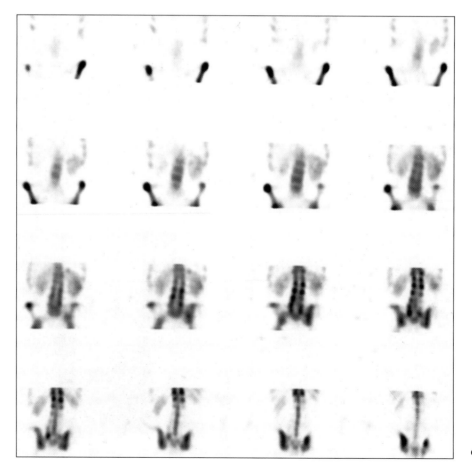

d

Psoriatic arthropathy

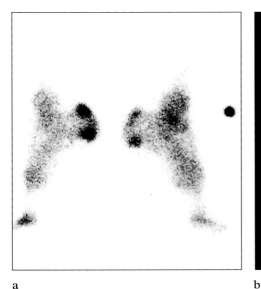

a

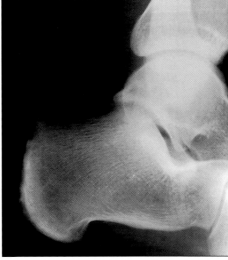

b

Figure 7.33

Psoriatic arthropathy. (a) DS, posterior foot, lateral. Abnormal uptake at the origin of the plantar fascia (calcaneal tubercle) and in the region of the posterior superior calcaneous. This latter uptake, more marked on the left than the right, is in the region of the retrocalcaneal bursa in addition to corresponding to the erosions seen on the X-ray in **(b)**. On the right side, which is less intense, the uptake extends more inferiorly to the region of the insertion of the Achilles' tendon. This emphasizes the involvement of enthesis by these seronegative spondyloarthropathies. **(b)** X-ray, left heel. Erosions on the posterior aspect of the calcaneous. Some overlying soft tissue thickening does not reproduce well.

Sacroiliitis

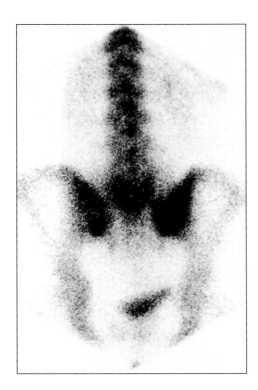

Figure 7.34

Crohn's disease and right sacroiliitis.
DS. Moderately intense increased tracer involving the lower half of the right SI joint when compared with the left. SI quantitation: right SI joint index 144, left SI joint index 110 (normal range 105–136).

Teaching point

Symmetrical increased uptake, especially in SI joint region, can be difficult to diagnose. Various semi-quantitative approaches using variations of the SI joint to adjacent bone uptake ratios have been used.

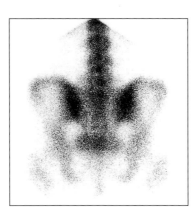

a

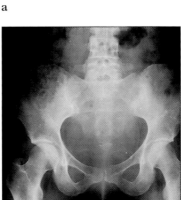

b

c

Figure 7.35

Sacroiliitis. (a) DS, lumbosacral spine and pelvis, posterior. Moderate intense uptake in SI joints bilaterally. SI quantitation: left SI joint index 142°, right SI joint index 148° (normal range 105–136°). **(b)** X-ray, pelvis, AP. Sclerosis of both SI joint regions. **(c)** Schematic SI joint quantitation technique.

Sacroiliac joint (SIJ) index

$$= \frac{\text{Uptake SIJ/unit area}}{\text{Uptake adjacent bone/unit area}}$$

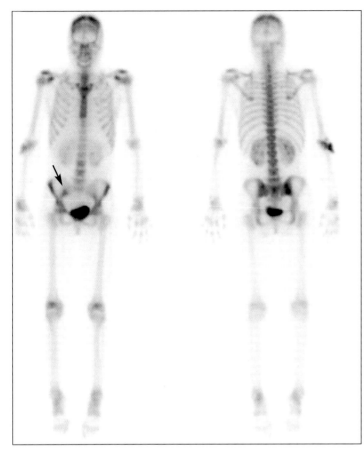

a

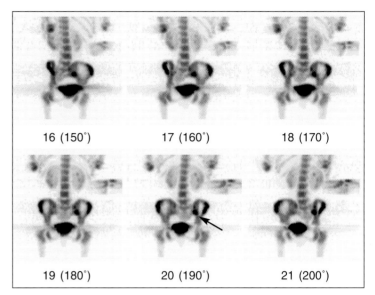

16 (150°)　17 (160°)　18 (170°)

19 (180°)　20 (190°)　21 (200°)

b

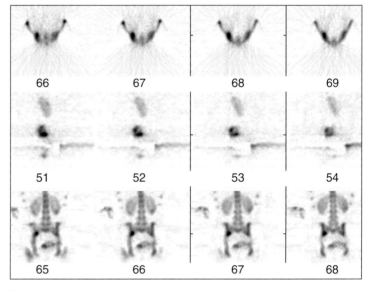

66　67　68　69

51　52　53　54

65　66　67　68

c

Figure 7.36

Sacroiliitis. (a) WB. Even on the anterior view, asymmetric focal increased tracer in the lower portion of the right SI joint can be seen (arrow). **(b)** 3-D volumetric reprojection images. Selected views from 150 to 200. The focal uptake in the lower portion of the right SI joint is well seen (arrow). **(c)** SPECT, triangulation display. All sections through the lower right SI joint. Exact localization of tracer is possible.

Teaching point

Although unilateral sacroiliitis is common in a variety of seronegative spondyloarthropathies, the SI joint is also a common site for infections, particularly in immunocompromised patients and intravenous drug abusers.

Infection and inflammation 8

Bone infection and inflammations in adjacent tissues that secondarily affect the underlying bone have been grouped together in this atlas. Named arthritic conditions, many of which have an initiating or associated inflammatory component, are discussed in Chapter 7. The scintigraphic findings in patients with bone infection are etiologically nonspecific. They reflect the pathophysiologic changes that are occurring: bone destruction, replacement of bone marrow by inflammatory tissue, and reparative new bone formation. However, as with other lesions, careful scintigraphic delineation of the location of abnormal tracer uptake, utilization of the physiologic information available on the RNA and BP phases of the three-phase scan, correlation with the patient's clinical presentation and more anatomic imaging studies will often yield a diagnosis or meaningful management information.

Osteomyelitis, simple (nonviolated bone)

The approach to scintigraphic diagnosis and image analysis in patients suspected of having osteomyelitis is affected by the presence or absence of pre-existing conditions associated with increased bone remodeling. When the plain X-ray is normal, or there is no antecedent history to suggest a coexisting process, we use the term 'nonviolated' bone. In these situations the three-phase scan is very sensitive with reasonable specificity.

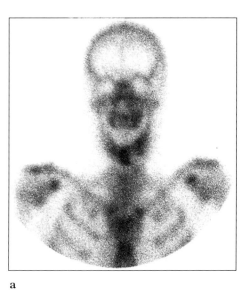

a

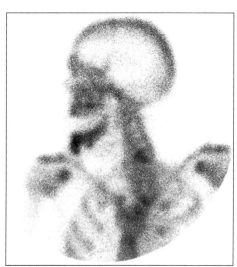

b

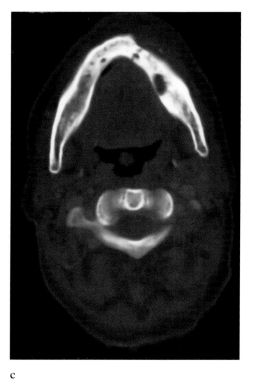

c

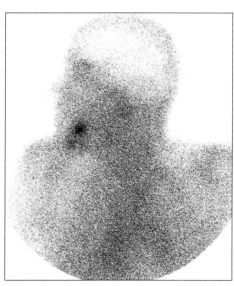

d   e

Figure 8.1

Bone abscess, mandible. (a) DS, mandible, anterior and (b) DS, mandible, left lateral. Focal increased tracer involving the left side of the mandible. A photon-deficient area within the zone of increased uptake corresponds to an area of more focal bone destruction on the CT scan. (c) CT, mandible, bone windows. Destruction and sclerosis are identified. (d) Gallium-67, head and neck, anterior and (e) ^{67}Ga, head and neck, left lateral. Focal increased uptake corresponding to the bone abscess.

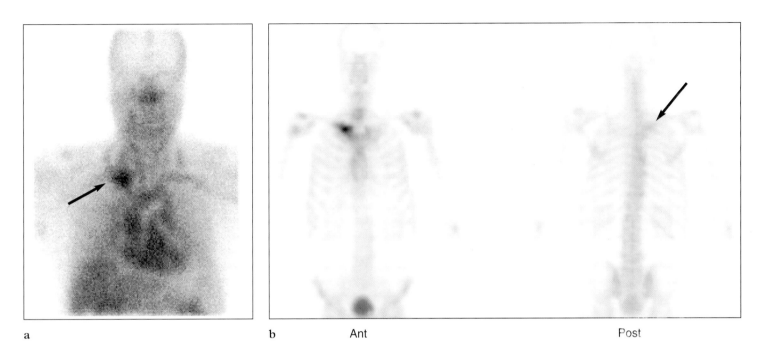

a   b   Ant   Post

Figure 8.2

Osteomyelitis, sternoclavicular joint. (a) BP, chest, anterior. Focal area of moderately intense increased tracer uptake (arrow) in the area of the right sternoclavicular joint represents increased relative vascularity. (b) DS, chest, anterior (left image) and posterior (right image) are taken from a WB study. The intense increased tracer on the anterior view is well seen, but is much less prominent (arrow) on the posterior view.

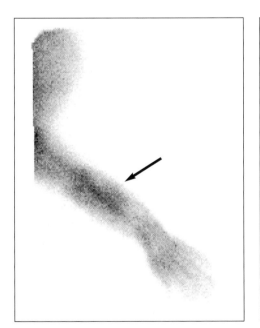
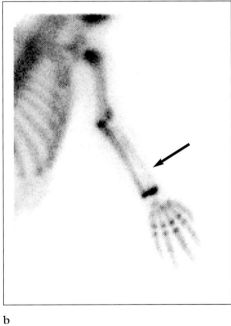

a   b

Figure 8.3 a and b

Osteomyelitis, right arm. 2½-year-old male, minimal soft-tissue swelling. (a) BP, right arm, posterior. Mild increased tracer uptake (arrow) in the mid-right forearm. (b) DS, right arm, posterior. Photon deficiency associated with the distal half of the right radius (arrow).

Teaching point

Hematogenous osteomyelitis, especially in infants and very young children, can often present as an area of photon deficiency. High-resolution images should be obtained in these patients.

continued

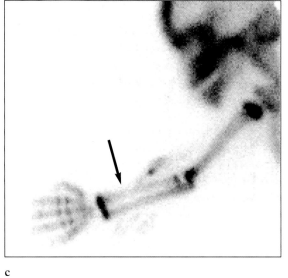

c

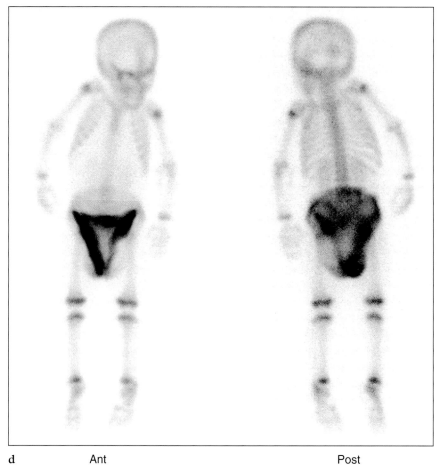

d   Ant   Post

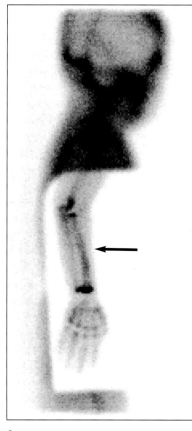

e

f

Figure 8.3 c–f

(c) DS, left arm, posterior. Normal left radius for comparison (arrow). (d) WB. The changes in the right forearm appreciated on the spot images are not appreciated on this WB study. Triangular intense activity over the right pelvis and perineum on the anterior view and well-defined shape of activity on the posterior view represent urine voided into the patient's diaper. (e) WB, anterior, follow-up study. Relative increased activity (arrow) without sharp anatomic definition involving the right forearm. (f) DS, right arm, lateral; follow-up study goes with WB bone scan in (e). The increased tracer uptake in the right radius (arrow) is associated with bone repair.

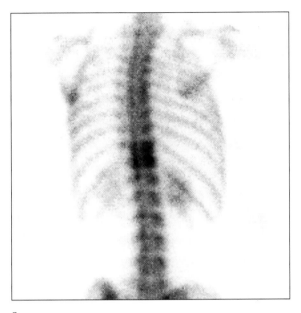

a

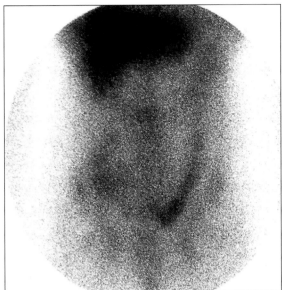

b

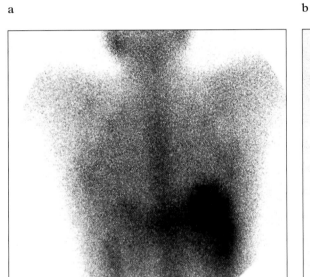

c

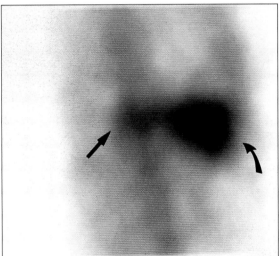

d

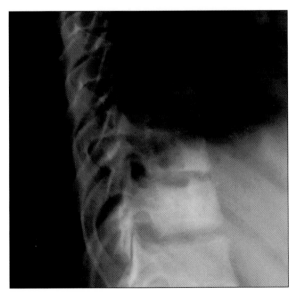

e

Figure 8.4

Osteomyelitis, thoracic spine, tuberculosis. 30-year-old woman who presented with back pain and no history of trauma. **(a)** DS, thoracolumbar spine, posterior. Increased tracer uptake, T10 and T11, with poor definition of intervertebral disk space. Compare with photon-deficient disk spaces at other levels. **(b)** ^{67}Ga, abdomen and pelvis, anterior and **(c)** ^{67}Ga, chest and upper abdomen, posterior. Because of overlying transverse colon on anterior view and additive effect of liver activity on posterior view, definite abnormal spinal uptake could not be diagnosed. **(d)** ^{67}Ga, SPECT, selected sagittal image. Activity involving the spine (straight arrow) is separated from the more anterior liver activity (curved arrow). **(e)** X-ray, lower thoracic spine, lateral. Follow-up X-ray demonstrates disk space narrowing and vertebral body endplate destruction.

Teaching point

When the normal photon deficiency of the intervertebral disk spaces is absent, infection should be considered. The disk spaces in the thoracic region are often more difficult to define on planar imaging than the disk spaces in the lumbar spine.

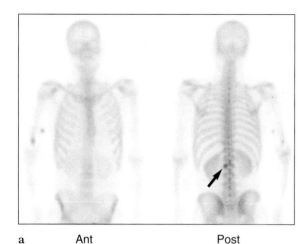

a   Ant   Post

Figure 8.5

Osteomyelitis, lumbar spine. 49-year-old male, HIV positive, intravenous drug abuser, back pain and fever. (**a**) WB. Activity projected over the left L2 pedicle region (arrow). Note that the linear scaling, with the most intense activity in the bladder, renders the bony uptake at a much lower intensity. (**b**) 3-D, volumetric reprojection. Selected images from 200° to 250°. The data for these images were obtained from a 180° posterior acquisition. Abnormal activity is visualized as more linear than the rounded appearance on the planar images. (**c**) SPECT, triangulation display. Transaxial images through the increased activity on the left side of the L2 region. Sagittal images are mid-line. The extension from the body into the pedicle region can be best appreciated on the transaxial images. (**d**) X-ray, lumbar spine, AP. Destruction of the L2 pedicle (arrow). Follow-up CT (not shown) demonstrated focal osteolysis involving the PS aspect of the L2 endplate with extension into the subchondral bone and adjacent left pedicle. There was hypodensity of psoas musculature centered on L2 but extending from L1 to L3. The scintigraphic diagnosis suggested that metastatic tumor should be strongly considered.

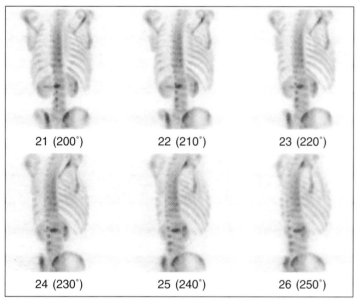

21 (200°)   22 (210°)   23 (220°)

24 (230°)   25 (240°)   26 (250°)

b

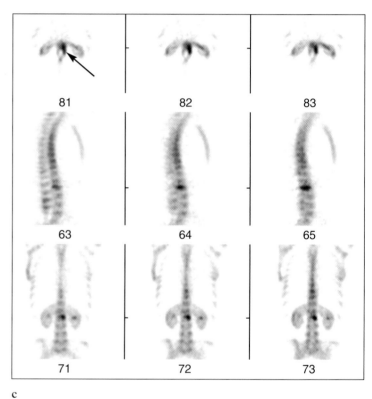

81   82   83

63   64   65

71   72   73

c

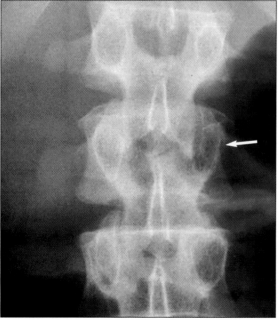

d

Teaching points

When a very intense area of abnormal uptake increases the count range of the linearly scaled image, contrast enhancement or window and leveling display manipulations should be considered to depict 'normal ribs' with a 'normal visual intensity'. This allows a better estimate of relative uptake in abnormal structures and also permits anatomic localization.

When SPECT imaging demonstrates abnormal tracer uptake in a vertebral body extending into the adjacent pedicle region, the finding is usually associated with metastatic disease. However, as illustrated in Figure 8.5, this is not an absolute specific finding.

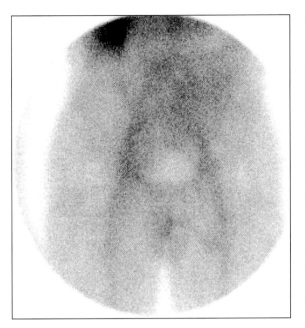

a

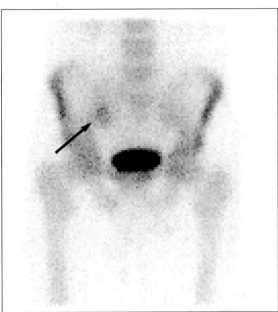

b

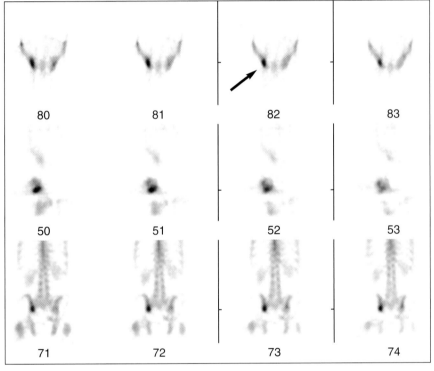

c

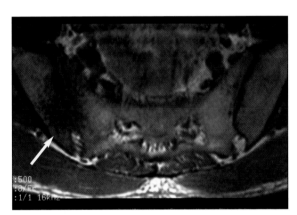

d

Figure 8.6

Pyogenic sacroiliitis (osteomyelitis of ilium and sacrum). 51-year-old male intravenous drug abuser with right hip pain and ulcers on anterior right thigh. (**a**) BP, pelvis, anterior. Minimal asymmetric increased tracer uptake, right SI region. (**b**) DS, pelvis, anterior. Faint focal increased tracer uptake, lower portion, right SI joint (arrow). (**c**) SPECT, pelvis, triangulation display. Transaxial images through lower SI joint. Focal increased tracer uptake (arrow) appears confined at this level to the lower-most portion of the iliac bone. (**d**) MR, T1-weighted image, coronal, pelvis. Decreased signal, iliac bone (arrow).

Figure 8.7

Staphylococcus aureus, sacroiliitis. 32-year-old female drug abuser, low back pain, tender to palpation over left SI joint. (a) RNA, posterior, five seconds per view. Focal increased perfusion to the area of the left SI joint (arrow). (b) BP, pelvis, posterior. Mild focal increased relative vascularity, left SI joint. (c) DS, pelvis. Posterior (left image) and LPO (right image). Focal increased tracer accumulation. (d) Ga, 96 hours post-injection. Posterior (left image) and LPO (right image). Relative uptake of tracer in abnormal regions compared with normal region is greater with Ga than on the ^{99m}Tc-MDP scan. This confirms infectious etiology. (e) CT, bone windows. SI joint region, transaxial. The left SI joint (arrow) is widened and shows cortical destruction on both sides. Anteriorly there is some periosteal new bone (arrowhead).

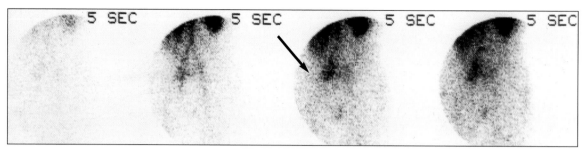

a

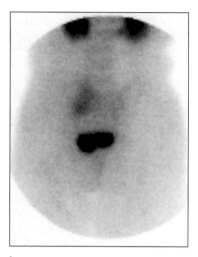

b

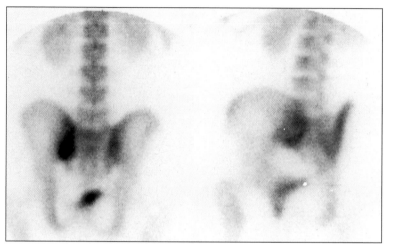

c

Teaching point

Correlating an abnormal three-phase RNB scan with an infection imaging study with ^{67}Ga or labeled white blood cells is often helpful in differentiating abnormal bone uptake associated with repair without any resultant infection. Although useful in nonviolated bone, it is especially important in dealing with violated bone (Chapter 8, page 327).

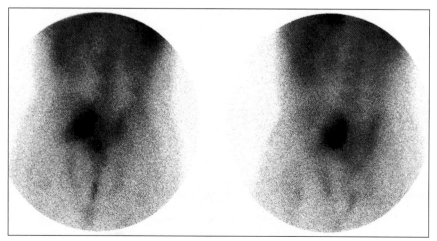

d

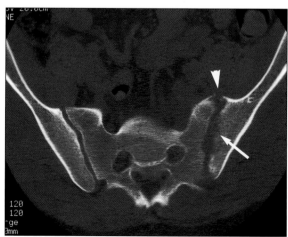

e

Osteomyelitis, complex (violated bone)

The presence of bone repair and remodeling secondary to any insult results in varying degrees of tracer accumulation during the RNA, BP and delayed phases of the three-phase bone scan, as well as uptake of gallium-67, labeled white blood cells (WBCs), and the accumulation of more or less sulfur colloid, which defines the presence of bone marrow. Such uptake is proportional to the stage and degree of the metabolism taking place and the state of the underlying bone marrow. The detection and diagnosis of superimposed infection often depend upon the relative uptake of these tracers. Many different protocols for so-called 'dual isotope' imaging are in use today.

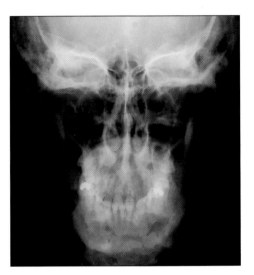

a

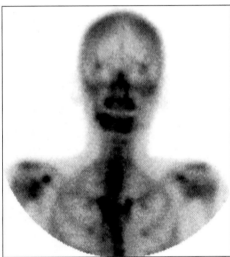

b

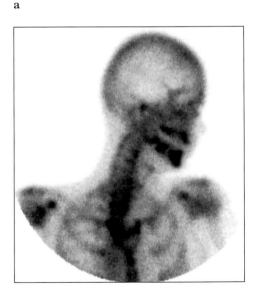

c

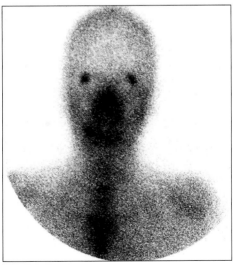

d

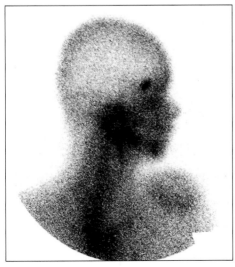

e

Figure 8.14

Mandible, healing fractures, no infection. 23-year-old man with pain and swelling eight months after segmental fracture. Cultures negative. (a) X-ray, face, AP. Nonunion of the right-sided fracture fragment. If osteomyelitis can be excluded, bone grafting is the treatment of choice in this setting. (b) DS, head and neck, anterior. (c) DS, head and neck, RL. Nonspecific moderately intense uptake about the fracture margins. Relative photopenic defect is at site of nonunion. (d) ^{67}Ga, head and neck, anterior and (e) ^{67}Ga, head and neck, RL. No significant uptake in the mandible.

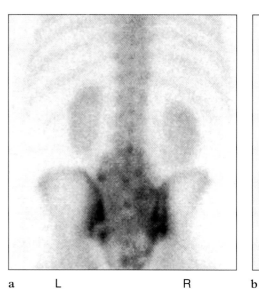

a   L   R

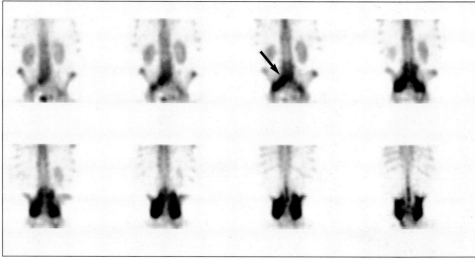

b

Figure 8.15

Pyogenic sacroiliitis, 72-year-old male with continued low back pain following L4 to S1 fusion. (**a**) DS, lumbosacral spine, posterior. In addition to irregular activity in the fusion mass, more marked on the left than on the right, there is intense abnormal increased tracer uptake in the SI joints. (**b**) SPECT, lumbosacral spine, coronal views. Moderate uptake in the right fusion mass (arrow) compared with the left; there is intense bilateral uptake in the SI joint regions. There was no surgery involving the SI joints.

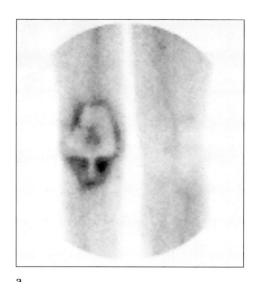

a

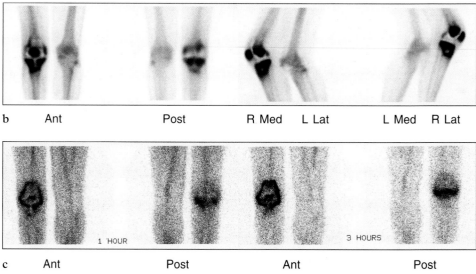

b   Ant   Post   R Med   L Lat   L Med   R Lat

c   Ant   Post   Ant   Post

Teaching point

Dual isotope imaging with indium-111 (^{111}In) WBC infection imaging, and ^{99m}Tc-sulfur colloid bone marrow scanning may be most sensitive and specific when evaluating prosthesis for infection.

Figure 8.16

Infected total knee arthroplasty. (**a**) BP, knees, anterior. Moderate increased tracer uptake surrounds portions of both the femoral and tibial components. Slightly more activity in medial proximal tibia. (**b**) DS, knees, multiple views. Intense abnormal activity in multiple areas, most marked in the proximal tibia. (**c**) ^{99m}Tc – WBC, knees, multiple views. One hour post-injection anterior and posterior (left images) and three-hours post-injection anterior and posterior (right images). Incongruence between activity in the ^{99m}Tc-WBC scan and bone scan is sign of infection.

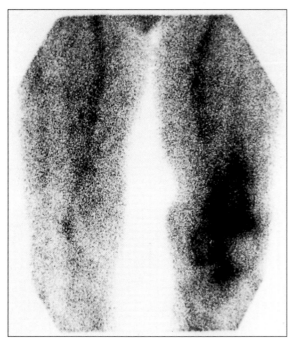

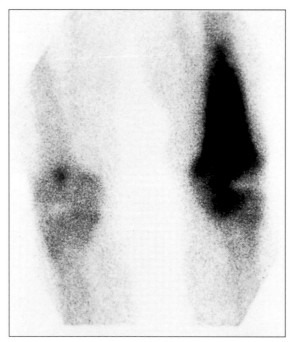

a   b

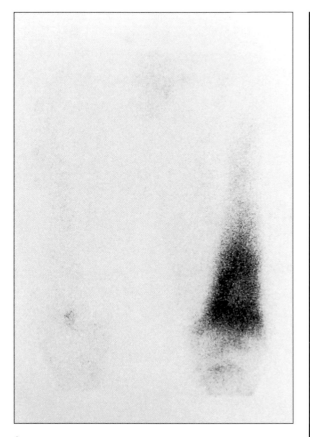

c

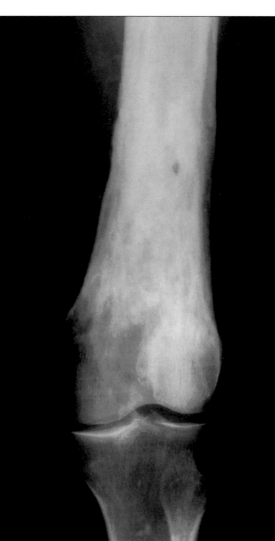

d

Figure 8.17

Acute exacerbation of chronic osteomyelitis. (a) BP, distal femur, anterior. Moderately intense, somewhat focal, irregularly distributed, increased uptake (relative vascularity) to distal femur. (b) DS, distal femur, anterior. Intense abnormal tracer involving distal third of femur. Focal increased uptake to medial tibial plateau. (c) DS, distal femurs, anterior. After antibiotic therapy. The intense abnormal uptake has decreased, representing improvement. (d) X-ray, distal femur, anterior. Changes of chronic osteomyelitis can sometimes be mistaken for Paget's disease.

Figure 8.18

Osteomyelitis, distal femur, post-fracture fixation. 21-year-old male with internally fixed open fracture began to drain pus at his wound site. (a) RNA, knees, anterior. Moderately intense, focal, increased tracer to the right knee. (b) DS, knee, anterior. Intense increased activity throughout the fracture site and distally. Photon deficiencies, medially, represent portions of the metallic external fixator. (c) ^{67}Ga, knees, anterior. Intense uptake involving the distal portion of the femur and knee is somewhat incongruent with the uptake on the bone scan. (d) RNA, knees, anterior. Four months following parenteral antibiotic therapy, the area of the right knee shows resolution of the focal increased perfusion seen in (a). The generalized decrease on that side probably represents some muscle wasting. (e) DS, much less intense tracer uptake than in (b). The photon deficiencies of metallic hardware have changed since the original study. (f) ^{67}Ga, knees, anterior. Even less relative intensity than on the earlier study.

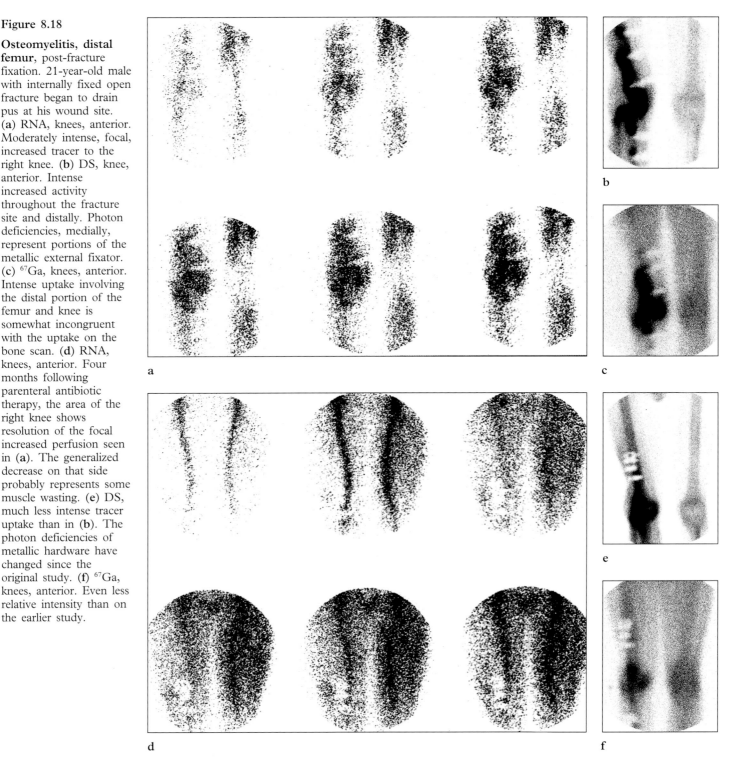

a

b

c

d

e

f

Teaching point

When acute osteomyelitis has been successfully treated, the gallium-67 scans will usually either return to normal or will show an abnormal to normal bone uptake ratio which is much less than the abnormal bone to normal bone uptake ratio on the ^{99m}Tc-MDP bone scan.

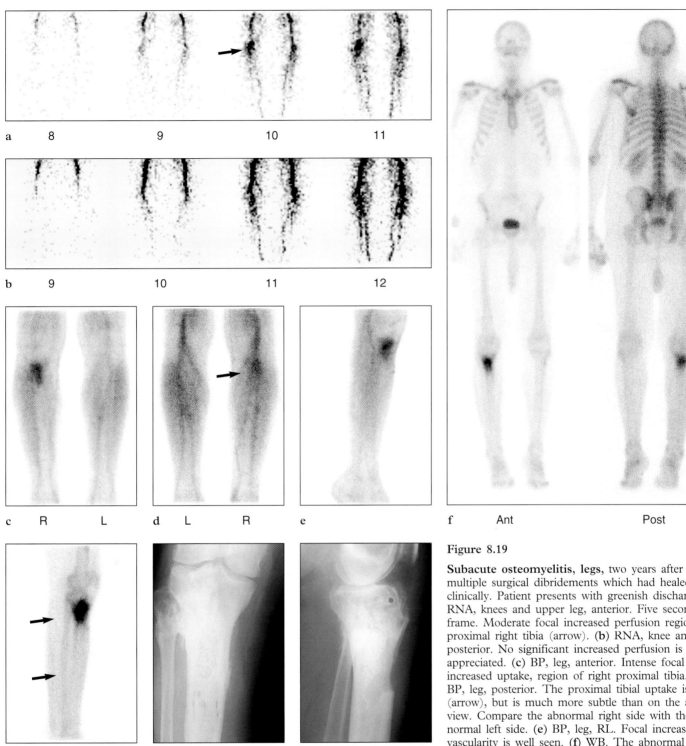

a 8 9 10 11

b 9 10 11 12

c R L d L R e

f Ant Post

Figure 8.19

Subacute osteomyelitis, legs, two years after multiple surgical dibridements which had healed clinically. Patient presents with greenish discharge. (**a**) RNA, knees and upper leg, anterior. Five seconds per frame. Moderate focal increased perfusion region of proximal right tibia (arrow). (**b**) RNA, knee and leg, posterior. No significant increased perfusion is appreciated. (**c**) BP, leg, anterior. Intense focal increased uptake, region of right proximal tibia. (**d**) BP, leg, posterior. The proximal tibial uptake is seen (arrow), but is much more subtle than on the anterior view. Compare the abnormal right side with the more normal left side. (**e**) BP, leg, RL. Focal increased vascularity is well seen. (**f**) WB. The abnormal increased activity in the proximal tibia was the only abnormal focus of increased tracer identified. The lower most legs and feet were imaged, but not reproduced. (**g**) DS, leg, RL. The intense abnormal tibial activity is seen. Note that on the lateral view the fibula is easily identified (arrows). (**h**) X-ray, upper leg, AP and (**i**) X-ray, right leg, lateral. The chronic bone changes with sclerosis and erosions are noted in both the tibia and fibula.

g h i

Teaching point

Lesion detection and localization require that the collimator be as close as possible to the abnormality. The differences between views taken from 180° opposite projections are often dramatic. When possible, both heads of dual detector cameras should be utilized.

Figure 8.20

Osteomyelitis and diabetic neuropathy, fifth metatarsal base. 45-year-old male with history of diabetes. Presents with necrotic right first toe and fever. (a) RNA, right foot, plantar view. Five seconds per frame. Moderate focal increased radiotracer activity at base of right fifth metatarsal (arrow), with minimal increase at the distal phalanx at the first toe (thin arrow). (b) BP, right foot, plantar. Moderate increased tracer uptake in the fifth metatarsal base region. A small area of more focal increase in the distal aspect of the first toe, which has a deformed-appearing tip after autoamputation. There is also some minimal increased uptake in the lateral portions of the tarsal–metatarsal joints. (c) BP, right foot, lateral. (d) DS, right foot, plantar. Areas of focal increased tracer uptake most marked in the area of the fifth metatarsal base, slightly less marked at the distal aspect of the first toe, and mild increase in portions of the MTP joints. (e) DS, right foot, lateral. (f) X-ray, right foot, AP with slight oblique. (g) X-ray, right foot, lateral. Neuropathic changes with destruction of the tarsal–metatarsal joints of the second through fifth rays compatible with neuropathic changes. A suggested healing fracture at the base of the fifth metatarsal. Patient received intravenous antibiotics with a good response.

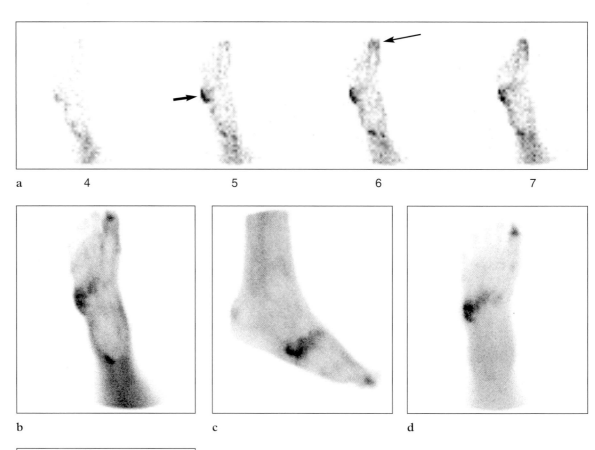

a 4   5   6   7

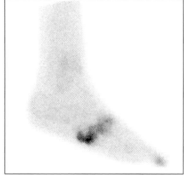

b   c   d

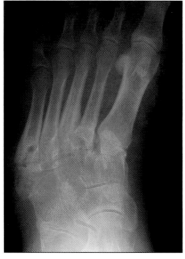

e

Teaching point

A positive three-phase bone scan is extremely sensitive for the detection of osteomyelitis; however, even when the classic findings of more intense, more focal, increased tracer on the delayed images, when compared with the BP images, are present, especially in the presence of 'violated' bone, the study is less specific and, depending on the clinical presentation and correlative images, 'dual isotope' imaging is often appropriate for precise differential diagnosis.

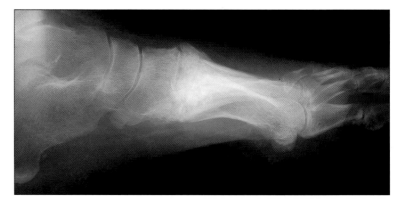

f   g

Miscellaneous lesions

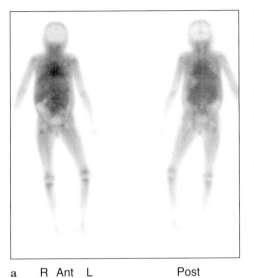

a   R Ant L   Post

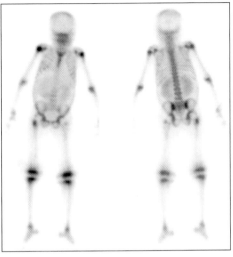

b

Figure 8.21

Septic arthritis and osteomyelitis, hips and femur. 8½-year-old female with sickle-cell anemia presents with fever and pain. (**a**) BP, WB. Acquired on WB table with speed of 16 cm/min. Slight focal increased uptake (relative vascularity), right proximal femur. Note the externally rotated position of the left hip. (**b**) WB. Moderately intense focal increased uptake, proximal right femur at intertrochanteric region. Represents osteomyelitis. Note photon deficiency of the left hip region with suggested increase in size of the joint. This was secondary to infected fluid with increased joint pressure.

Teaching point

Acute septic arthritis and blood-borne osteomyelitis, especially in infants and young children, often present as a photon deficiency because marrow packing or tense joints filled with fluid prohibit any tracer from reaching the bone crystal surface.

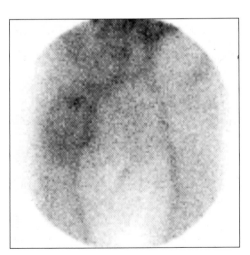

a

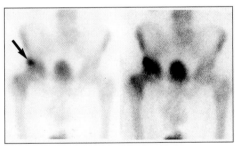

b

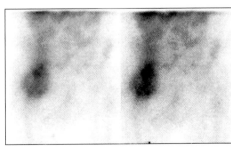

c

Figure 8.22

Septic right hip superimposed on chronic osteoarthritis. 83-year-old male four weeks more acute pain. Culture: coagulase-positive *Staphylococcus aureus*. (**a**) BP, hips, anterior. RNA was technically unsatisfactory. Mild, diffuse, increased tracer uptake (relative vascularity) around right hip region. (**b**) DS, hips, anterior. Standard display (left image) and contrast-enhanced image (right image). The most intense area of abnormal tracer corresponded to a large osteophyte (arrow). The contrast-enhanced image demonstrates some activity extending throughout the joint region. (**c**) Ga, 72 hours post-injection. Anterior pelvis. Standard display (left image) and contrast-enhanced image (right image). The extent of abnormal uptake corresponds to the joint capsule. The incongruence between the Ga and the bone tracer image as well as the anatomic extent of the Ga abnormality suggest the correct diagnosis.

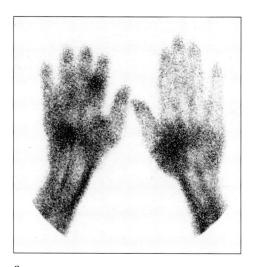
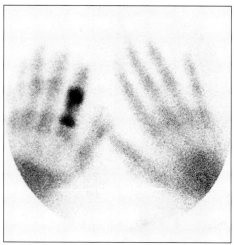
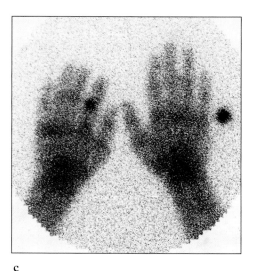

a   b   c

Figure 8.23

Septic arthritis. X-ray (not shown) three weeks following penetrating injury to left second PIP joint showed only soft-tissue swelling. **(a)** BP, hands and wrist, palmar. Mild, generalized, increased tracer uptake throughout the left hand, most pronounced at the left second PIP joint region. This represents increased relative vascularity. **(b)** DS, hands, palmar. Increased uptake at the PIP joint region as well as the base of the proximal phalanx. **(c)** Ga, palmar. Focal uptake in the PIP joint is discordant or incongruent when compared with the abnormal uptake on the ^{99m}Tc-MDP bone scan. Joint aspiration confirmed septic arthritis.

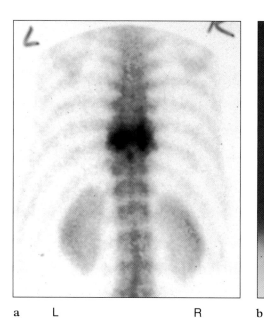
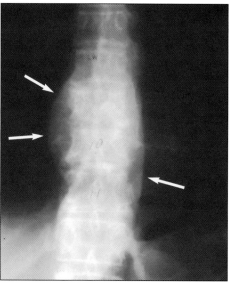

a   L   R   b

Figure 8.24

Diskitis, vertebral osteomyelitis, and paraspinal abscess. (a) DS, thoracic spine, posterior. Activity obliterates the T10–T11 intervertebral disk space, extends into the adjacent vertebra, and bulges laterally. **(b)** X-ray, lower thoracic, AP, overpenetrated technique. The soft-tissue shadows (arrows) outline the paraspinal mass.

Teaching points

- Abnormal increased activity involving the intervertebral disk space (often with increased relative vascularity on the BP images) suggests disk inflammation or infection. Any abnormal increased uptake in the adjacent vertebral bodies generally precludes ability to scintigraphically exclude associated vertebral osteomyelitis.
- The presence of photopenia in the spine has more frequently been associated with vertebral osteomyelitis.
- Labeled WBCs are less sensitive than ^{67}Ga citrate imaging in excluding spine infections.
- 48 and 72 hour post injection Ga images should be considered if 4 or 24 hour images are normal.

Correlative imaging comment

When radicular signs and symptoms are present or there is an extremely high clinical suspicion for epidural abscess, MR imaging, if available, should be considered as the first diagnostic imaging modality.

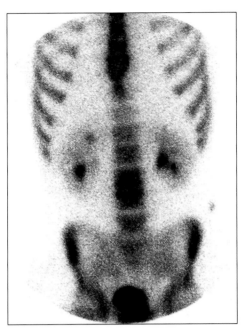

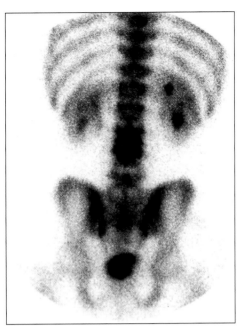

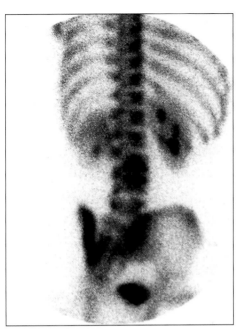

a b c

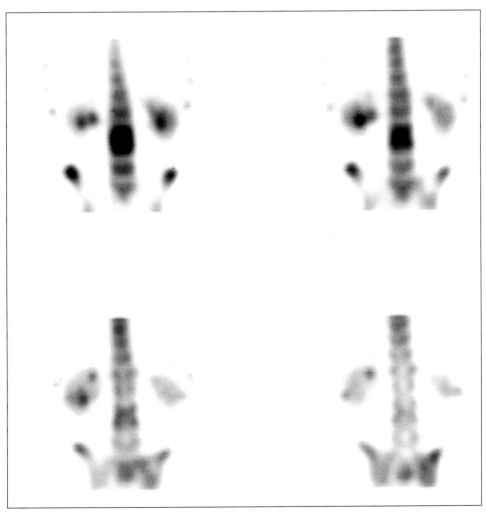

d

Figure 8.25

Diskitis, secondary to *Aspergillus* in a 32-year-old male, intravenous drug abuser. (a) DS, abdomen, anterior, (b) DS, lumbar spine, posterior, and (c) DS, lumbar spine, RPO. Moderately intense increased tracer uptake at the vertebral body endplates adjacent to the L2–L3 intervertebral disk spaces. Less pronounced increased tracer uptake is seen within the vertebral bodies. (d) SPECT, lumbar spine, selected coronal images. The abnormal increased tracer activity is localized to the vertebral bodies, without resolution of the intervertebral disk space at the level of involvement.

Teaching points

- Inability to resolve disk spaces as areas of photon deficiency especially in the clinical setting of possible infection usually indicates diskitis. BP images are often helpful when abnormal.
- The 'typical' appearance of vertebral body endplate fractures may be mimicked by discitis. Correlation with the clinical presentation, plain radiographs X-rays, or even aspiration biopsy may be necessary for differential diagnosis.

Periostitis

Periosteal new bone formation is a response of bone which can occur after a wide variety of insults. Some examples of periosteal new bone have been illustrated in association with tumors in Chapter 3 and in relation to shin splints in Chapter 4. It is our view that inflammation does not equal infection, and further that infection of the periosteum can be treated before organisms enter the marrow space and osteomyelitis develops.

Figure 8.26 a–d

Leg ulcer and periostitis, 54-year-old male, intravenous drug abuser with 1½-year history of leg ulceration, increasing pain, and odor for one week. X-ray demonstrated minimal periosteal new bone formation. (a) RNA, leg, anterior. Five seconds per frame. Mild-to-moderate increased tracer appearance (relative perfusion) to the medial aspect of the left lower leg. (b) BP, leg, anterior. Increased tracer uptake (relative vascularity) is present medially in the lower leg. (c) DS, knees and legs, anterior and posterior. Mild increased metabolic activity medially in the distal left lower leg. (d) DS, lower leg, left medial view. Linearly oriented increased tracer in the anterior tibial cortex of the lower leg has varying intensity.

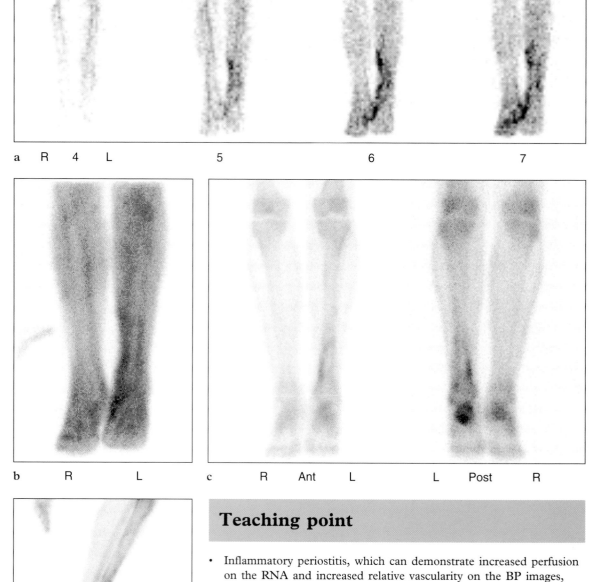

a   R   4   L   5   6   7

b   R   L   c   R   Ant   L   L   Post   R

d

Teaching point

- Inflammatory periostitis, which can demonstrate increased perfusion on the RNA and increased relative vascularity on the BP images, can be contrasted with the periostitis associated with shin splints which almost never has increased tracer activity on the RNA or BP images.
- Activity of ^{67}Ga accumulation is often related to the relative intensity of uptake in the liver, as appreciated on WB imaging. When spot images are obtained, the location of even minimal amounts of tracer uptake can be seen if the time of acquisition is increased, but judging the significance is more difficult.

continued

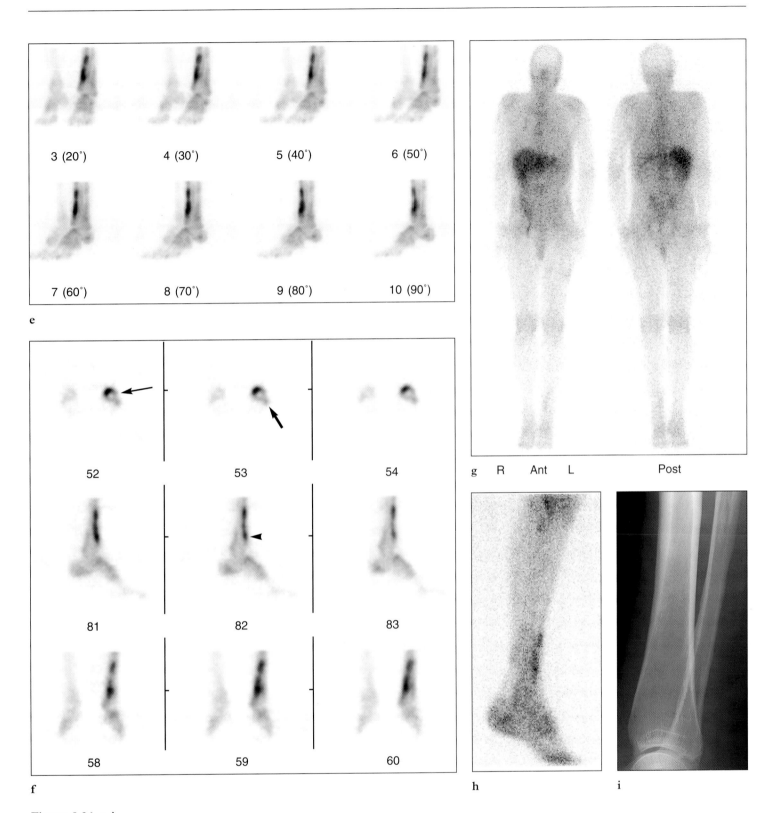

Figure 8.26 e–i

(e) 3-D volumetric reprojection images. Selected views from 20° to 90°. The anterior location of the irregular linear increased tracer is well seen. (f) SPECT, lower leg, triangulation display. Transaxial slices (upper row) are obtained through the lower-most part of the periosteal uptake at the level indicated by the arrowhead. The relative size of the fibula (regular arrow on mid-transaxial slice) is contrasted to the larger-diameter tibia (thin arrow). The abnormal increased activity anteromedially does not encroach into the central marrow space. (g) Ga, WB, 24 hour post-injection image. Study done four days following bone scan. The most minimal asymmetric increased uptake in the medial aspect of the distal left tibia. (h) Ga, left leg, medial view. Linear increased uptake has a somewhat congruent pattern when compared with the bone scan images, but the relative activity in the abnormal area to the normal area is less than on the bone study. (i) X-ray, lower left leg, lateral periosteal changes are minimal.

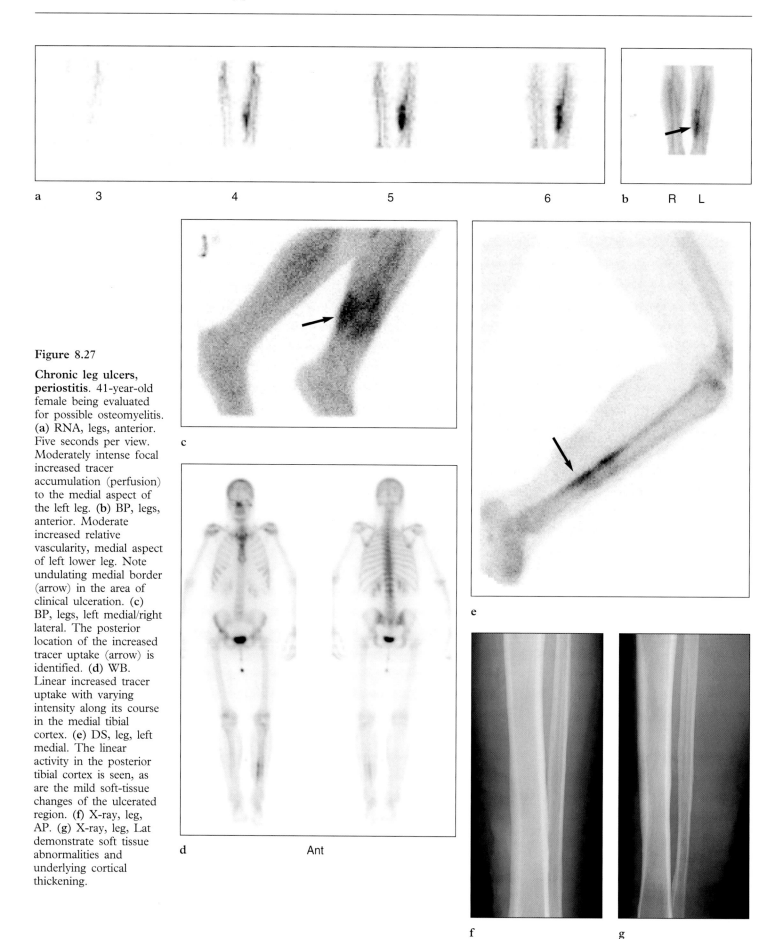

a   3   4   5   6   b   R   L

c

e

Figure 8.27

Chronic leg ulcers, periostitis. 41-year-old female being evaluated for possible osteomyelitis. (a) RNA, legs, anterior. Five seconds per view. Moderately intense focal increased tracer accumulation (perfusion) to the medial aspect of the left leg. (b) BP, legs, anterior. Moderate increased relative vascularity, medial aspect of left lower leg. Note undulating medial border (arrow) in the area of clinical ulceration. (c) BP, legs, left medial/right lateral. The posterior location of the increased tracer uptake (arrow) is identified. (d) WB. Linear increased tracer uptake with varying intensity along its course in the medial tibial cortex. (e) DS, leg, left medial. The linear activity in the posterior tibial cortex is seen, as are the mild soft-tissue changes of the ulcerated region. (f) X-ray, leg, AP. (g) X-ray, leg, Lat demonstrate soft tissue abnormalities and underlying cortical thickening.

d   Ant

f   g

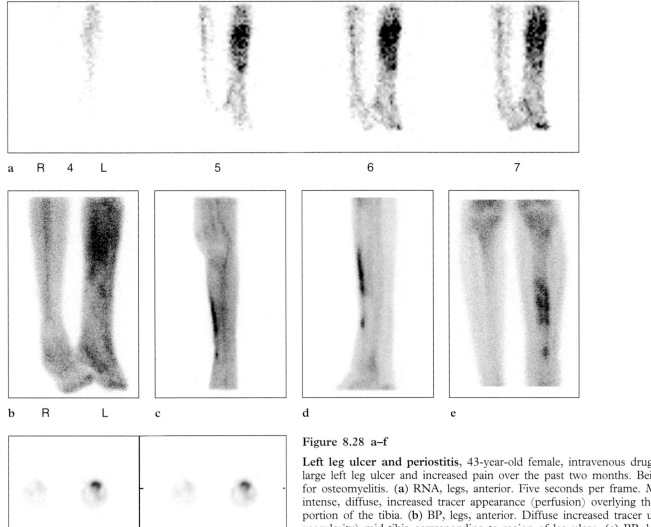

a R 4 L   5   6   7

b R   L   c   d   e

Figure 8.28 a–f

Left leg ulcer and periostitis, 43-year-old female, intravenous drug abuser, with large left leg ulcer and increased pain over the past two months. Being evaluated for osteomyelitis. (a) RNA, legs, anterior. Five seconds per frame. Moderately intense, diffuse, increased tracer appearance (perfusion) overlying the lower portion of the tibia. (b) BP, legs, anterior. Diffuse increased tracer uptake (relative vascularity) mid-tibia corresponding to region of leg ulcer. (c) BP, left leg, lateral. The linear very anteriorly located increased tracer with varying intensity along its course. This spot BP image was taken 15 minutes after the injection and 12 minutes after the anterior BP, so that there is a degree of 'early fixation' phase activity. (d) DS, left leg, lateral. The linear anterior activity is noted. (e) DS, legs, anterior. There is some activity involving the medial cortex as well as the lateral tibial cortex. (f) SPECT, legs, triangulation display. The linear activity is again identified.

continued

77   78

94   95

94   95

f

Teaching points

- Images obtained 10–30 minutes post-injection of bone tracer have a significant component of 'early fixation' phase of bone uptake. This results because of the 30-minute half-time for tracer movement from the extravascular, extracellular spaces to the hydration shell of the bone crystal surface.
- Congruent Ga and MDP bone images are considered indeterminate for the ability to diagnose infection.
- Linear superficial uptake of tracer on delayed images is strongly suggestive of periostitis. On delayed images alone, the underlying bone insult leading to periosteal new bone formation cannot be determined.

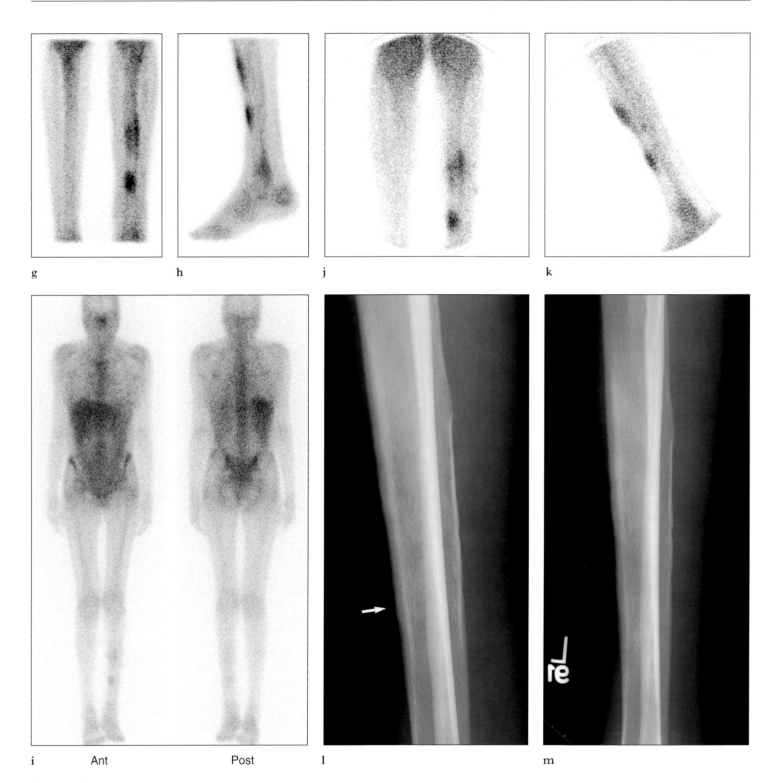

g   h   j   k

i   Ant   Post   l   m

Figure 8.28 g–m

Follow-up examination (**g–k**) obtained six months after the initial examination (**a–f**). (**g**) DS, legs, anterior. The smaller inferior focus of increased tracer appears larger than on the early study while the more superior lesion appears smaller. (**h**) DS, left leg, lateral. Although larger, the inferior lesion is still very anterior and superficial. (**i**) Ga WB, 24 hours post-injection. Performed eight days following the follow-up bone scan images (**g** and **h**). Minimal increased relative tracer uptake in the lower of the two tibial lesions when compared with the activity in the liver. (**j**) Ga, legs, anterior spot and (**k**) Ga, left leg, lateral spot, 48-hours post-injection. Relative congruence of the lesions (compare spot in (**j**) with bone spot in (**g**)). Although a superimposed osteomyelitis was considered for the lower lesion because of the increasing size and relative prominence on the Ga study, the congruence and the linear anterior superficial appearance on the bone scan were more suggestive of periostitis. (**l**) X-ray, leg, 8/90. (**m**) X-ray, leg, 11/97. Chronic changes (arrow).

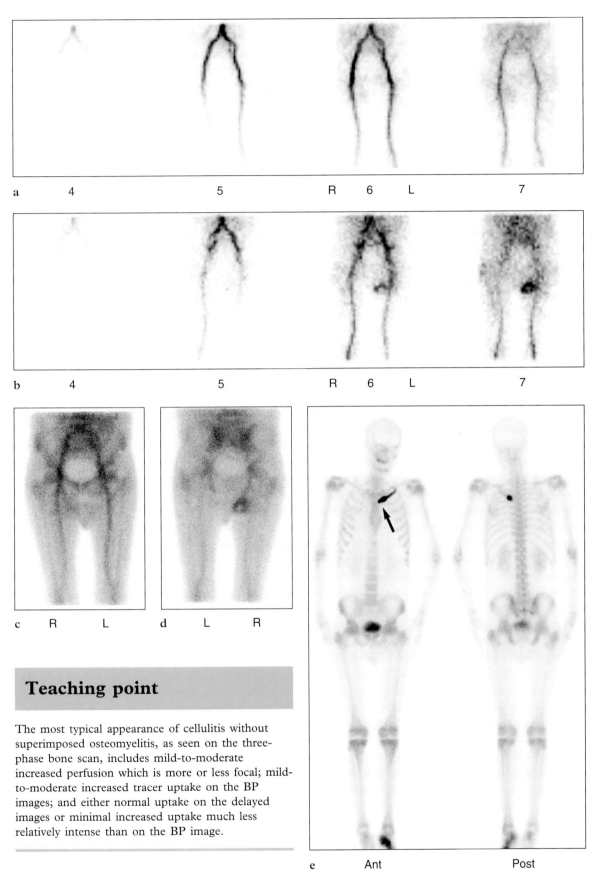

Soft tissue ulcer, right buttocks. This multi-trauma patient developed a bedsore. (a) RNA, pelvis, anterior. Five seconds per frame. Minimal asymmetry with only the slightest increased tracer visualization (relative perfusion) is seen on the right when compared with the left. (b) RNA, pelvis, posterior. Intense round focus of increased tracer over the right buttocks. There is a central photopenic defect. (c) BP, pelvis, anterior. The most minimal asymmetric increase in the right hip when compared with the left. (d) BP, pelvis, posterior. The focal round area of moderate increased tracer with a photopenic center is again seen. (e) WB. No abnormal increased tracer in the bones of the pelvis. Injection port for Hickman catheter seen over the left chest. This projects as an intense round focus of activity on the posterior view.

Teaching point

The most typical appearance of cellulitis without superimposed osteomyelitis, as seen on the three-phase bone scan, includes mild-to-moderate increased perfusion which is more or less focal; mild-to-moderate increased tracer uptake on the BP images; and either normal uptake on the delayed images or minimal increased uptake much less relatively intense than on the BP image.

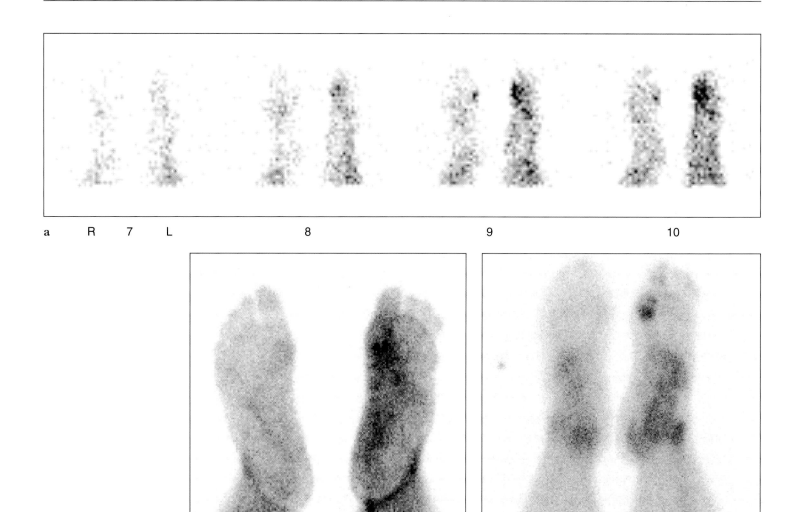

a   R   7   L   8   9   10

b

c

Figure 8.30

Cellulitis over first MTP joint region in a patient
with underlying neuropathic arthritis. **(a)** RNA, foot,
plantar. Mild, poorly defined, increased tracer uptake
in the area of the medial MTP joint regions. **(b)** BP,
foot, plantar. The mild diffuse increase throughout
the lower leg, ankle, and foot is seen, as is the more
prominent, but still poorly marginated, activity at the
first MTP joint region. **(c)** DS, foot, plantar. Mild
activity at the first MTP joint region.

Teaching point

The diagnosis of osteomyelitis on three-phase bone
imaging requires that the abnormal increased activity
on delayed images be more intense and more focal
than activity in a similar area on the BP or tissue-
phase image.

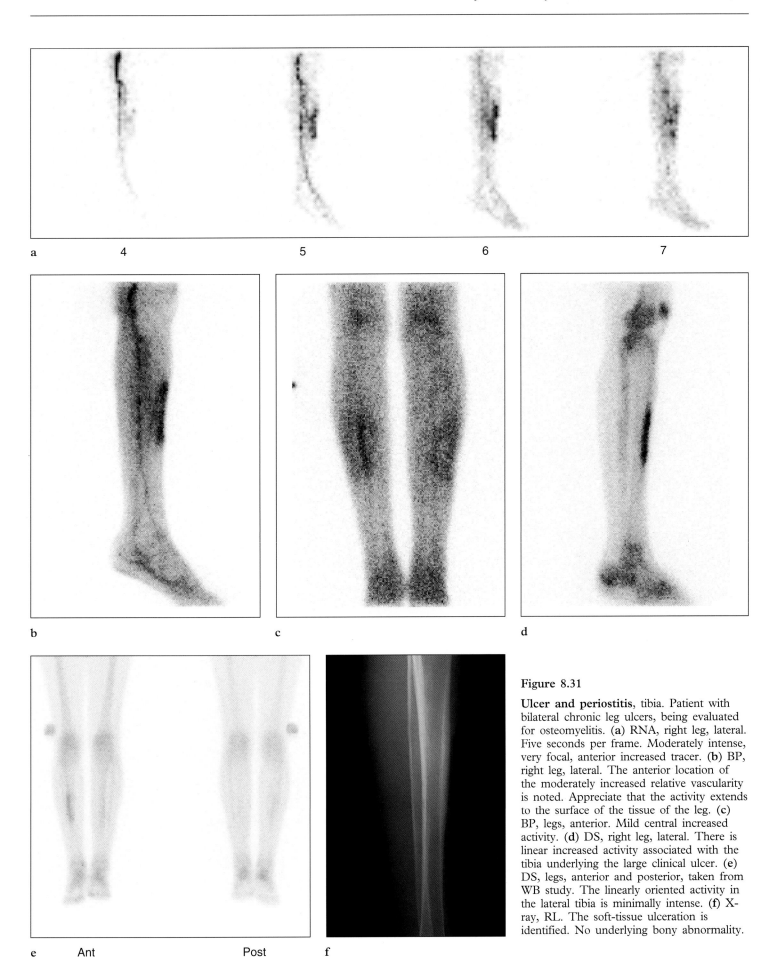

a   4   5   6   7

b

c

d

e   Ant   Post   f

Figure 8.31

Ulcer and periostitis, tibia. Patient with bilateral chronic leg ulcers, being evaluated for osteomyelitis. (**a**) RNA, right leg, lateral. Five seconds per frame. Moderately intense, very focal, anterior increased tracer. (**b**) BP, right leg, lateral. The anterior location of the moderately increased relative vascularity is noted. Appreciate that the activity extends to the surface of the tissue of the leg. (**c**) BP, legs, anterior. Mild central increased activity. (**d**) DS, right leg, lateral. There is linear increased activity associated with the tibia underlying the large clinical ulcer. (**e**) DS, legs, anterior and posterior, taken from WB study. The linearly oriented activity in the lateral tibia is minimally intense. (**f**) X-ray, RL. The soft-tissue ulceration is identified. No underlying bony abnormality.

Figure 8.32

Insertional tendonitis, medial capsular insertion on ulna, 27-year-old male, pain in right elbow, tender to palpation. (**a**) Elbow. Bony spur (arrow). (**b**) DS, elbow, anterior, palms up. Moderately intense focal area of increased uptake (arrow) corresponds to spur. Uptake represents bony repair from excessive traction at the insertion.

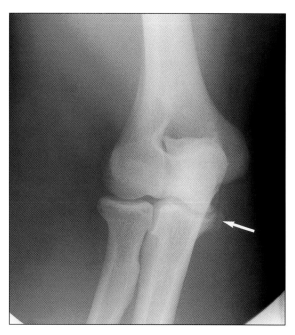

a

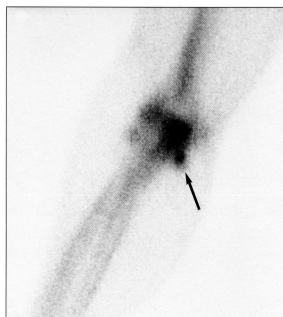

b

Teaching point

Although most 'tendonitis' lesions are related to work or recreational trauma, often of the repetitive stress type, the clinical presentation and referral are often in the context of an infection or inflammation evaluation.

Metabolic bone disease

Metabolic bone disease is the general term for a category of systemic diseases in which normal bone metabolism is altered. In most of these conditions there are changes in the bone mass, which is usually decreased, and fractures occur commonly. Osteopenia is the general term for decreased bone mass. Osteoporosis is secondary to abnormal mineralization of normal osteoid. In osteomalacia the serum calcium and phosphorus are usually normal, with the abnormality being in the osteoid that is not normally mineralized. There is an excess of osteoclastic over osteoblastic activity.

Scintigraphic features of metabolic bone disease

The patterns of osseous uptake of tracer illustrated in this section are nonspecific. They are often seen when there is increased skeletal metabolism (see Metabolic features present on bone scan, page 91).

Table 9.1 Bone scan in metabolic bone disease (MBD)

Disease	*Cause +ve bone scan*	*Differentiating features*	*Comment*
Renal osteodystrophy	Hyperparathyroidism	Metabolic features Absence of tracer in bladder	May find the most dramatic images seen in MBD
Primary hyperparathyroidism	Hyperparathyroidism	Metabolic features Uncommon: brown tumors, ectopic calcification	Bone scan usually normal
Osteomalacia	Hyperparathyroidism Uptake in osteoid	Metabolic features Pseudofractures (PF)	May not be possible to differentiate PF and metastases
Aluminum (Al)-induced osteomalacia	–	Low bone uptake High background activity	Al is a bone poison that blocks mineralization
Osteoporosis	Fracture	Intense linear uptake at site of vertebral fracture May be low/patchy uptake in axial skeleton	Bone scan usually normal When there is fracture the bone scan cannot differentiate other causes, e.g., tumor, on basis of scan alone Activity at site of fracture fades over subsequent 1–2 years

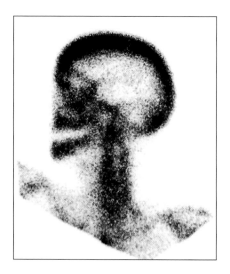

Figure 9.1

Calvarial uptake. DS, head and neck, lateral. Increased tracer uptake throughout the calvaria and mandible.

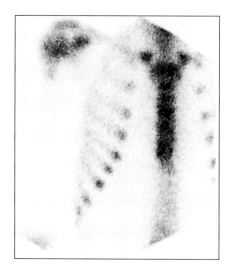

Figure 9.2

Costochondral junctions (beading). DS, chest, anterior. Increased tracer at all the costochondral junctions.

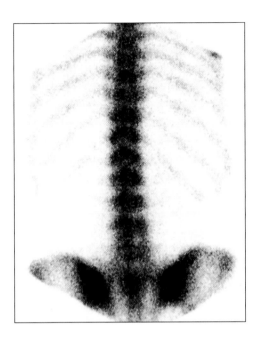

Figure 9.3

Superscan. DS, thoracolumbar spine, posterior. Intense uptake throughout the axial skeleton with high contrast between bone and soft tissue. The kidneys are not visualized at these standard display settings.

Teaching point

The so-called 'superscan' with intense abnormal skeletal uptake and no visualization of excreted activity in the kidneys is not specific for either metabolic bone disease or diffuse metastasis.

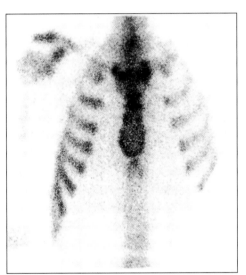

a

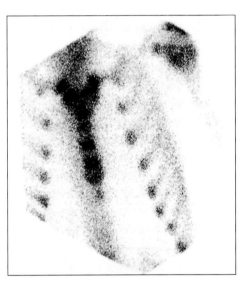

b

Figure 9.4

Sternum, tie sign. (a) DS, chest, anterior. Increased tracer uptake throughout the sternum. (b) DS, chest, anterior. In another patient, a 'striped' tie sign.

Pseudofractures are zones composed of osteoid and fibrous tissue and are thought to represent healing changes of microfractures. Pseudofractures have been described in osteomalacia, rickets, Paget's disease, fibrous dysplasia, and hyperphosphatasia. These may progress to complete fractures.

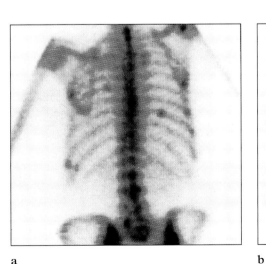

a

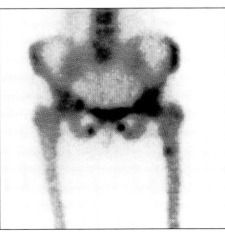

b

Figure 9.5

Pseudofractures. 50-year-old female with osteomalacia who complained of pain in ribs and difficulty on walking. (a) DS, thoracolumbar spine, posterior. Foci of abnormal tracer in the ribs. Renal activity not visualized. (b) DS, pelvis, anterior. Foci of abnormal increased activity in the pubic rami, left femoral neck, and proximal diaphysis.

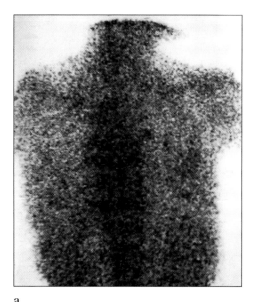

a

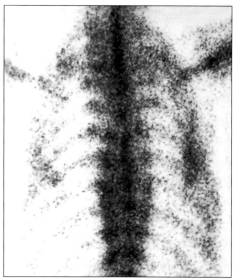

b

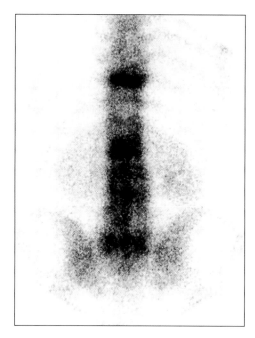

Figure 9.12

Osteomalacia, secondary to aluminum toxicity. This complication of renal dialysis is rarely seen today. (**a**) DS, thoracic spine, posterior. High background activity with poor delineation of bone. (**b**) DS, thoracic spine, posterior. Following desferrioxamine therapy. Image quality dramatically improves.

Figure 9.13

Pathologic vertebral fractures secondary to osteoporosis. DS, thoracolumbar spine, posterior. Several areas of linear increased tracer uptake seen at T10, L1, and L5, with nonhomogeneity of tracer uptake throughout the remainder of the spine. Such scan appearances with lesions of varying intensity of tracer uptake are often seen in patients with severe osteoporosis who have multiple vertebral fractures, which have occurred at different time intervals.

Figure 9.14

Thyrotoxicosis with osteoporosis. 80-year-old female. WB. There is prominent WB uptake. Typical vertebral compression fractures at T11 and T12. Incidental mild uptake, left greater trochanter.

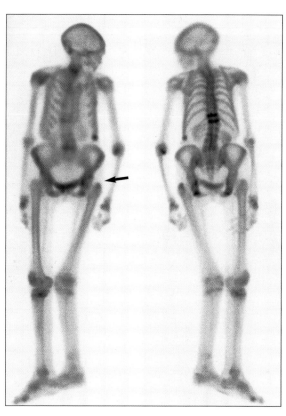

Ant   Post

Teaching point

In extreme old age, thyrotoxicosis may not be clinically apparent and can on occasion present with vertebral fractures.

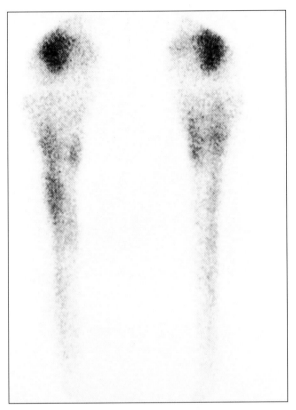

a

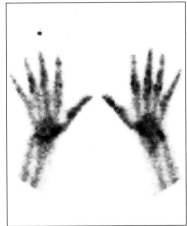

a

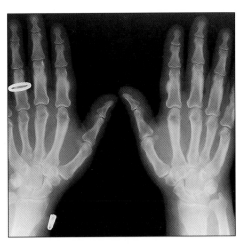

c

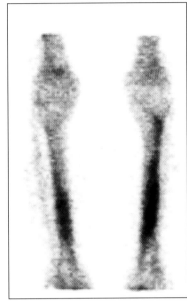

b

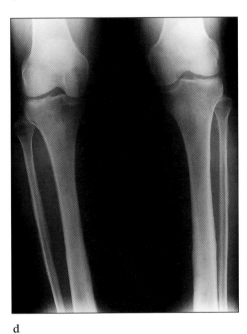

d

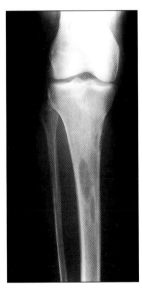

b

Figure 9.15

Brown tumors. Patient with primary hyperparathyroidism. (**a**) DS, legs, anterior. Mild areas of increased tracer uptake in both upper tibias. (**b**) X-ray, proximal leg, anterior. Lytic areas represent the brown tumor.

Figure 9.16

Thyroid acropachy. This patient has severe Graves' disease, with eye changes and pretibial myxedema. (**a**) DS, hands, palmar view. (**b**) DS, legs, anterior. Increased patchy accumulation of tracer. Most marked in the mid-tibia. (**c**) X-ray, hands, PA and (**d**) X-ray, legs, AP. Cortical sclerotic changes.

Teaching point

The brown tumor is a giant cell reparative granuloma which is brown because of hemosiderin deposition. The intensity of lesion uptake on delayed bone images is variable. Most brown tumors seen in developed countries today are associated with secondary hyperparathyroidism.

Figure 9.17

Thyroid acropachy. DS, hands and wrists, palmar.

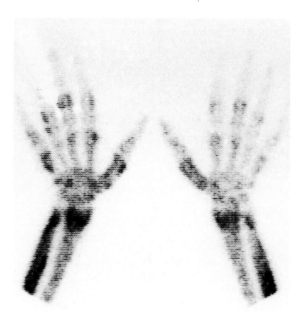

Teaching point

In most patients with thyrotoxicosis the bone scan is entirely normal.

Miscellaneous lesions 10

With the widespread use of CT scanning and the rapid introduction and development of MR imaging to problems of the musculoskeletal system, the role of RNBI has also been modified. Because of their anatomic specificity MR and CT are often used as the first imaging examination after plain X-rays have been obtained. RNBI is used either in very specific situations, or as a problem-solving tool when the clinical symptomatology is confusing or the anatomic image is diagnostically unrewarding. It is in this latter context that this chapter is particularly important.

Although in this atlas we have grouped images according to disease entities or clinical referral areas, very often the underlying etiology of the presenting problem is unclear. Knowledge of the scintigraphic appearance of a variety of lesions, many represented here, will be important for diagnosis or to direct further imaging. The findings during careful review of the RNA and BP images, and of the pattern of renal excretion of tracer, should also be an integral part of study interpretation.

Osseous lesions

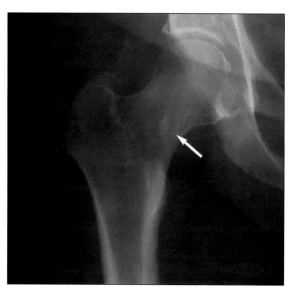

a

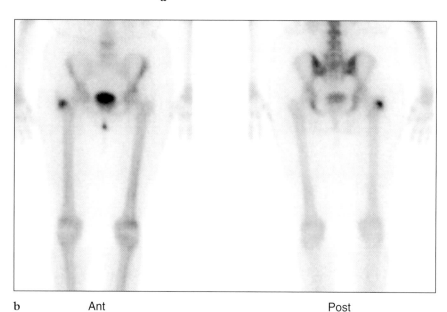

b   Ant   Post

Figure 10.1

Bone island with no abnormal tracer uptake. **(a)** X-ray, right hip, AP. The homogeneous oval density in the medial aspect of the right femoral neck is typical for bone island. **(b)** DS, pelvis and hips, anterior and posterior from WB study. The medial femoral neck shows no area of abnormal increased tracer accumulation. Small, well-defined focus of intense increased tracer at the lateral aspect of the greater trochanter represented atypical greater trochanteric bursitis in this 54-year-old female being evaluated for osseous metastasis from breast cancer. Its atypical location (bursitis is usually more SL) required follow-up since a metastasis was a strong consideration.

Teaching point

- RNBI continues to be the primary means of differentiating bone islands from more aggressive or malignant bone lesions. An occasional bone island, usually the 'giant bone island', may show some minimal increased tracer uptake.
- Osteopoikilosis, an uncommon hereditary bone disease, consists of hundreds of symmetric lesions, each of which is histologically and radiographically a bone island (enostosis).

Correlative imaging point

A bone island can usually be diagnosed with certainty by plain radiography. These present as a well-defined homogeneous round or oval radiodensity in the medullary canal, usually in the metaphysis with sharply circumscribed margins. Occasionally there is a feathered or brush border.

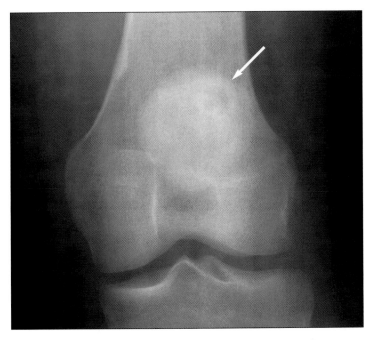

a

b

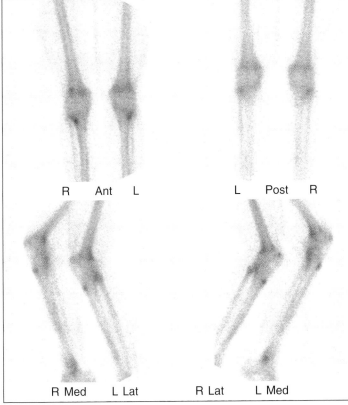

c

Figure 10.2

Dorsal defect of the patella. The dorsal defect is most likely an anomaly of ossification and of little clinical significance. (**a**) X-ray, knee, AP and (**b**) X-ray, knee, oblique. The round, radiolucent lesion surrounded by a zone of sclerosis located on the SL aspect of the dorsal surface of the patella (arrows) is typical. (**c**) DS, knee, multiple views. There is no abnormal increased metabolic activity associated with the left patella.

Teaching point

Providing information about the relative vascularity and metabolic activity of lesions seen incidentally on anatomic imaging studies is an important use for RNBI. Such information aids in patient management.

Figure 10.3

Engelmann's disease (progressive diaphyseal dysplasia). DS, selected views. (**a**) Right lateral skull. (**b**) Right anterior chest. (**c**) Left anterior chest. (**d**) Anterior pelvis. (**e**) Anterior femurs. (**f**) Anterior tibia. (**g**) Increased patchy tracer uptake throughout the diaphyseal areas of all long bones and the skull. The bones are spindle-shaped with under-tubulated appearance.

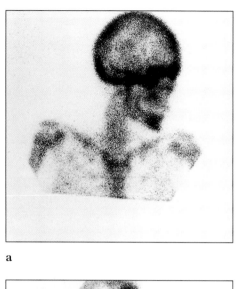

a

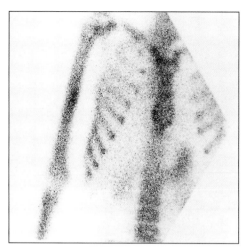

b

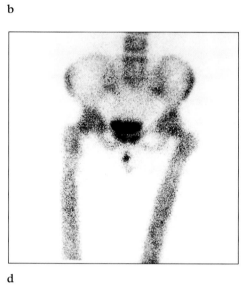

c

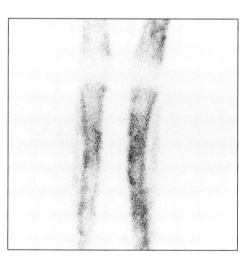

d

e

f

Bone infarct

Osteonecrosis describes the histologic changes that follow bone death, which occurs from disturbances in blood circulation. Osteonecrosis in association with a variety of clinical conditions has historically been termed bone infarct, and several examples will be included under this heading. These conditions included alcoholism, steroid therapy, decompression sickness, sickle-cell anemia, Gaucher's disease and pancreatitis.

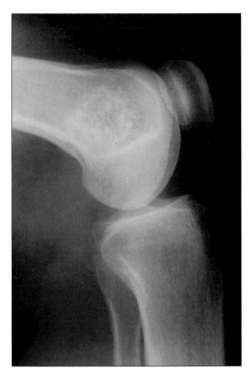

a

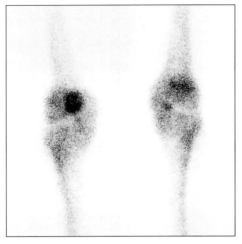

b

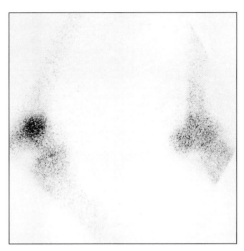

c

Figure 10.4

Bone infarct, distal femur. (a) X-ray, right knee, lateral. This mature infarct demonstrates a calcified area in the medullary cavity. Although some infarcts have a sharper sclerotic border, this is a well-defined lesion. (b) DS, knees, anterior and (c) DS, knee, right medial. Single area of mild-to-moderate, well-defined, increased tracer in the distal femur. On the anterior view alone the scan appearance could be mistaken for the normal variation termed 'hot patellar sign'.

Teaching point

- Most bone infarcts appear normal on RNBI. The degree of metabolic activity relates to the stage of infarct. During the early stages there may be photon deficiency, slight increase during repair, and then a more normal metabolic appearance, which may be related to the size of the lesion with overlying uptake in normal bone obscuring the photon deficiency.
- The radiographic differential diagnosis always includes enchondroma.

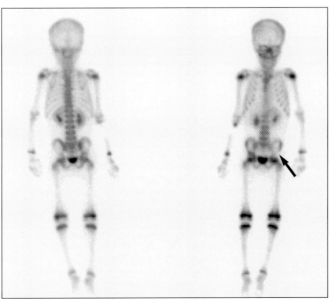

Post   Ant

Figure 10.5

Sickle-cell anemia, infarct left ilium. Five-year-old male. WB. Obtained with 1.25 acquisition zoom. Photon deficiency involving the lower half of the left ilium (arrow).

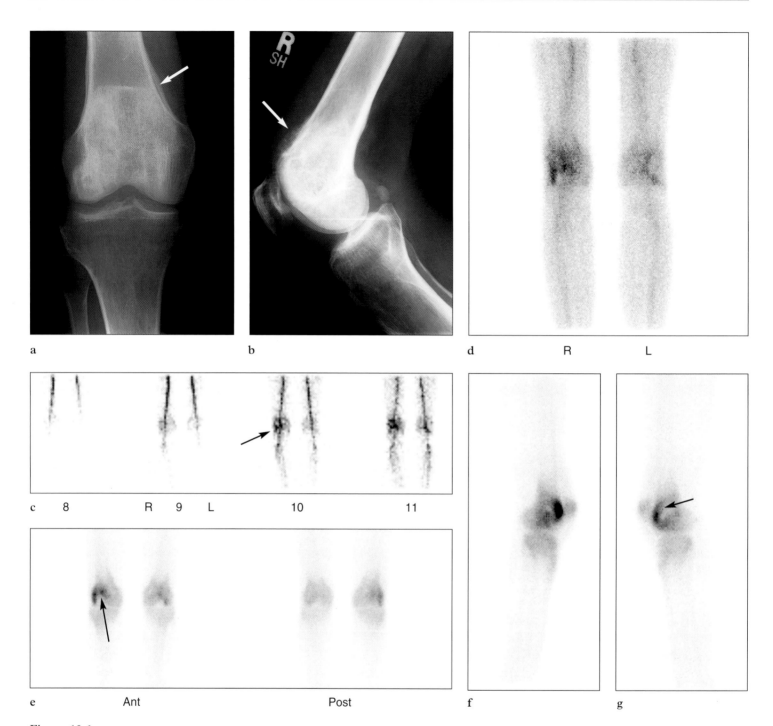

a   b   d   R   L

c   8   R   9   L   10   11

e   Ant   Post   f   g

Figure 10.6

Idiopathic bone infarct, with superimposed fracture. 44-year-old male
presented with pain. (a) X-ray, right knee, anterior and (b) X-ray, right knee,
lateral. Density in the distal femur with periosteal reaction, anterior and medial
(arrows). (c) RNA, knees, anterior. Five seconds per view. Mild, somewhat focal,
increased perfusion to the right distal femur. The third image demonstrates
slightly more activity lateral than medial (arrow). (d) BP, knees, anterior.
Somewhat linear increased uptake laterally, with mild photon deficiency just
medial. (e) DS, knees, anterior and posterior (from WB study, the rest of which
was normal). Moderate increased uptake, somewhat linearly oriented laterally at
the distal femur with photon deficiency medially (arrow). (f) DS, right knee,
lateral and (g) DS, right knee, medial. The activity anteriorly associated with a
healing fracture is somewhat inferior to the larger area of periosteal reaction on
the X-ray, which suggests that periosteal reaction may be from a more distant
insult. The photon deficiency associated with the main portion of the infarct is
best appreciated on the medial view (arrow).

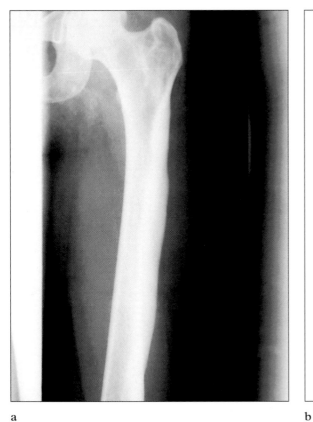

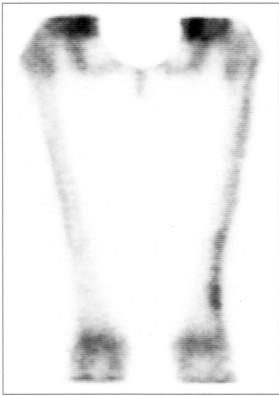

a

b

Figure 10.7

Melorheostosis. (a) X-ray, left femur, AP. Irregular cortical hyperostosis involving the entire shaft of the femur is the result of periosteal new bone, which has matured into lamellar bone. (b) DS, femurs, anterior. The increased tracer uptake throughout the femur corresponds to the increased volume of cortical bone present.

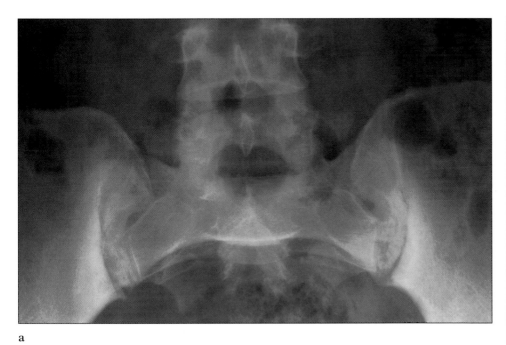

a

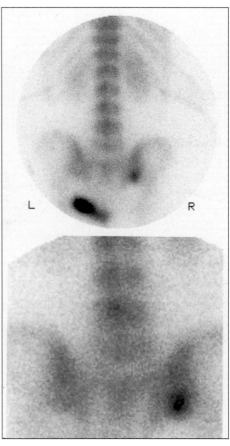

b L   R

Figure 10.8

Osteitis condensans ilii. (a) X-ray, SI joints, AP. Bilateral sclerosis on iliac aspect of the SI joints. The sclerosis is more marked in the inferior portion of the bone. (b) DS, sacrum, posterior. Standard display (upper image) and magnified view (lower image). Focal sclerosis more marked in the inferior portion of the ilium. This probably represents more focal stress remodeling secondary to mechanical stress at this level. (Images courtesy of M. Magiotti, Berlin, MD, and A Curcin, Baltimore, MD.)

Osteonecrosis

Under this heading are illustrated a variety of lesions characterized by bone death. Although infarcts were placed under their own heading because of historic descriptive considerations that continue in common use, avascular necrosis (AVN) and aseptic necrosis, terms that are less frequently used, have been consolidated here. Similarly, osteochondritis dissecans, in which an osteochondral fragment is detached from the bone with death of the bony portion, is included here. AVN following gross fracture was discussed in Chapter 4.

Figure 10.9

Avascular necrosis, left femoral head in avascular phase, six-year-old with pain. (a) DS, pelvis and hips, anterior (left image) and posterior (right image). Photon deficiency in the lateral half of the left femoral head epiphysis (arrow). (b) X-ray, hips, frog leg lateral. The deformity of the PL half of the epiphysis for the femoral head on the left (arrow) can be compared with the more normal right side.

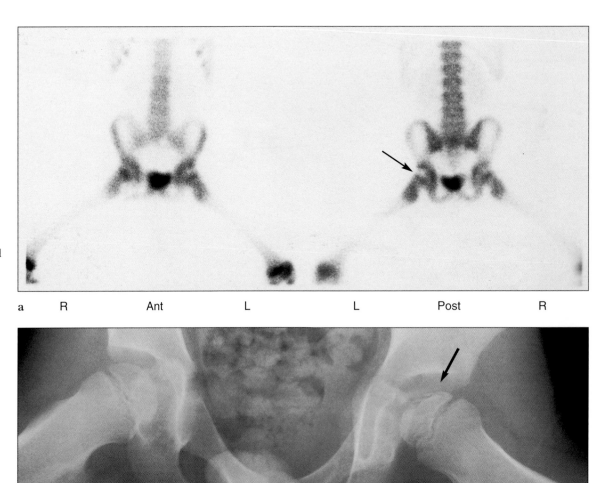

a R   Ant   L   L   Post   R

b R   L

Teaching point

In contrast to the adult patient, in children avascular necrosis of the femoral head (Legg–Calvé–Perthes disease) is easily diagnosed. Scanning is often done to detect early AVN of the contralateral asymptomatic side since the disease can be bilateral in 10–15% of children. MR imaging provides excellent anatomic detail.

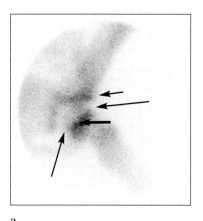

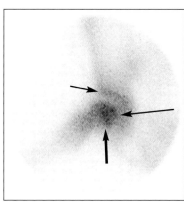

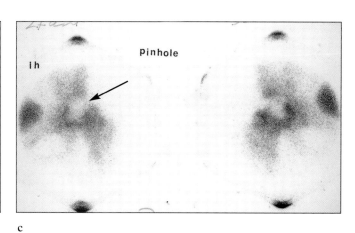

a   b   c

Figure 10.10

Avascular necrosis, pinhole collimator views. **(a)** DS, left hip, pinhole collimator, anterior view. Eight-year-old female. Normal. The acetabulum (short arrow), femoral head (long thin arrows), and normal increased tracer associated with the growth plate (regular arrow). **(b)** DS, right hip, pinhole collimator, anterior view. Eight year old. Mid-stage AVN with revascularizing, medial portion, femoral head epiphysis Acetabulum (short arrow), revascularizing femoral head (long arrow), and adjacent growth plate (regular arrow). **(c)** DS, left hip, pinhole collimator, anterior, 24-year-old treated for asthma with steroids. AVN, left hip. The femoral head region is photon deficient (arrow).

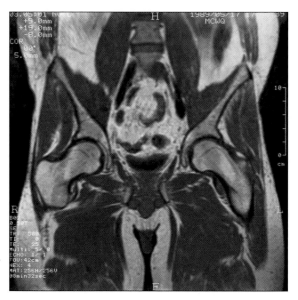

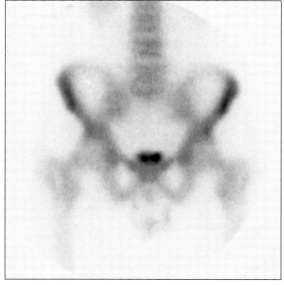

a   b

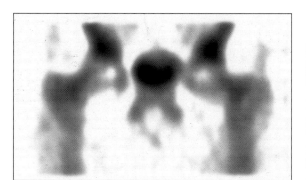

c

Figure 10.11

Bilateral AVN femoral heads, early avascular phase, 46-year-old male with vasculitis, treated with steroids. **(a)** MR, T1-weighted images. Hips, coronal. Normal marrow signal in both hips. **(b)** DS, pelvis and hips, anterior. Symmetric normal uptake. Acetabular activity mildly increased but normal. **(c)** SPECT, hips, selected coronal image. Sharply defined photon deficiency in femoral heads bilaterally.

Teaching point

In adults, with a strong index of suspicion for the presence of AVN, MR imaging, when available, is the diagnostic modality of choice. SPECT is particularly valuable when imaging the pelvis and hips, as are pinhole collimator images.

Figure 10.12

AVN, right femoral head, 91-year-old female, two weeks status post fall. Also right proximal humeral fracture, right distal radial fracture, and right second and third rib fractures. (**a**) WB. Intense activity associated with healing fractures. Photon deficiency of the avascular right femoral head. (**b**) X-ray, right hip, anterior. Subcapital fracture with slight impaction.

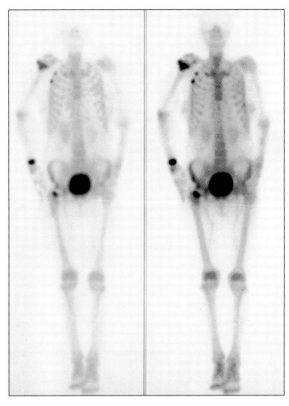

a

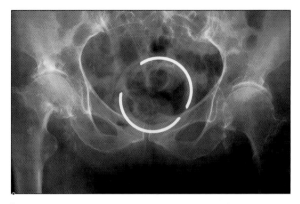

b

Teaching point

Although in adults steroid-induced or idiopathic AVN of the femoral head may be difficult to diagnosis because of overlying activity in the acetabulum, when the entire head is avascular following trauma that diagnosis is usually straight-forward.

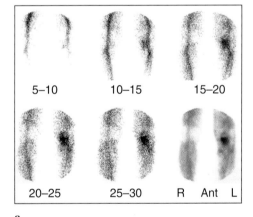

a

Figure 10.13

Osteochondritis dissecans, proximal left tibia. (**a**) RNA, knees, anterior. Focal moderately intense increased perfusion to the medial aspect of the left knee. (**b**) BP, knees, multiple views. Activity in the area of the medial aspect of the proximal tibia is moderately intense. (**c**) DS, knees, multiple views. Mild activity in the left patella. Intense activity in the posteromedial aspect of the proximal tibia at the articular and subarticular location. There is no significant increase in the supra-adjacent distal femur.

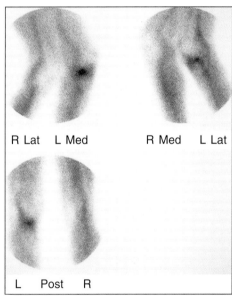

b

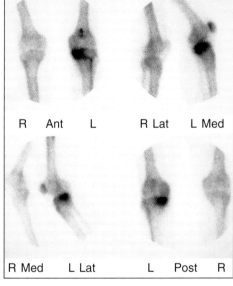

c

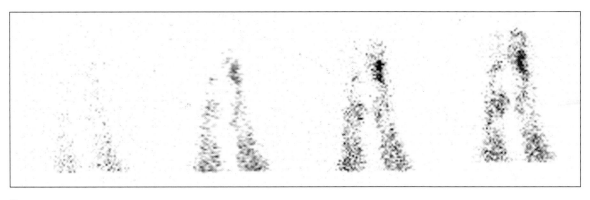

a

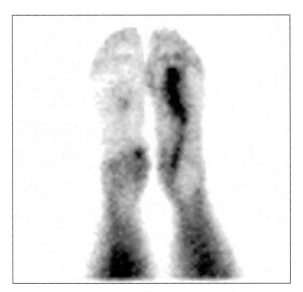

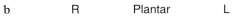

b   R   Plantar   L

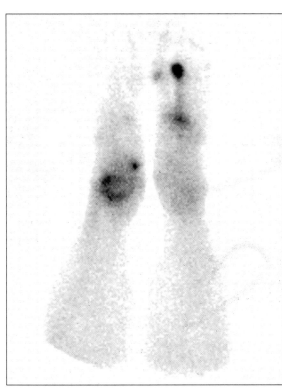

c

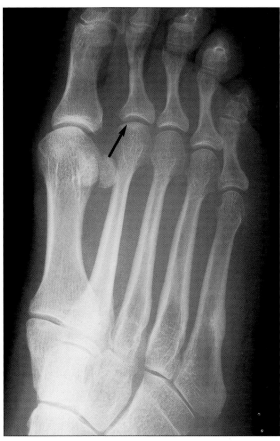

d

Figure 10.14

Freiberg's disease (osteochondrosis of second metatarsal head). (a) RNA, foot, plantar, five seconds per view. Focal increased perfusion to second metatarsal. (b) BP, foot, plantar, intense increased uptake (relative vascularity) in the second metatarsal region. (c) DS, foot, plantar, the most activity in the area of the second metatarsal head. (d) X-ray, foot, slight oblique. There is flattening of the second metatarsal head with subchondral sclerosis (arow). The X-ray and scan findings are typical for AVN of the second metatarsal head with the scan in the active revascularization phase.

Figure 10.15

AVN, revascularizing phase, right talus, 42-year old male renal transplant recipient with right ankle pain. Long-term steroid therapy. (a) X-ray, right ankle, right lateral and (b) X-ray, right ankle, AP. Sclerosis and subchondral deformity (arrows). (c) RNA, ankle, posterior, five seconds per view. Mild focal increased perfusion to the area of the distal tibia (arrow). (d) BP, posterior (left image) and anterior (right image). Moderate focal increased uptake (relative vascularity), area of right talus. (e) DS, ankle and foot, anterior (left image) and right lateral (right image). Standard display. Intense uptake localized to the talus. (f) DS, ankle and foot, anterior (left image) and right lateral (right image). Background subtracted technique. This technique better defines an individual tarsal bone.

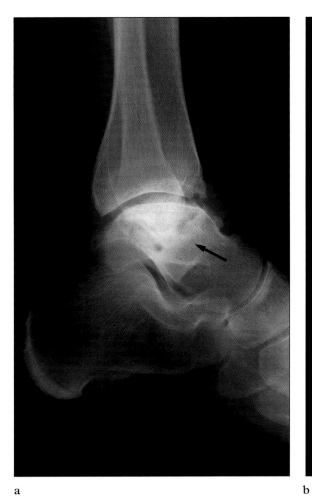

a

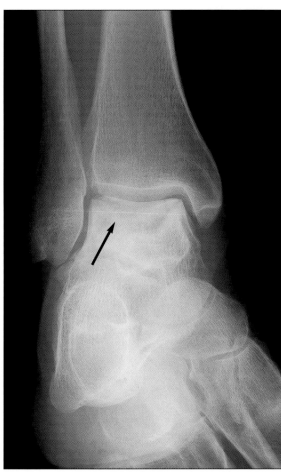

b

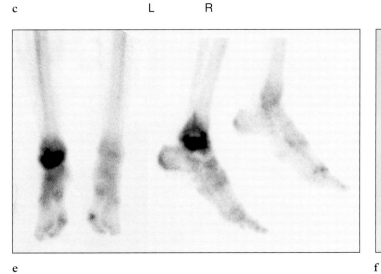

c

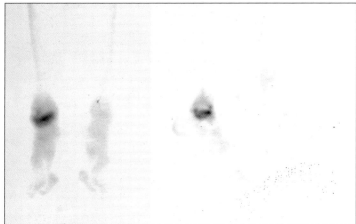

d

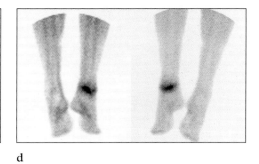

e

f

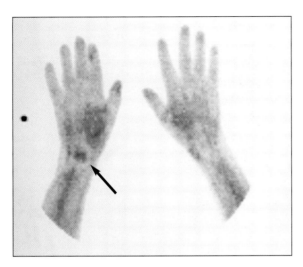

a

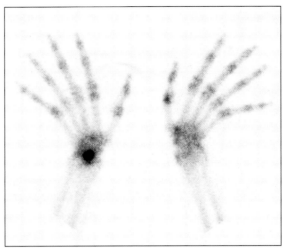

b

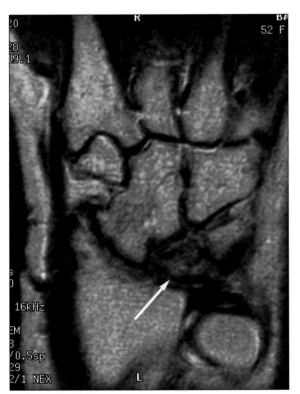

c

Figure 10.16

AVN lunate. (a) BP, hand and wrist, palmar view. Mild focal increased tracer uptake (relative vascularity) involving the right lunate region (arrow). (b) DS, hand and wrist, ulnar deviation. Intense tracer uptake associated with the lunate. (c) MR, proton density image, coronal section through wrist. Abnormal signal in lunate compared with distal radius and other carpal bones.

Teaching point

When patients with a history of trauma are imaged for unexplained pain, focal uptake in the lunate should raise the question of AVN (Kienböck's disease) and MR imaging suggested.

Paget's disease

Paget's disease is a condition of unknown etiology, characterized by bone remodeling. Three phases of the disease have distinct, but overlapping, histologic, radiographic, and scintigraphic features. The initial phase of rapid bone resorption and the intermediate phase, in which there is markedly increased osteoblastic activity, have very intense abnormal uptake on the delayed bone scan. Occasionally increased perfusion on the RNA and often, especially in the intermediate phase, increased uptake (relative vascularity) on the BP images can be seen. Activity on all three phases of the bone scan reflects the physiologic status of the disease process. The hallmark of scintigraphic uptake is whole bone involvement. In the long bones lesions begin near the ends of the bone and progress into the shaft. Osteoporosis circumscripta often presents with only a rim of increased tracer uptake on the delayed image. The third phase, often called late or cold, occurs when active remodeling slows or ends. Tracer uptake on delayed bone imaging is variable in these patients. The radiographic diagnosis is most obvious.

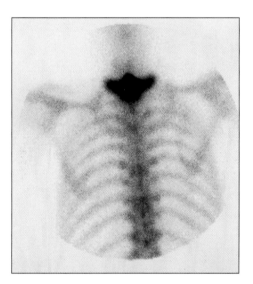

Figure 10.17

Paget's disease. Cervical spine, isolated vertebra. WB. Intense abnormal uptake involving all portions of a single bone is typical of Paget's disease.

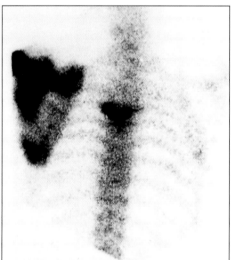

Figure 10.18

Paget's disease involves the left scapula and T5. DS, shoulder.

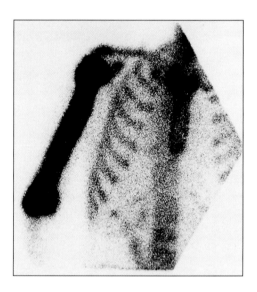

Figure 10.19

Paget's disease involving the right humerus. DS, humerus.

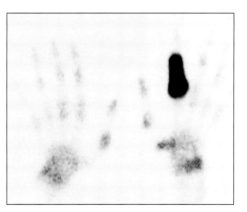

Figure 10.20

Paget's disease involving the left first proximal phalanx of the left hand. DS, hand.

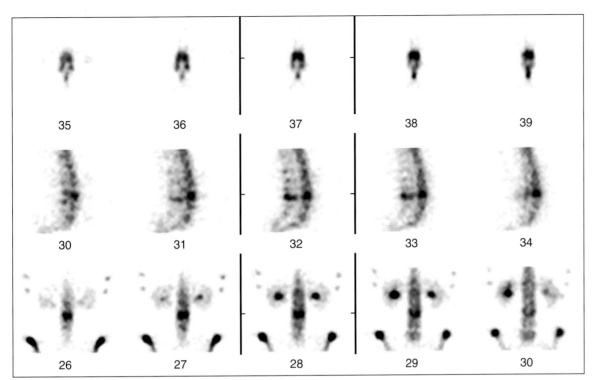

35   36   37   38   39

30   31   32   33   34

26   27   28   29   30

Figure 10.21

Paget's disease, lumbar vertebrae. SPECT, triangulation display. Less intense uptake than in most early stages of the disease. The SPECT technique demonstrates involvement of all portions of the vertebrae.

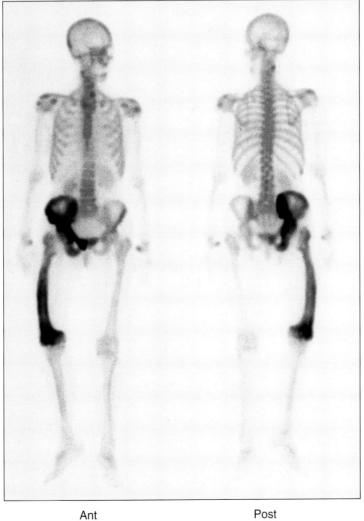

Ant   Post

Figure 10.22

Paget's disease. WB. Involvement of the entire ilium and pubis, as well as involvement of the entire femur with bowing, are typical appearances of Paget's disease.

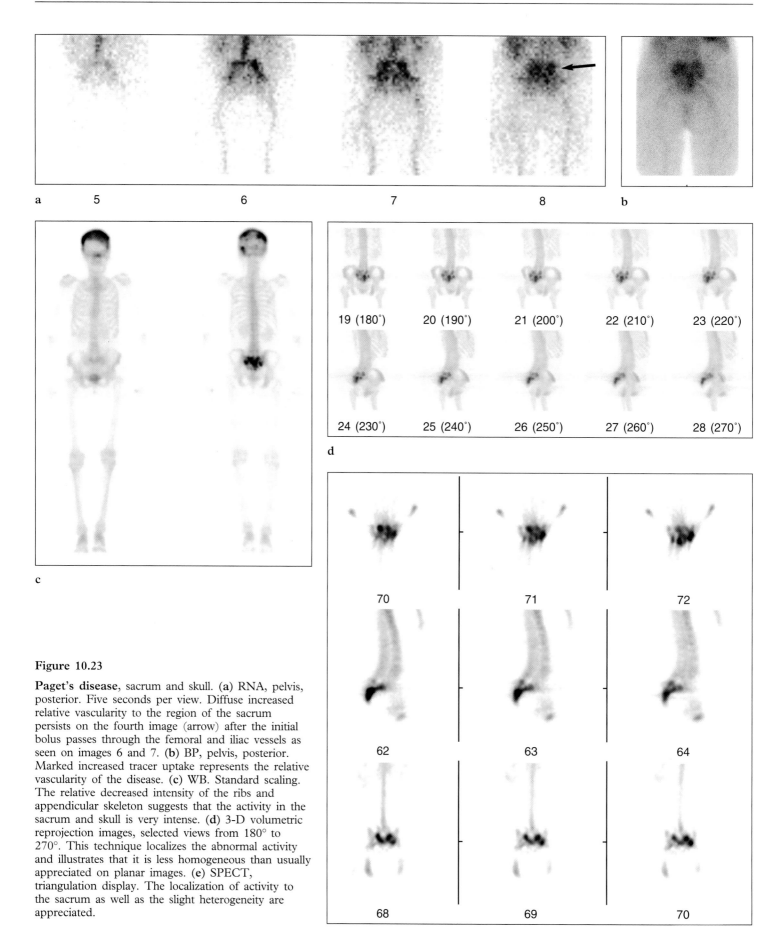

a   5   6   7   8   b

c

d   19 (180°)   20 (190°)   21 (200°)   22 (210°)   23 (220°)
24 (230°)   25 (240°)   26 (250°)   27 (260°)   28 (270°)

70   71   72
62   63   64
68   69   70
e

Figure 10.23

Paget's disease, sacrum and skull. (**a**) RNA, pelvis, posterior. Five seconds per view. Diffuse increased relative vascularity to the region of the sacrum persists on the fourth image (arrow) after the initial bolus passes through the femoral and iliac vessels as seen on images 6 and 7. (**b**) BP, pelvis, posterior. Marked increased tracer uptake represents the relative vascularity of the disease. (**c**) WB. Standard scaling. The relative decreased intensity of the ribs and appendicular skeleton suggests that the activity in the sacrum and skull is very intense. (**d**) 3-D volumetric reprojection images, selected views from 180° to 270°. This technique localizes the abnormal activity and illustrates that it is less homogeneous than usually appreciated on planar images. (**e**) SPECT, triangulation display. The localization of activity to the sacrum as well as the slight heterogeneity are appreciated.

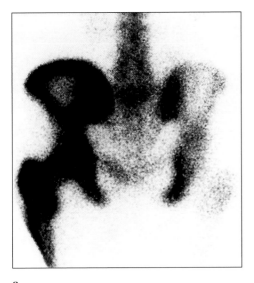

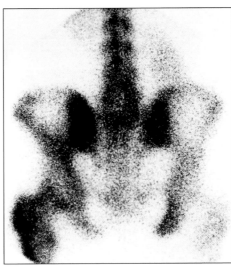

a

b

Figure 10.24

Paget's disease, response to therapy. 63-year-old woman. (a) DS, pelvis, posterior. Pre-therapy. (b) DS, pelvis, posterior. Nine months post-treatment with oral bisphosphonate. Striking decrease in abnormal tracer uptake in the hemipelvis and proximal femur.

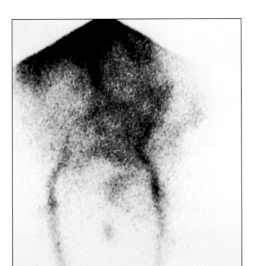

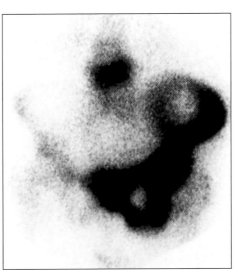

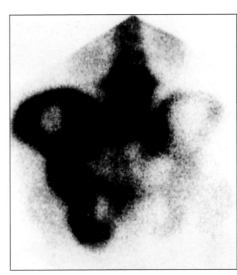

a

b

c

d

Figure 10.25

Paget's disease, pelvis, demonstrating vascularity of pagetic bone. (a) RNA, anterior, selected frame. Diffuse increased perfusion to the left hemipelvis. (b) DS, pelvis, anterior and (c) DS, pelvis, posterior. Abnormal uptake involving the entire hemipelvis and the L5 vertebra. (d) X-ray, pelvis, AP. Enlargement of bone with prominent trabecula, typical of Paget's disease.

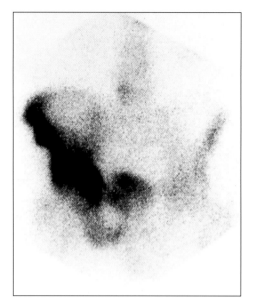

a

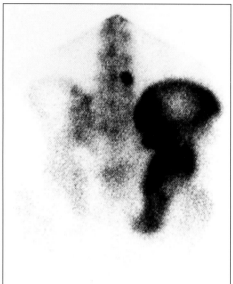

b

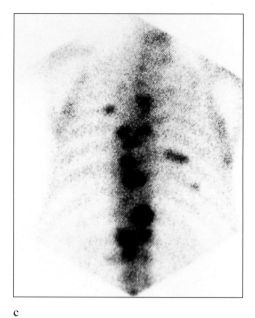

c

Figure 10.26

Coexistent Paget's disease and metastatic disease. (a) DS, pelvis, anterior, (b) DS, pelvis, posterior, and (c) DS, thoracic spine, posterior. Typical pagetic changes in the right hemipelvis, with activity involving the entire bone. The spine and rib lesions, however, are more typical of metastasis. (d) X-ray, pelvis, AP. Enlarged bone with prominent trabecula, typical of Paget's disease. (e) X-ray, thoracolumbar spine, lateral. The sclerotic densities in the spine are more typical of metastasis.

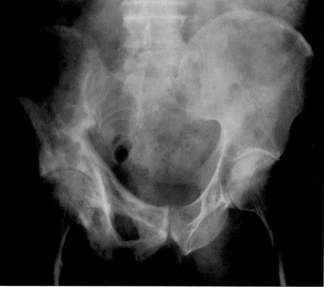

d

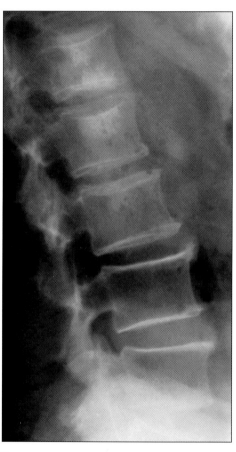

e

Teaching point

Although Paget's disease and metastasis usually show characteristic scan patterns of abnormality and can usually be easily differentiated, when the pattern is atypical, radiographic examination is required for more certain differential diagnosis.

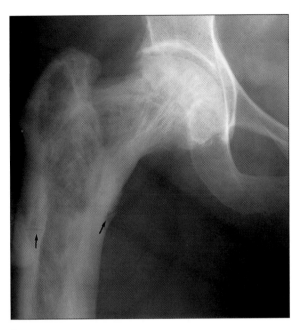

a

Teaching point

Correlative X-rays are usually required to diagnose superimposed lesions when changes in signs or symptoms occur in patients with long-standing Paget's disease. The intense, abnormal, increased tracer uptake associated with the initial and intermediate phases of the disease obscures the increased tracer accumulation associated with healing fractures or sarcomatous degeneration.

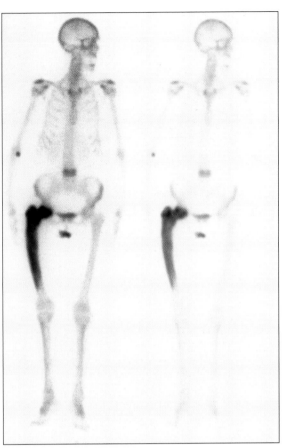

b

Figure 10.27

Paget's disease, femur, with superimposed stress fracture. (a) X-ray, proximal femur, AP. Bone enlargement, prominent large trabecula, and mixed sclerotic and lytic lesions have appearance typical of Paget's disease. Linear radiolucency (arrows) represents stress fracture. Patient presented with exacerbation of pain. (b) Anterior, standard display (left image) and background subtracted display (right image). Abnormal increased tracer uptake, usually associated with healing fracture, cannot be seen within the intense uptake of the pagetoid bone.

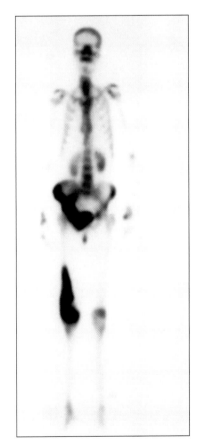

Figure 10.28

Osteogenic sarcoma and Paget's disease. Patient presented with new pain in right leg. WB. Focal photopenic defect at medial aspect of right lower tibia. Destructive changes were identified at this site by radiography. Additional pagetic changes throughout the pelvis.

Figure 10.29

Paget's disease of the patella. This was a monostotic lesion. **(a)** DS, knees, anterior. **(b)** X-ray, knee, lateral.

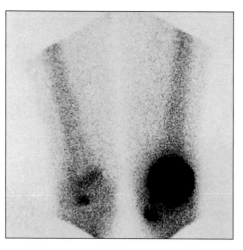

a

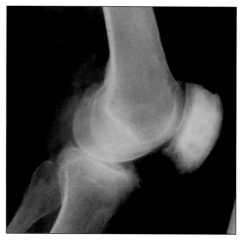

b

Teaching point

Monostotic Paget's disease is not uncommon, and accounts for approximately 20% of cases.

Figure 10.30

Paget's disease, tibia, pre- and post-therapy. **(a)** DS. Tibia, anterior. The very intense abnormal increased tracer with a typical wedge or flame-shaped area of uptake extending from the metaphysis, distally into the diaphysis, is present. **(b)** Same patient, six months after pamidronate therapy. Reduction in the intensity of bone uptake.

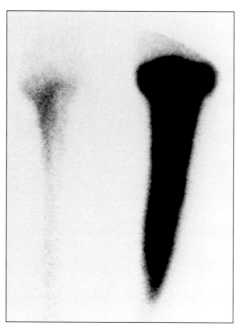

a

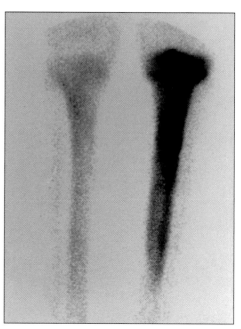

b

Teaching points

The bone scan can demonstrate changes in disease activity following therapy and there is the potential to utilize changes in activity in evaluating requirements for further therapy.

Early Paget's disease can be detected on bone scanning, prior to radiographic changes. In long bones, a flame-shaped lesion beginning in the metaphysis and extending toward the diaphysis is very suggestive of Paget's disease.

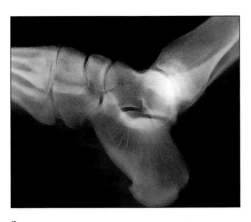
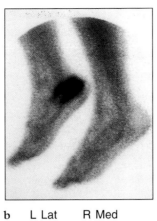
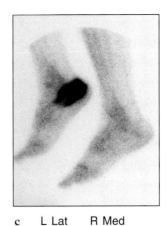
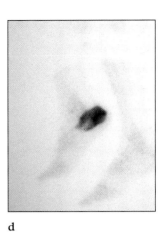

a

b   L Lat   R Med

c   L Lat   R Med

d

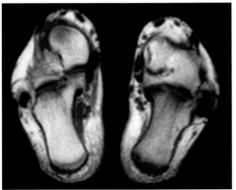

e

Figure 10.31

Paget's disease of the calcaneous, 32-year-old female presents with unexplained foot pain. (**a**) X-ray, ankle and foot, lateral. Interpreted as normal. (**b**) BP, ankle and foot, lateral. Intense increased relative vascularity in the calcaneous. (**c**) DS, ankle and foot, lateral, standard display and (**d**) DS, ankle and foot, lateral, display manipulation with background subtraction. These images define areas of intense abnormal uptake most marked posteriorly. (**e**) MR, T1-weighted images. Long axis of the foot. Subtle decrease in signal in the right calcaneous was the only finding. Open biopsy was required for diagnosis.

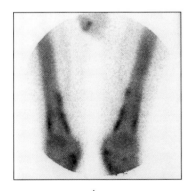
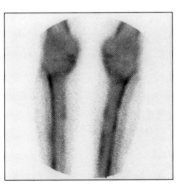
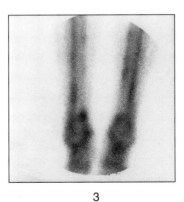

1   2   3

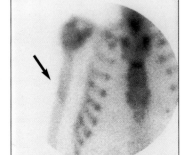
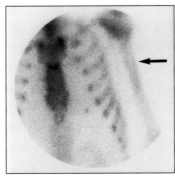

4   5

Figure 10.32

Hypertrophic osteoarthropathy. DS, multiple views, anterior. Femurs (1), knees and proximal legs (2), distal legs and ankles (3), proximal right humerus (4), and proximal left humerus (5). Linear peripheral activity, typical of periosteal location best seen in distal femur (1) and tibias (2). The detail of the abnormal activity in the proximal humeri (arrows) is less obvious because these body parts were further from the camera surface with resultant loss of resolution.

Primary hypertrophic osteoarthropathy is a rare disorder, whereas secondary hypertrophic osteoarthropathy is much more common, occurring in about 5–10% of patients with bronchogenic carcinoma and a variety of other disease states. The clinical syndrome consists of clubbing of the digits of the hands and feet, enlargement of the extremities secondary to periosteal bone deposition, and painful, swollen joints.

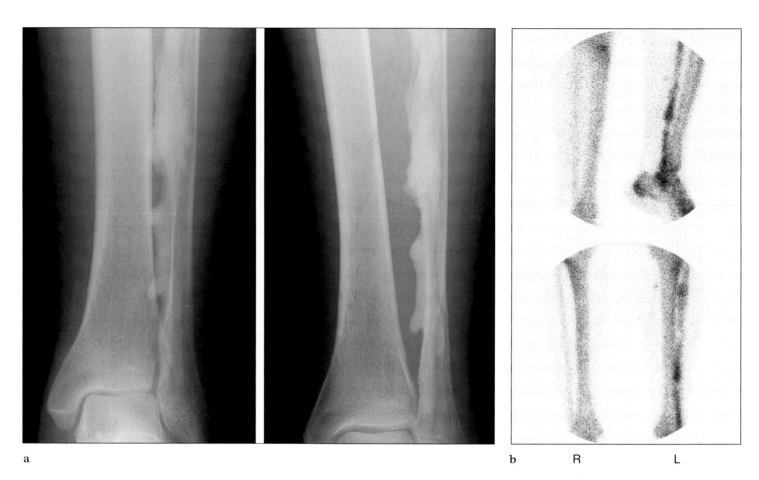

a   b   R   L

Figure 10.33

Chronic benign periostitis. (a) X-ray, leg, AP and slight oblique. Think linear undulating osseous change. **(b)** DS, leg, left lateral (left image) and anterior (right image). Nodular superficial uptake involves the fibula as seen best on the lateral view.

Figure 10.34

Periostitis, benign, in eight-month-old female with one-week history of pain on extension of lower extremity. Periostitis throughout the long bones. The differential diagnosis given for the periostitis on the X-ray emphasizes the nonspecificity of these findings. That differential included infantile cortical hyperostosis, vitamin A or vitamin D intoxication, Goldbloom's syndrome, infection, healing rickets, and hypertrophic osteoarthropathy. DS, lower extremities. Fusiform-type uptake throughout the long bones including femur and leg. There is also activity appreciated in the proximal humerus and radius at the upper aspect of the image. This is an outside examination and orthogonal or high-resolution spot views were not available.

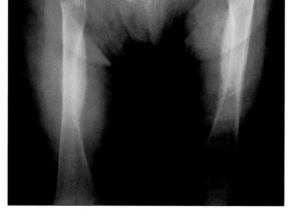

a

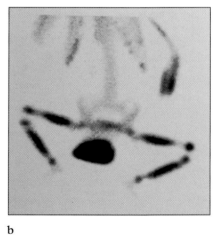

b

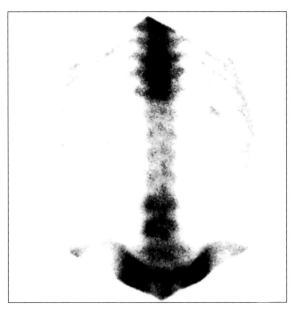

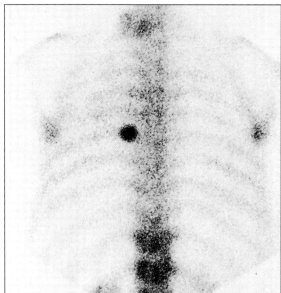

Figure 10.36

Radiation therapy effect and fracture. DS, thoracic spine, posterior. Differential uptake between the bones within the radiation port in the upper thoracic spine, which shows decreased tracer uptake and the nonradiated bone in the lower thoracic spine, which shows more normal uptake. The round focus of intense uptake in the left seventh posterior rib was due to a fracture demonstrated on radiography.

Figure 10.35

Radiation therapy effect. DS, thoracic spine, posterior. The generalized reduced tracer uptake throughout the thoracic spine with a sharp cut-off between radiated and nonradiated bone. In this case the extreme difference results from metastatic involvement of the nonradiated bone.

Teaching point

Following radiotherapy, a fracture of the ribs may occur spontaneously. This is most often seen in carcinoma of the breast.

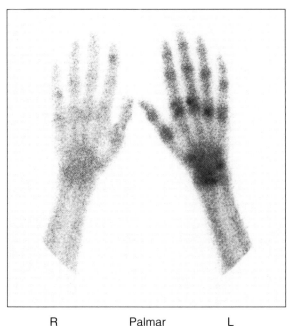

R   Palmar   L

Figure 10.37

Reflex sympathetic dystrophy (RSD), left hand and wrist, 53-year-old female, six months' post fracture distal radius. DS. Hand and wrist, palmar view. Diffuse tracer uptake throughout the forearm, wrist, and hand with juxta-articular accentuation. This image illustrates that uptake may extend proximally to involve the radius and ulna in the forearm.

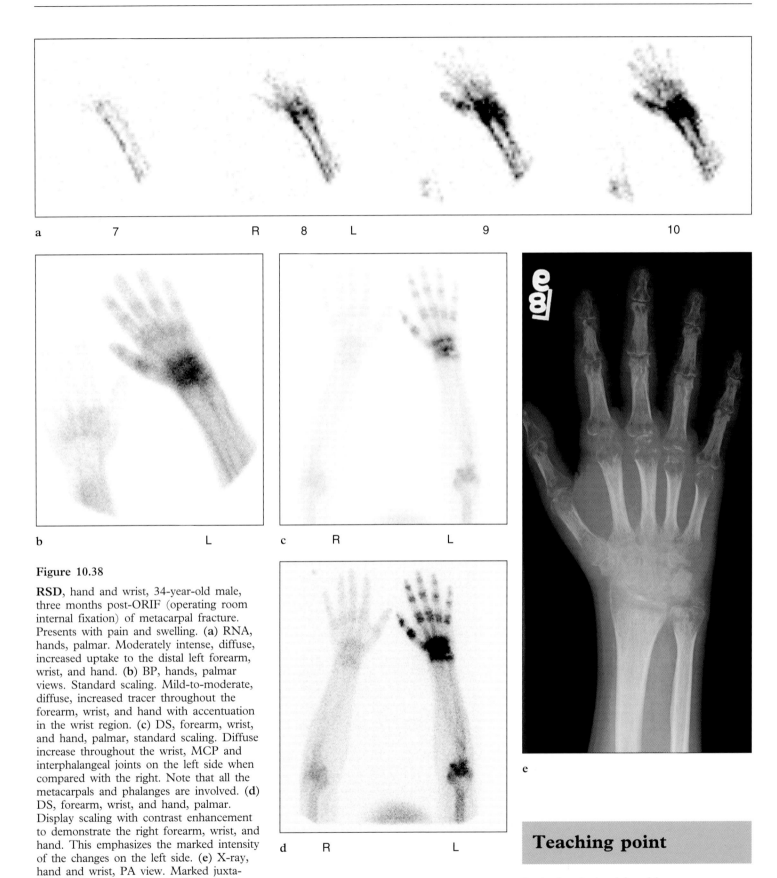

a   7   R   8   L   9   10

b   L   c   R   L

Figure 10.38

RSD, hand and wrist, 34-year-old male, three months post-ORIF (operating room internal fixation) of metacarpal fracture. Presents with pain and swelling. (**a**) RNA, hands, palmar. Moderately intense, diffuse, increased uptake to the distal left forearm, wrist, and hand. (**b**) BP, hands, palmar views. Standard scaling. Mild-to-moderate, diffuse, increased tracer throughout the forearm, wrist, and hand with accentuation in the wrist region. (**c**) DS, forearm, wrist, and hand, palmar, standard scaling. Diffuse increase throughout the wrist, MCP and interphalangeal joints on the left side when compared with the right. Note that all the metacarpals and phalanges are involved. (**d**) DS, forearm, wrist, and hand, palmar. Display scaling with contrast enhancement to demonstrate the right forearm, wrist, and hand. This emphasizes the marked intensity of the changes on the left side. (**e**) X-ray, hand and wrist, PA view. Marked juxta-articular osteoporosis. There is poor definition of the carpus.

d   R   L

e

Teaching point

In the hand, the delayed images are more sensitive and more specific for reflex sympathic dystrophy than the RNA or BP images.

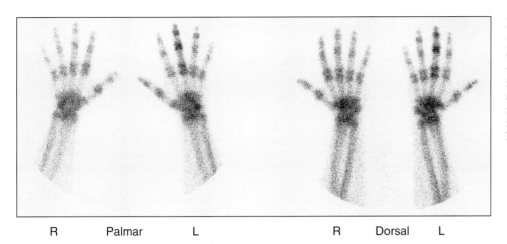

R   Palmar   L   R   Dorsal   L

Figure 10.39

RSD, segmental, involving the third ray of the left hand. This is a very uncommon variant. DS. Hand. Abnormal uptake involves shafts and there is juxta-articular accentuation of uptake. Compare with regional RSD in Figure 10.38, which involves all the rays and is the 'classic' lesion.

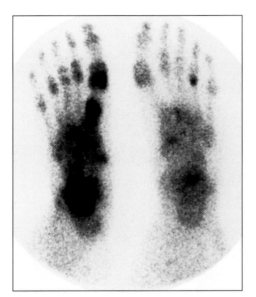

Figure 10.40

RSD of the right foot, and healing fracture at the base of the first metatarsal. DS, foot, plantar. Diffuse increased tracer throughout the hind, mid-, and fore-foot with juxta-articular accentuation. There is also some nonspecific uptake, possible DJD involving the right first MTP and left fourth MTP joints.

Teaching point

The specificity of the scintigraphic pattern for RSD in the foot is less than in the hand, since it can be mimicked by patients with significant foot infections, particularly if there is underlying diabetes mellitus. This is, however, not usually a clinical dilemma since the history of infection is known and these patients are not usually imaged to evaluate for the presence of RSD.

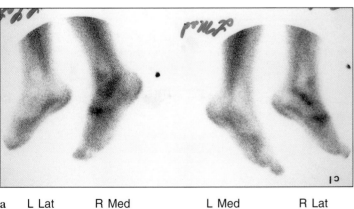
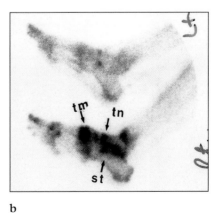

a   L Lat   R Med   L Med   R Lat   b

Figure 10.41

Subtalar coalition. (a) BP, ankle and foot, left lateral/right medial (left image) and left medial/right lateral (right image). Increased tracer uptake (relative vasculartity) in the subtalar and talonavicular joint regions. (b) DS, ankle and foot, right medial. Increased tracer uptake in the talonavicular, subtalar, and tarsal–metatarsal joints. Uptake on bone scan in this condition is nonspecific. Uptake usually occurs in the bone adjacent to the coalition, reflecting the abnormal biomechanics at that location. Early on, however, during the development of the osseous bridge, activity can be found at the point of actual coalition. MR imaging allows visualization of both bony and soft-tissue bridging.

Nonosseous lesion accumulation

Examples of uptake of tracer in soft-tissue lesions have been presented in other portions of this atlas based primarily on the potential underlying etiology. These include traumatic soft-tissue lesions in Chapter 4; heterotopic ossification after nonsurgical trauma in Chapter 4; heterotopic ossification postsurgical trauma in Chapter 4; by primary nonosseous tumor in Chapter 5; by extraosseous metastasis in Chapter 6; and secondary to metabolic disorders leading to hypercalcemia (metastatic calcifications) in Chapter 9. Recognizing non-osseous accumulation of tracer can result in serendipitous diagnosis of an unsuspected problem, but can also aid in differential diagnosis of osseous lesions with which such accumulation may be associated.

Dystrophic calcification

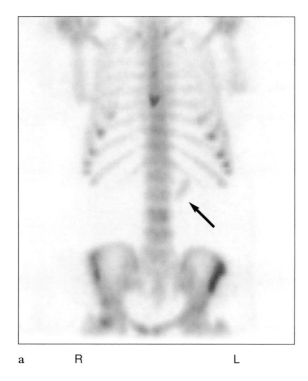

a   R   L

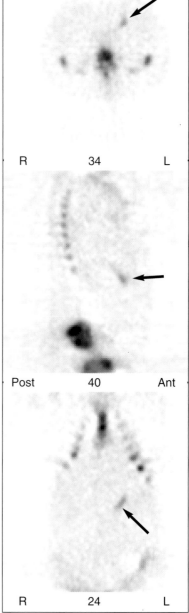

b

Figure 10.42

Dystrophic calcification in an abdominal scar. (a) 3-D volumetric reprojection. Abdomen, anterior image. Mild-to-moderate, curvilinear, increased uptake to the left of the L1 and L2 vertebrae. (b) SPECT, triangulation display, abdomen. Transaxial (top image), sagittal (middle image), and coronal (lower image). Localization of the uptake in the anterior scar is well appreciated on tomographic imaging (arrows). Note absent renal activity in this patient with end-stage renal disease.

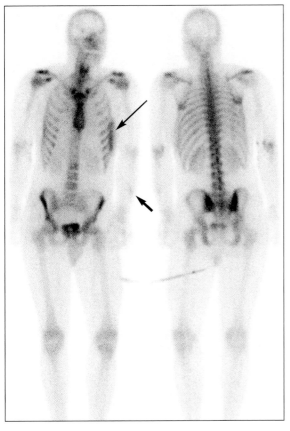
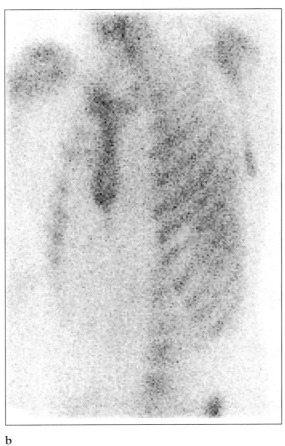

a   b

Figure 10.43

Dystrophic calcification in chest wall muscle. Electrician sustained electrical injury at work. **(a)** WB. Anterolateral activity is most marked at the exit site (long arrow) and faintly at the entry site (short arrow). **(b)** DS, chest, LAO. The uptake in the injured soft tissue blurs the detail of rib activity.

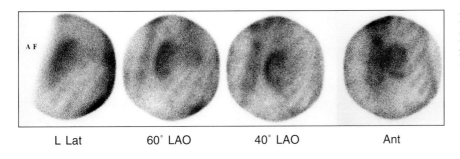

L Lat   60° LAO   40° LAO   Ant

Figure 10.44

Dystrophic calcification in anterolateral myocardial infarction. DS, chest, multiple views. Obtained approximately 90 minutes post-injection.

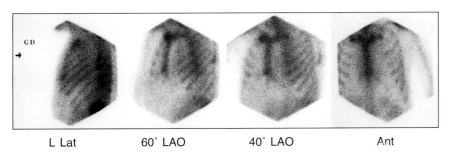

L Lat   60° LAO   40° LAO   Ant

Figure 10.45

Dystrophic calcification in lateral myocardial infarction. DS, chest, multiple views. Much less obvious myocardial uptake when compared with Figure 10.44. In a patient who may have chest discomfort, poor definition of ribs overlying myocardium could suggest this diagnosis. The finding, however, is nonspecific. SPECT imaging is more sensitive in detecting myocardial tracer uptake.

Figure 10.46

Dystrophic calcification in a splenic infarct. Six year old with sickle-cell anemia. DS, abdomen, anterior and posterior from a WB examination. The abnormal uptake in the spleen (arrow) seen best on posterior view has the same relative intensity as the kidney.

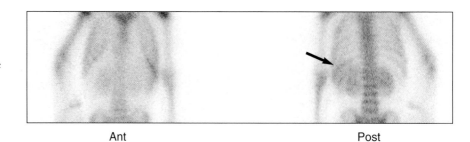

Ant   Post

Figure 10.47

Dystrophic calcification in a splenic infarct. DS, abdomen, anterior and posterior views from a WB examination. The intense round area of increased tracer (arrow) seen best on posterior view has a greater intensity of uptake than the subadjacent kidney.

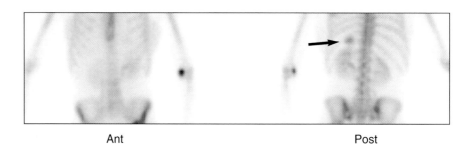

Ant   Post

Teaching point

The shape and intensity of uptake in infarcted spleen are extremely variable.

Figure 10.48

Dystrophic calcification in a portion of a calcified uterine fibroid. (a) DS, pelvis, anterior. The increased tracer uptake is located at the right SL aspect of the fibroid, just beneath the right SI joint. The bladder is displaced inferolaterally to the right. (b) X-ray, pelvis, anterior. The calcification is seen just to the right of the lower SI joint.

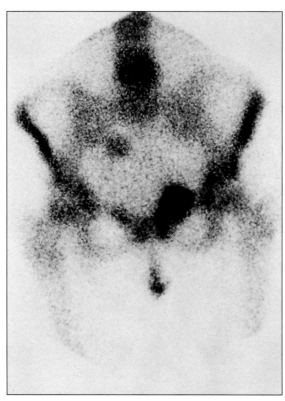

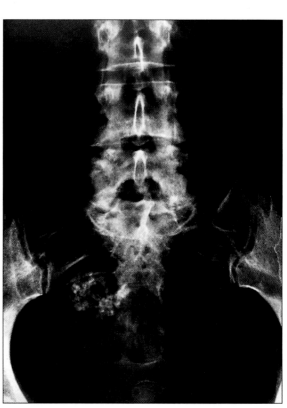

a   b

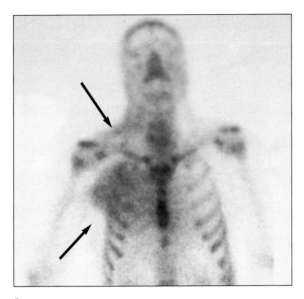

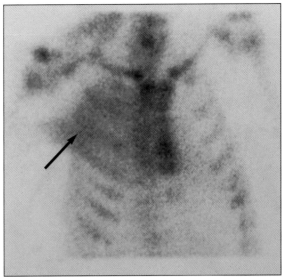

a

b

Figure 10.49

Minimal burns injury, 27-year-old struck by lightning. Significant muscle necrosis would have much more intense activity than that in the ribs. WB. The activity in the right neck region (thin arrow) and over the right chest (arrow) represents exit wounds. The entry was in the head, which is not seen on these views. (Reprinted with permission from *Skeletal Nuclear Medicine*, Figure 14–22.)

Teaching point

- ^{99m}Tc–PYP rather than ^{99m}Tc–MDP is the agent of choice for evaluating soft-tissue injury.
- Although tracer uptake defines the extent of muscle damage, the severity can only be estimated from the relative uptake of tracer. Intense uptake supports the referring physician's decision to débride, whereas minimal uptake would support a decision to support the patient and allow for natural healing.

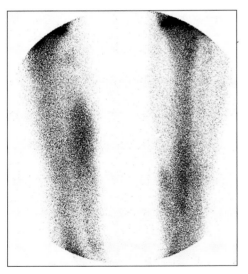

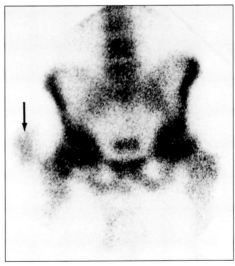

a

b

Figure 10.50

Dystrophic calcification. Soft-tissue, calf musculature secondary to high-voltage electric line burns. DS, legs, anterior. Moderate uptake medial aspect of right calf and less uptake at a slightly inferior location, left calf.

Figure 10.51

Dystrophic calcification in thigh muscles secondary to intramuscular injections. (a) DS, pelvis, anterior and (b) DS, pelvis, posterior. Abnormal tracer uptake lateral to the right hip (arrows).

Figure 10.52

Dystrophic calcification around the distal phalanges in a patient with systemic sclerosis and calcinosis. (a) DS, hands, palmar view. Areas of focal moderately intense increased tracer correspond to calcium seen in (b). (b) X-ray, hands, palmar view. The focal calcifications are best appreciated on the right first and second and left first rays.

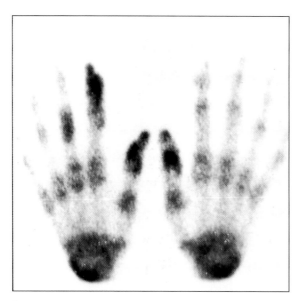

a

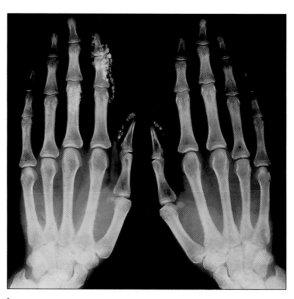

b

Figure 10.53

Sarcoma, soft tissue. (a) RNA, thigh, anterior, five seconds per view. Mild increased perfusion to the left thigh (arrow). (b) BP, thigh, anterior. Increased uptake (relative vascularity) is irregularly distributed (arrow). (c) WB. A portion of an anterior WB image. Very faint medial soft-tissue uptake can barely be seen (arrow). The underlying bone appears normal.

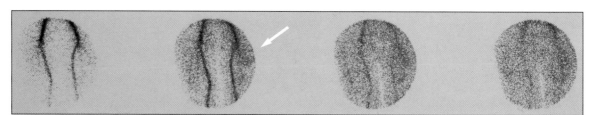

a

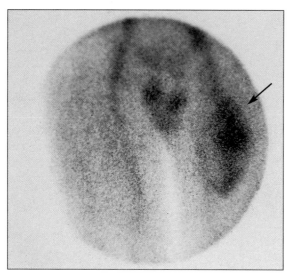

b

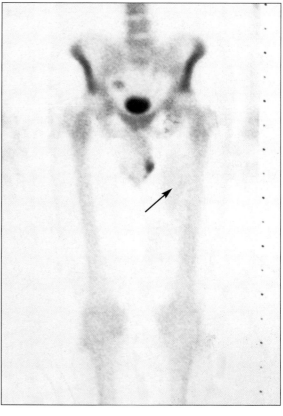

c

Teaching point

Abnormal tracer accumulation on RNA and/or BP images should be investigated even if the underlying bone is normal on delayed images.

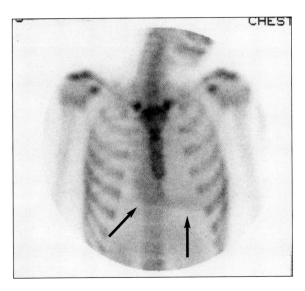

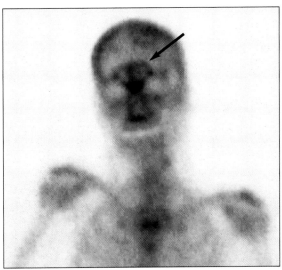

Figure 10.54

Pericardial effusion, 40-year-old patient with
mucinous papillary carcinoma. DS, chest, anterior. The
faint uptake in the pericardial region (arrows). This
uptake is probably similar to that associated with pleural
effusions (Figure 6.24) and ascites (Figure 6.25).

Figure 10.55

Frontal sinusitis. Incidental finding. DS, head and
neck, anterior. Activity outlines frontal sinuses
(arrow). (Images courtesy of Dr Masanori Ichesi,
Toronto, Canada.)

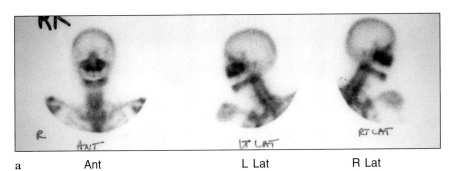

a   Ant   L Lat   R Lat

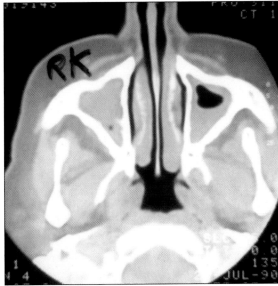

b

Figure 10.56

Maxillary sinusitis, bilateral. Patient being
evaluated for osteomyelitis following dental surgery.
(a) DS, multiple views. Intense abnormal activity
outlines and fills the entire maxillary sinus. (b) CT,
transaxial view. Soft-tissue windows. The right
maxillary sinus is completely opacified with a small
amount of air still present in the left maxillary sinus.
(c) SPECT, head, selected transaxial images. The
definition of the maxillary sinus corresponds to the
CT image in (b).

c

Figure 10.57

Maxillary pyocele and sinusitis. (a) DS, Water's view of the face. This view is obtained by angling either the patient's face or the camera to project the frontal and maxillary sinus regions on to a plane different from the central facial structures. The definition of the maxillary sinus is excellent. (b) X-ray, face, Water's view. This right maxillary sinus is opacified. The X-ray can be directly compared with the delayed bone image.

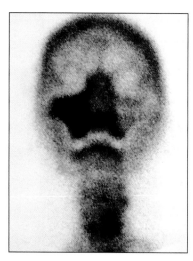

a

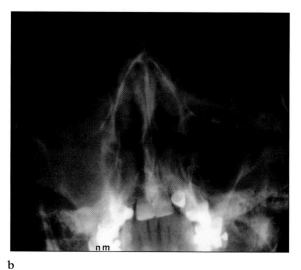

b

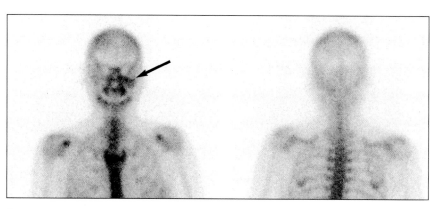

a

Figure 10.58

Maxillary sinusitis. (a) DS, face, anterior and posterior from WB study. Asymmetry is appreciated (arrow) with mild increased activity in the region of the left maxillary sinus. (b) SPECT, triangulation display, face. Transaxial (upper image) obtained through the mid-portion of the maxillary sinus as appreciated on the sagittal and coronal views. The anterior and PL involvement of the sinus wall can be appreciated on all three views (arrows).

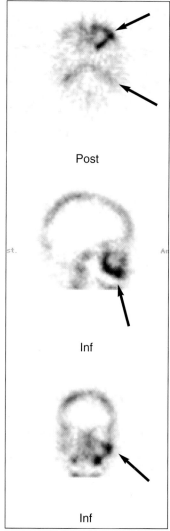

b

Genitourinary system

The evaluation of bone tracer uptake and excretion via the urinary tract should be an integral part of the analysis of every bone imaging study. When the three-phase technique is utilized and the kidneys are in the field of view, the initial arterial perfusion through the major vessels into the kidney can be evaluated, as can the relative vascularity and early function on the BP or tissue phase images. Delayed images demonstrate asymmetry, mass lesions, obstructions or dilatations, changes in size, and displacement by adjacent structures. Although examples of genitourinary tract pathology are present throughout this atlas, we have grouped some lesions in this section to emphasize the importance of these changes in everyday practice.

Kidneys

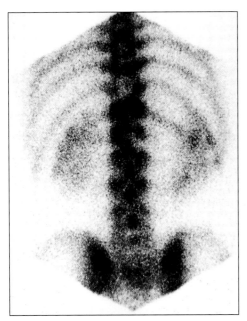

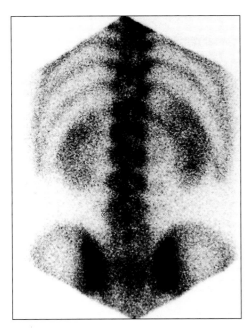

a

b

Figure 10.59

Displaced kidney secondary to lymph node involvement with lymphoma. **(a)** DS, thoracolumbar spine, posterior. The right kidney is displaced laterally and the upper pole rotated slightly clockwise. A photon deficiency is associated with the left side of T11 vertebra. **(b)** DS, thoracolumbar spine, posterior. Four months following therapy. The orientation of the right kidney is now normal and the photon deficiency in T11 is less prominent.

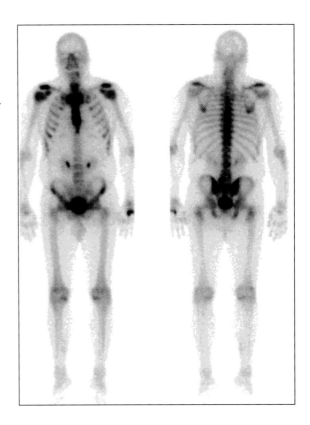

Figure 10.60

Horseshoe kidney. WB. Anterior and posterior. Note the better visualization of the kidneys on the anterior image, as well as the orientation of the kidneys.

Teaching point

Always look at the kidneys.

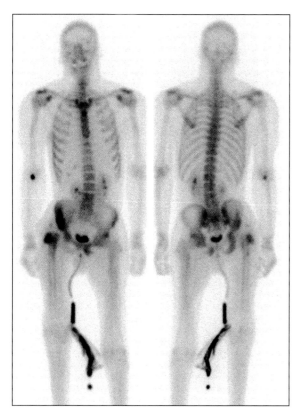

a

Figure 10.61

Horseshoe kidney. (a) WB. In this patient, the kidney orientation and visualization on the anterior image are less obvious than on Figure 10.60. An incidental lesion in the right ilium is noted in this patient who is being evaluated for metastatic disease. (b) RNA, pelvis, anterior view, five seconds per image. The increased perfusion to the typical horseshoe appearance of the kidneys with perfusion to the isthmus tissue in the mid-line is well seen. (c) RNA, pelvis, posterior, five seconds per image. The perfusion to the isthmus tissue, which is attenuated by the spine, is not appreciated. (d) BP, abdomen/pelvis, anterior. The appearance and orientation of the horseshoe kidney. (e) BP, abdomen/pelvis, posterior. Again the attenuation of isthmus tissue by the spine is seen. (f) SPECT, triangulation display. Abdomen and pelvis. Transaxial section through the mid-portion of the kidney (arrow). Sagittal image through the mid-line with only faint visualization of renal tissue (arrow). The coronal image is anterior to the spine and demonstrates some activity in a right upper pole calyx (arrow).

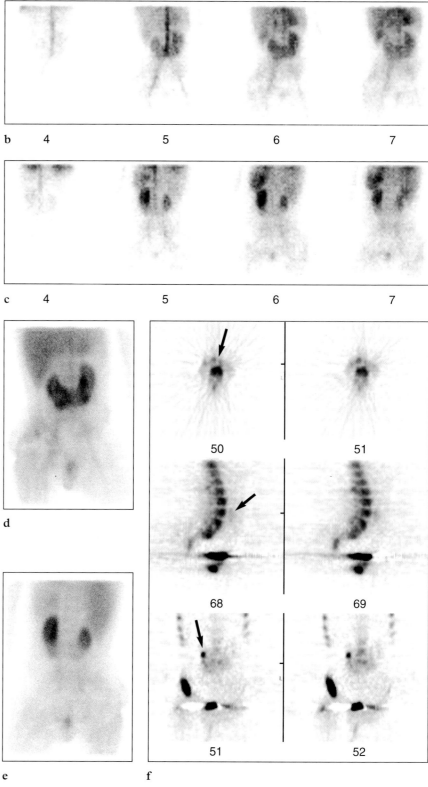

b 4   5   6   7

c 4   5   6   7

d

e   f

Teaching point

When available and technically feasible, both detectors of dual-headed cameras should be utilized for RNA, BP, and DS images.

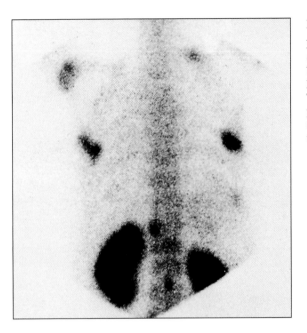

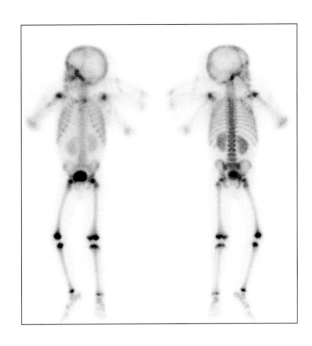

Figure 10.62

Nephrocalcinosis, 67-year-old female with breast cancer and hypercalcemia. DS. Thoracolumbar spine, posterior. Intense, abnormal, increased tracer in the kidneys.

Teaching point

Diffuse increased uptake more intense than lumbar spine uptake on delayed images is always abnormal, while diffuse uptake of similar intensity to osseous structures, especially if the kidneys are enlarged, should also raise the question of abnormality. The diffuse abnormal renal uptake includes liver sclerosis, anemias, anti-cancer therapy, and iron overload.

Figure 10.63

AIDS nephritis, four-year-old HIV-positive patient being evaluated for possible osteomyelitis. Diffuse increased uptake in enlarged kidneys.

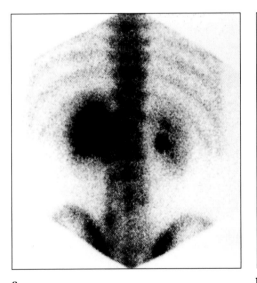

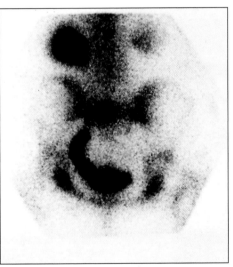

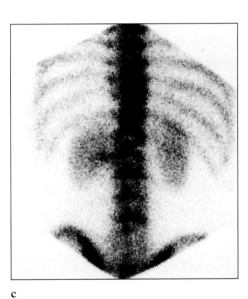

a   b   c

Figure 10.64

Calices, functional dilatation. (a) DS, thoracolumbar spine, posterior and (b) DS, squat view. Marked accumulation in the left renal pelvis and lower ureter. (c) DS, thoracolumbar spine, posterior. Image following diuretic. The tracer has cleared from the left collecting system.

Teaching point

A dilated collecting system is not necessarily obstructed. Imaging following additional attempts at voiding or walking around, or after Lasix administration, can be obtained.

Figure 10.65

Transplanted kidney in right iliac fossa. (a) RNA, abdomen and pelvis, anterior, five seconds per view. Increased perfusion to the transplanted kidney is seen on the bottom of the large field of view image (short arrow). The right iliac artery (thin arrow) can be used for anatomic orientation. (b) RNA, abdomen and pelvis, posterior. The perfusion to the transplanted kidney is not convincingly seen (arrow). (c) WB. The transplant kidney with activity in the calices is seen in the right iliac fossa. There is still some native kidney activity.

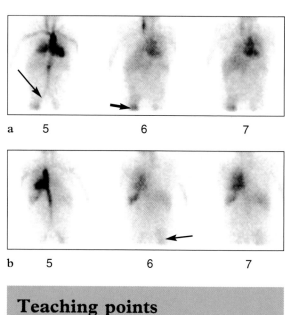

a   5   6   7

b   5   6   7

Teaching points

- There is often some retained function in native kidneys following transplantation.
- Calyceal activity in the transplanted kidney should not be mistaken for an iliac bone lesion.

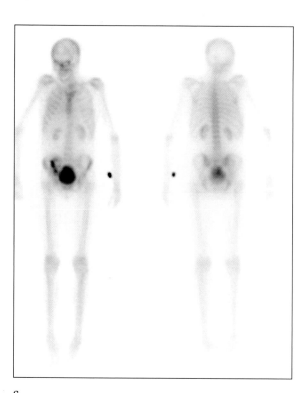

c

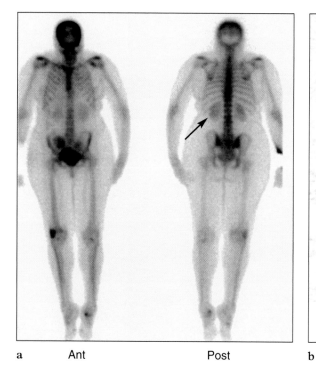

a   Ant   Post

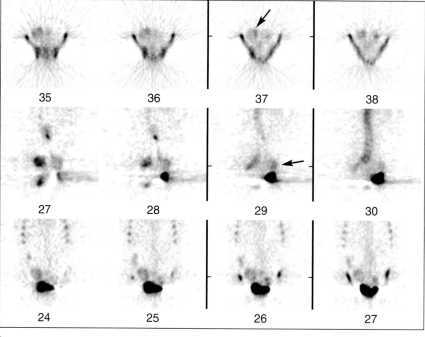

b

35   36   37   38

27   28   29   30

24   25   26   27

Figure 10.66

Renal transplantation. (a) WB. The transplant is seen in the right iliac fossa. There is still some activity in native kidneys. (b) SPECT, triangulation display, pelvis. The activity in the transplanted kidney (arrows) is seen medial to the iliac bone on the transaxial image and above the bladder on the sagittal image.

Ureters

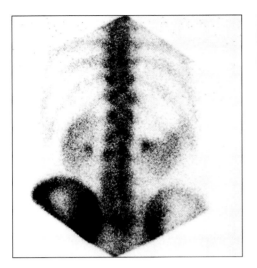

Figure 10.67

Cyst in right kidney. DS. Lumbar spine, posterior. Photon deficiency above a deformed and rotated right kidney represents nonfunctioning tissue. This is a nonspecific finding.

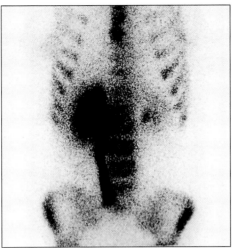

Figure 10.68

Ureterovesical junction obstruction. DS, lower thorax and abdomen, anterior. Marked increased tracer uptake in the right kidney and ureter ending sharply at the vesicoureteral junction.

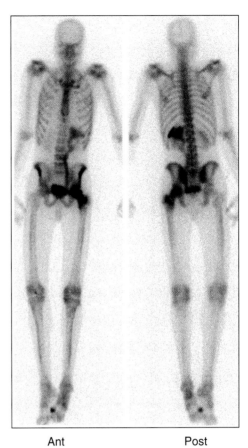

Ant   Post

Figure 10.69

Duplicated left renal collecting system with obstruction of upper pole ureter. WB. The dilated upper collecting system drapes over the normal lower pole, best seen on the posterior view. The dilated filled distal ureter to the level ureterovesical junction is best seen on the anterior view.

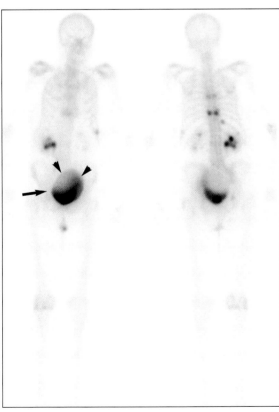

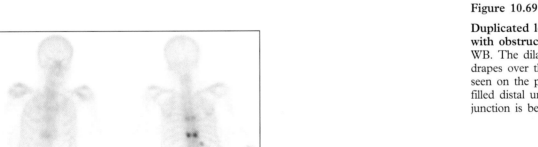

Teaching point

Patients with obstructed ureters may often present with back pain.

Figure 10.70

Large cystic pelvic mass obstructs distal third of ureter. The large mass causes an extrinsic imprint on the bladder. The more completely filled PI portion of the bladder has the most discrete imprint (arrow), with the more anterior, less filled, superiorly displaced bladder accounting for the larger, less intense, rounded appearance seen best on the anterior view (arrowheads).

Bladder

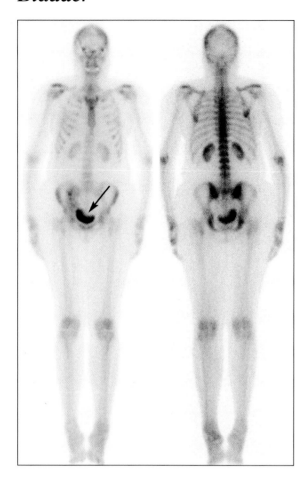

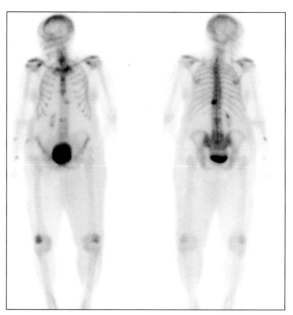

Figure 10.72

Displaced bladder. Patient with known renal cancer being restaged. (**a**) WB. Osseous lesions in the spine, absent left kidney, and large full bladder on anterior view. On posterior view only the lower half of the bladder appears as dense as it does on the anterior view and its superior border has a relatively sharp horizontal appearance. (**b**) DS, pelvis, anterior. With data manipulation on the anterior view, two different densities of tracer within the bladder. (**c**) 3-D volumetric reprojection images. Selected views from 40° to 90°. The upper portion of the bladder is displaced anteriorly by a large pelvic mass. Less volume in the upper half of the bladder accounts for the decreased density seen on the anterior and posterior projections.

a

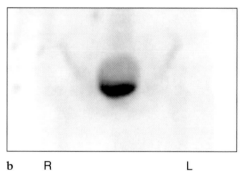

b   R   L

Figure 10.71

Extrinsic imprint. Patient is status after combined renal and pancreas transplantation. When first introduced, this surgery consisted of the pancreas being sewn into a bowel loop, which is then sewn on to the bladder. WB. Extrinsic imprint on the bladder (arrow) is nonspecific. Renal transplant in the right iliac foss.

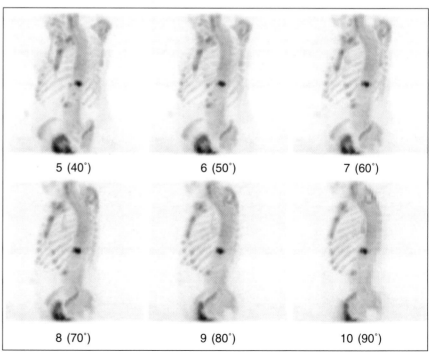

5 (40°)   6 (50°)   7 (60°)

8 (70°)   9 (80°)   10 (90°)

c

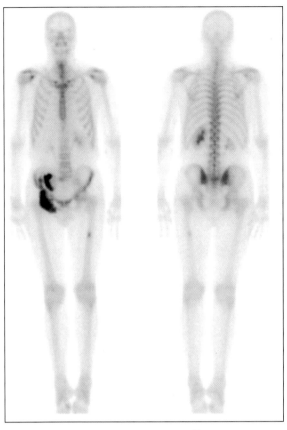

a   Ant   Post

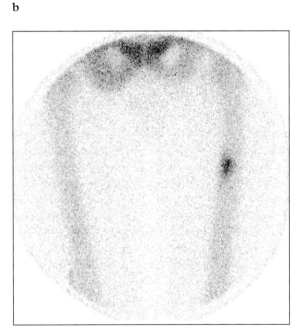

4 (30°)   5 (40°)   6 (50°)

7 (60°)   8 (70°)   9 (80°)

b

c

Figure 10.73

Ileal loop diversion. (a) WB. The ileal loop is seen in the right pelvis and an external bag filled with radioactive urine is seen overlying the right hip. Incidentally noted was a small focus of mildly increased tracer in the proximal left mid-femur. (b) 3-D volumetric reprojection images demonstrate the anterior location of the urine-filled bag. Alternatively, additional planar imaging after physically moving the bag could have been done. Abnormal focus on plain film is within the femur. (c) DS, anterior, 24 hours post-injection. This spot view was obtained to exclude completely the possibility of urine contamination. The abnormal uptake in the mid-femur is still present. Diagnosis: bladder cancer.

Figure 10.74

Caecocystoplasty.
Caecocystoplasty performed for carcinoma of the bladder. (a) DS, pelvis, anterior and (b) DS, pelvis, posterior. Marked tracer uptake is seen in the caecocystoplasty which obscures part of the bony structures of the pelvis.

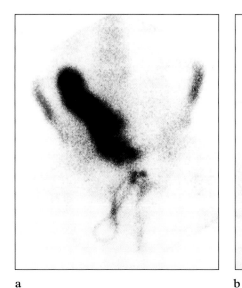

a

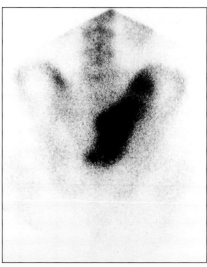

b

Figure 10.75

Neobladder with stone. Patient with bladder cancer who had cystectomy 8 years prior to this examination. (a) WB, standard display. Absent right kidney, no abnormal osseous uptake, but very large tracer collection in the pelvis filling the 'bladder'. (b) WB, window, and level display manipulations. Within the 'bladder' is a circular area of relatively intense tracer accumulation with a less intense center. (c) DS, pelvis, anterior. Magnified view of the pelvic activity shows that the larger, less intense, rounded area is not as smoothly shaped as a normal bladder. (d) CT, through lower portion of neobladder. There is a radiodense calculus (arrow) within the neobladder. The intense activity on the WB scan is thought to represent the tracer accumulating on the exposed crystal surface of the calculus.

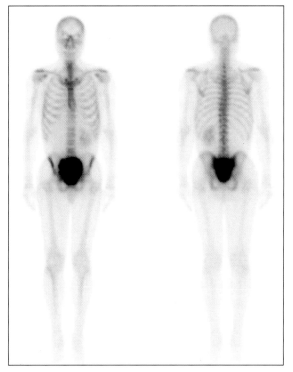

a

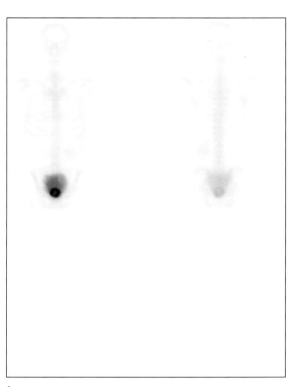

b

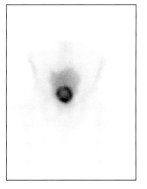

c

d

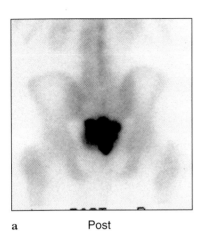

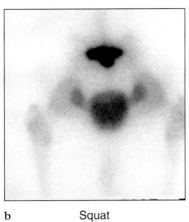

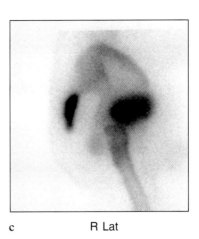

a Post   b Squat   c R Lat

Figure 10.76

Sacral lesion. (a) DS, pelvis, posterior. Intense activity centrally, could be misinterpreted as all representing the bladder. Note the somewhat irregular shape. (b) DS, squat view. The anterior bladder is less intense than the intense abnormal activity posteriorly. (c) DS, RL. The intense abnormal uptake in the sacrum is well separated from the bladder on this orthogonal view.

Scrotum

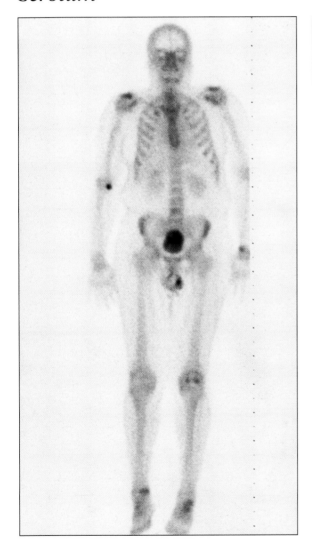

Figure 10.77

Hydrocele and 'urine contamination'. WB, anterior. The activity in the scrotal region is identified with a photon deficiency in the left half of the scrotum. The more lateral activity represented urine contamination.

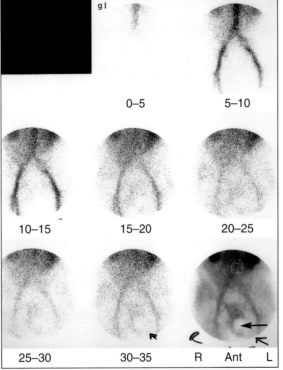

0–5   5–10

10–15   15–20   20–25

25–30   30–35   R Ant L

Figure 10.78

Hydrocele. Patient being evaluated for hip pain. RNA and BP. RNA showed normal perfusion through the lower abdominal aorta and iliac vessels. There was some faint perfusion to the upper scrotum. BP image (lower right) demonstrated photon deficiency in the left half of the hemiscrotum (arrow). This is not the rim sign of the delayed phase of testicular torsion, which would be much more intense.

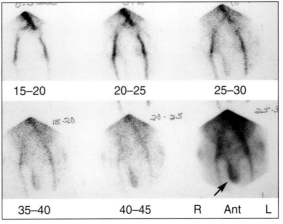

15–20   20–25   25–30

35–40   40–45   R Ant L

Figure 10.79

Acute epididymitis. Patient presents with right-sided hip pain, imaged to rule out fracture. RNA and BP. There was mild curvilinear increased perfusion to the lateral half of the right hemiscrotum on the RNA. The BP image (lower right) shows typical lateral curvilinear increased tracer (arrow).

Miscellaneous vascular lesions

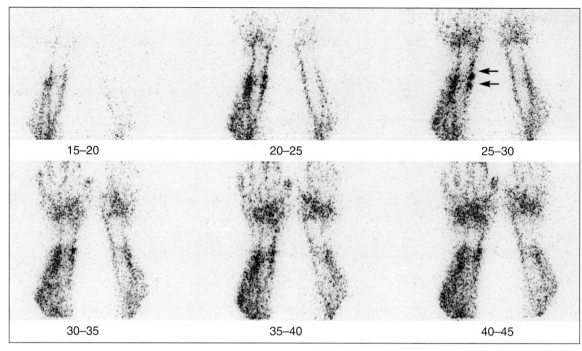

a

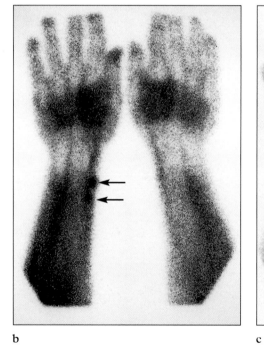

b

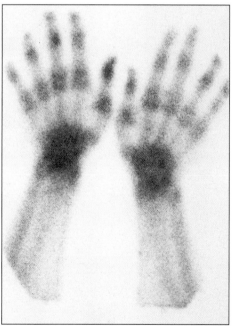

c

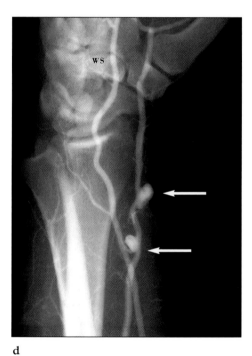

d

Figure 10.80

Aneurysm, traumatic. Four months prior to this examination being performed, the patient had received hemodialysis during the course of treatment for multi-trauma following a motor vehicle crash. He presented with pain and a soft-tissue mass. (**a**) RNA, forearm, wrist and hand, palmar view. Two small foci of round increased tracer uptake in the early arterial phase in the area of the distal radial artery (arrows). (**b**) BP, forearm, palmar. The round foci of increased tracer uptake are better seen (arrows). (**c**) DS, forearm, wrist and hand, palmar. No abnormal tracer uptake identified. (**d**) Contrast angiogram, forearm, arterial phase. Two traumatic aneurysms with well-defined necks are seen (arrows).

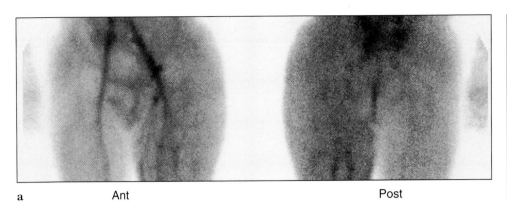

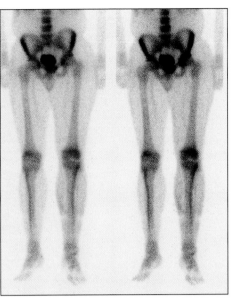

a   Ant   Post

Figure 10.81

Congenital arterial venous malformation (AVM), 30-year-old male with hypertrophy of left leg. (a) BP, pelvis and proximal thigh, anterior and posterior. Enlargement of the aberrant veins. (b) WB. Enlarged left lower extremity, particularly the thigh.

b   R   L

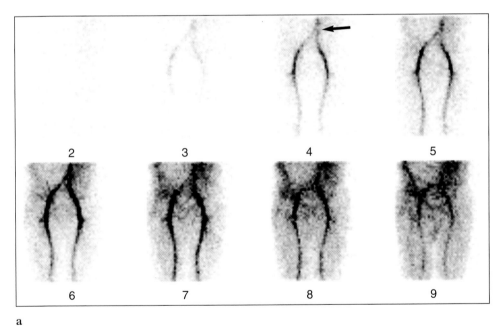

a

Figure 10.82

Displaced aorta, IVC, and right kidney. 53-year-old male with retroperitoneal sarcoma. (a) RNA, abdomen and pelvis, anterior. The lower abdominal aorta is displaced from right to left by a large photon-deficient mass. (b) BP, abdomen and pelvis, anterior. Both the IVC and the aorta are displaced from right to left by the large photon-deficient mass (arrow). (c) WB. The right kidney is displaced superolaterally and there is dilatation of the right upper pole collecting system.

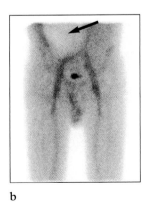

b

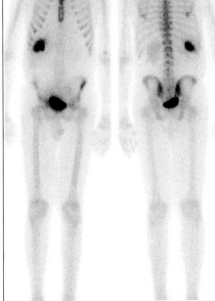

c   Ant   Post

Figure 10.83

Frostbite. Severe bilateral frostbite with only the left fourth ray viable. DS, plantar views, left foot (upper left image) and right foot (upper right image). Cobalt string gel markers outline the anatomic extent of the toes in the lower images. Only the left fourth toe has metabolic activity.

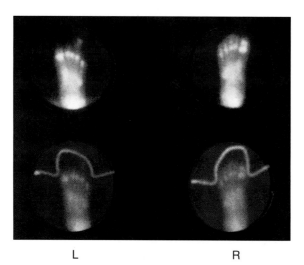

L　　　　　　　R

Teaching point

Markers should be routinely utilized to define anatomic structures.

Figure 10.84

Hemangioma. Patient presented with mass. (a) DS, hands and wrist, palmar (left image) and (b) BP, hands and wrist, palmar (right image). There is increased tracer accumulation on the BP images in the region of the fourth and fifth distal metacarpals. On the delayed image, there is only the most minimal activity associated with the head of the fourth metacarpal. This delayed activity was thought to represent a nonspecific pressure response from the mass, rather than tumor invasion. (c) Angiogram, venous phase image. Vascular malformation overlying the fourth and fifth MCP regions, with puddling of contrast (arrow).

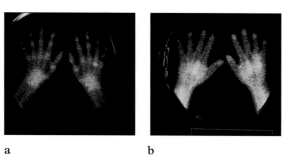

a　　　　　　　b

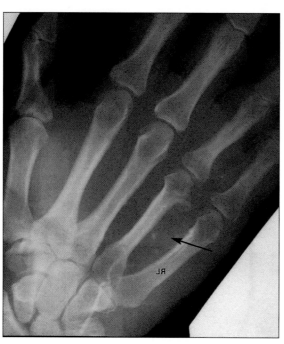

c

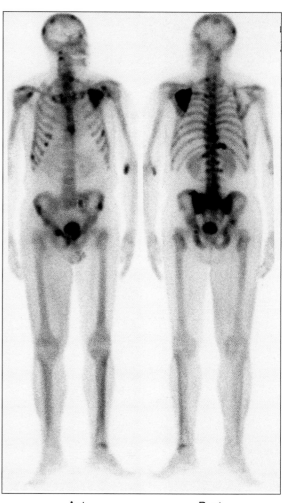

Ant　　　　　　　Post

Figure 10.85

Swollen right lower extremity, secondary to lymphedema. WB. Increased size of the right lower extremity. Widespread osseous metastasis and a belt buckle artifact overlying the left SI joint on anterior view. This scintigraphic pattern in the lower extremity can also be seen secondary to deep vein thrombosis.

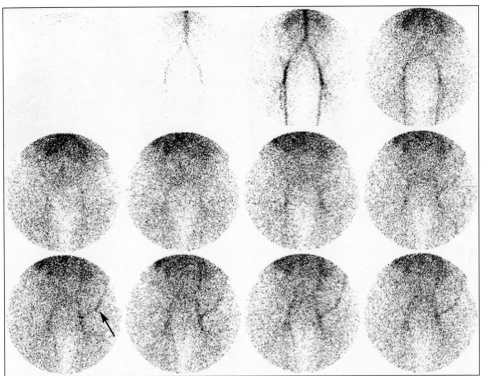

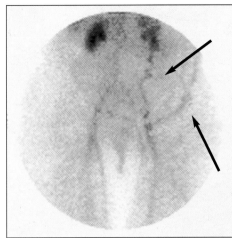

b

a

Figure 10.86

IVC, occlusion secondary to deep vein thrombosis. 49-year-old female with history of pulmonary embolus. Bone scan performed to evaluate hip pain. (**a**) RNA, pelvis and hips, anterior, five seconds per view. Early arterial perfusion is normal through abdominal aorta and iliac arteries. Later venous phase images demonstrate left-sided collaterals (arrow). (**b**) BP, pelvis and thighs, anterior. Left-sided collaterals well defined (arrows).

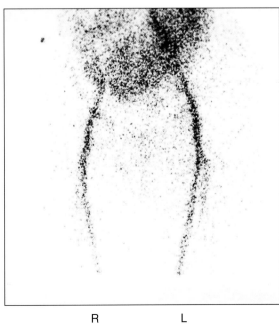

R   L

Figure 10.87

Occlusion of the right common iliac artery. RNA, pelvis and hips, anterior, selected frame. The absent visualization of the right common iliac artery in the pelvis. Subtle increase in flow through the left common iliac, with slightly earlier visualization of the bifurcation on the left side compared with the abnormal right side.

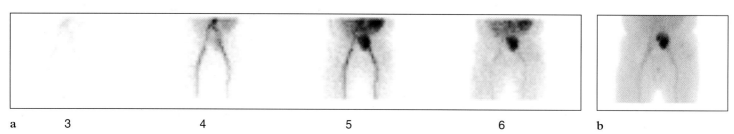

a   3   4   5   6   b

Figure 10.88

Pelvic kidney. Patient with pain after Girdlestone's procedure. (**a**) RNA, pelvis, anterior view. Five seconds per frame. Focal increased perfusion with rounded shape overlies the left common iliac artery. (**b**) BP, pelvis, anterior. The somewhat more reniform shape of the accumulation is now appreciated. (**c**) WB. Dental caries in the left maxilla, some heterotopic bone associated with Girdlestone's procedure, and left leg shortening are demonstrated. The left kidney is not seen in the normal position. A postoperative, traumatic iliac artery aneurysm was considered until a correlative CT examination was reviewed, which demonstrated the pelvic kidney.

Teaching point

History and correlative images are always important.

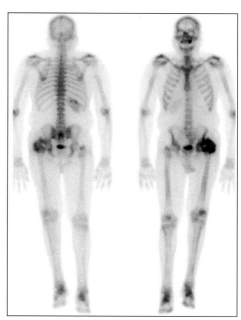

c

Figure 10.89

Congenital venous malformation. 20-year-old male evaluated for nonspecific knee pain. (**a**) RNA, knee, anterior, five seconds per view. Capillary and venous phase accumulation of tracer in the lateral aspect of left distal thigh. (**b**) BP, anterior (left image), and left lateral (right image) demonstrate anterior, lateral, and posterior components of malformation. Delayed image (not shown) was entirely normal. (**c**) X-ray, contrast venogram, left lower thigh and knee, lateral view. The venous malformation in the distal thigh is well defined and can be correlated with the BP images.

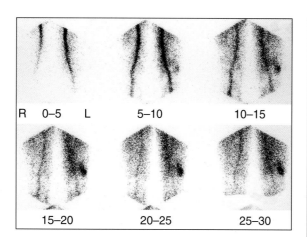

R   0–5   L   5–10   10–15

15–20   20–25   25–30

a

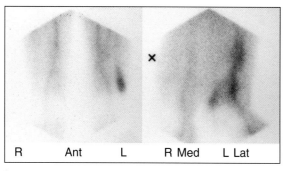

R   Ant   L   R Med   L Lat

b   c

Index

Pediatric patients

Sports-related injuries